BEHAVIORAL SCIENCE AND DENTAL PRACTICE

BEHAVIORAL SCIENCE AND DENTAL PRACTICE

SAMUEL F. DWORKIN, D.D.S., Ph.D.

Professor of Oral Surgery, School of Dentistry; Adjunct Professor of Psychiatry, School of Medicine, University of Washington, Seattle, Washington

THOMAS P. FERENCE, Ph.D.

Associate Director of Executive Programs; Director, Masters Degree Program for Executives, Graduate School of Business, Columbia University, New York, New York

DONALD B. GIDDON, D.M.D., Ph.D.

Professor of Behavioral Sciences and Community Health, College of Dentistry; Professor of Anesthesiology, School of Medicine; Professor of Psychology in the Faculty of Arts and Sciences, New York University, New York, New York

with 55 illustrations

THE C. V. MOSBY COMPANY

Saint Louis 1978

Printed in the United States of America

The C. V. Mosby Company
11830 Westline Industrial Drive, St. Louis, Missouri 63141

Library of Congress Cataloging in Publication Data

Dworkin, Samuel F.
Behavioral science and dental practice.

Bibliography: p.
Includes index.
1. Dentistry—Psychological aspects.
2. Dentist and patient. I. Ference, Thomas P., 1941- joint author. II. Giddon, Donald B., 1930- joint author. III. Title. [DNLM: 1. Dentist-patient relations. 2. Interpersonal relations. 3. Behavior. WU61 D993b]
RK53.D88 617.6′001 77-26634
ISBN 0-8016-1484-8

GW/CB/CB 9 8 7 6 5 4 3 2 1

To

Mona, Adam, and Teddy
who are around all the time
S. F. D.

Ellie, who even typed it all
T. P. F.

My wife and children
D. B. G.

PREFACE

Dentistry has matured through several eras. Early dentistry in this country was characterized by mechanics, technical procedures, and surgery to remove infected parts. Then came the recognition of a need for greater biological sophistication, a kind of belated awareness that since teeth and other oral structures are connected to the rest of the body's physiology, dentists should know the principles and facts of human biology and pathology. Now dentistry has grown ready to manage patients holistically, incorporating into diagnosis and treatment considerations of how the patient as a person responds to dentists and dental treatment.

Real and pragmatic ways are available to the practicing dentist for responding to a spectrum of patient needs reaching beyond technically well-executed restorations or surgical procedures. The dental profession has taken seriously the oft-quoted euphemism that it has the responsibility to treat people, not just teeth. Dentists have recognized that they must treat all kinds of people, even if they act or look strange or if they cannot see, hear, or walk. The era of the dentist as a practitioner largely for the able and the affluent is coming to an end.

The overall purpose of this book is to analyze how people become dental patients or dentists. The organization of this book is by concepts, with liberal use of case material. The concepts applied are those from the science of behavior that are relevant to the providing or receiving of dental health care.

The text is divided into three major parts. The first is informational, providing a backdrop for the following two. These last two parts provide principles and strategies for the dentist-patient interaction. We begin with the concept of a psychological contract and end with specific situations that typify dentist-patient interactions. Each part starts with an introductory section providing an overview of the topic. This is followed by individual chapters on the specific psychosocial dimensions involved.

Part one sets the stage for dental treatment. It provides the context in which dentistry occurs. As we shall discuss, a number of factors affect people's perception of dentistry before they ever become patients or dentists. Part one provides background information related to different psychosocial aspects of dentistry and includes the psychological significance of the face and mouth, psychological factors relating to a patient's need for dental care, the evidenced need for dental care, the utilization of dental care, and factors involved in becoming a dentist.

Part two provides the basic principles of interpersonal behavior. It is designed to give dental students or practitioners an opportunity to explore and practice a number of the basic psychological principles that will assist them in the delivery of dental care. The principles that will be discussed and experienced include psychological contracting, learning styles, motivation, perception, group and individual approaches to problem solving, conflict, communications and the helping relationship, and interpersonal influence and the change process.

Part three explores ways of applying the basic psychological principles discussed earlier to the actual dentist-patient interaction. In this part a number of specific concepts and management strategies are discussed. They include the process of behavior change; stress, anxiety, and fear; pain; maintenance of healthy behaviors; and life cycle changes.

This text is intended for students of dentistry, whether dentist or paraprofessional. Although primarily intended for use in dental schools, it is equally suitable for postdoctoral education, whether for graduate work or in continuing education.

We believe that the concepts discussed in this book are best understood if they are connected to dynamic processes of behavior that are experienced by the reader and then reflected on, preferably in small-group sessions. In Part two we encourage the reader to experience what is being read, for example, the resolution of conflicts that arise within the dentist over "problem patients," by incorporating suggested methods for structuring such experiences so they may allow for reflection and assimilation, probably best accomplished in a classroom setting. We believe these experiential opportunties make real for the dentist the underlying psychosocial dynamics of behavior that might often otherwise be acknowledged only intellectually. We also believe that it is important to take a stand—to present a text that integrates certain established principles of behavior with a pragmatic set of strategies for action. We have chosen as our theoretical point of departure an interpersonally oriented, psychosocial approach to behavioral analysis, borrowing heavily from Maslow, Sullivan, and McClellan, with a liberal sprinkling of learning theory. Our own teaching experiences confirm the usefulness of this approach.

Thus this text serves the dual purpose of providing an informational base about the psychological and social makeup of the patient, the dentist, and their interactions and of suggesting strategies that allow the reader, student, or graduate to experience and manage concrete human experiences relevant to a health professional. We hope to have at least touched on all the major issues, well recognizing that in many instances we have been too brief. Our readers can help us tremendously if they care to comment on the relative weight we have given to different issues or problems.

A serious attempt has been made to organize the contents of this text to prove suitable in instructional situations that differ in (1) course format (seminar, small-group sessions, lectures, etc.), (2) placement in the educational sequence (beginning, middle, or end of dental, postgraduate, or continuing education), and (3) length of course.

A suggested sequence for a brief lecture course might incorporate Part one, Chapters 1, 2, and 4 as background information; Part two, Chapters 8, 9, 11, and 13 as basic principles of psychological need formation, the nature of conflict, and its resolution; and Part three, Chapters 14, 15, 16, and 18 as examples (positive and negative) of dentist-patient interactions and their appropriate modification. A seminar or small-group discussion course format could include, in addition, Chapters 5, 6, 7, and 17, emphasizing the dentist's role as an active participant, or Chapters 5, 6, 7, 10, and 12, emphasizing the fundamental principles of interpersonal psychology.

As a convenient description of the dental health professional, we consistently use the term "*dentist*" in this book. The concepts are equally applicable for use by any dental health professional, dental student, general practitioner, specialist, hygienist, assistant, receptionist, or educator.

Finally, we note that more than one practicing dentist has observed that feelings of technical competence come relatively quickly. The challenges that emerge for dentists in their daily work, providing both rewards and frustrations, come undeniably from people—the patients who accept or reject treatment and who respond well or poorly; the decision to "do it over or not"; the staff that does or does not get along; and the ability or inability to deal confidently with other health professionals. We recognize that these challenges are lifelong cues and that their resolution comes slowly, if at all. It is our goal to accelerate this process of becoming a total health professional.

Sustained interest in the work-a-day world for dentists, to their credit, involves, perhaps to a greater extent than the public realizes, an intense commitment to respond to these challenges as dentists struggle to be increasingly effective health care providers. This book is dedicated to this commitment and to this struggle.

Each of us is deeply indebted to the many teachers, colleagues, students, and friends who have contributed directly or indirectly to this book.

Perhaps the only virtue of a book authored by three people is that the failure, by any one of us, to cite all those who helped can be attributed to the other two. However, Sam Dworkin wishes to acknowledge the unfailing encouragement of Dr. Bernard Kalinkowitz and the faculty of the New York University Programs in Clinical and Social Psychology, especially the late Dr. George Klein. Much of the opportunity to test ideas expressed in the book were effected by Dr. Irwin Mandel and Dr. Bernard Soloerberg of Columbia University.

Tom Ference expresses a special debt to James A. F. Stoner of Fordham University for 10 years of working together on many segments of his part of the book and to David Kaplan of Columbia University who got us started.

Don Giddon is indebted to James Dunning, Professor Emeritus, Harvard University, and to Paul Goldhaber, Dean of the Harvard School of Dental Medicine, for their confidence and encouragement of concepts exposed in this book and to the late Dr. Abraham Maslow, Brandeis University, who provided the wisdom and inspiration to pursue the dual profession of psychology and dentistry.

Collectively, we wish to thank individuals too numerous to mention at Columbia University, Harvard University, New York University, and the University of Washington for generously permitting us use of research facilities and materials and for offering perceptive comments while the book was in progress.

We also owe a collective debt of gratitude to Carol Bikofsky, Deborah Diserens, Barbara Freitas, Leah Soltar, June Mendelson, Joan Moritz, Sharry Pollock, Jane Moosbruker, and Elizabeth Adler for their contributions to the preparation of this book and for keeping us all together.

Judy Morton acted as our principal editor, and her ability and patience must be uniquely acknowledged. We are pleased to share with all these people the positive contributions this book may represent, although we take full responsibility for its inadequacies.

Samuel F. Dworkin
Thomas P. Ference
Donald B. Giddon

CONTENTS

Part one

SETTING THE STAGE

Facts and figures about patients and dentists

The stage is already set before two individuals ever meet as dentist and patient. In Part one questions that set the stage for the dentist-patient interaction will be considered.

OBJECTIVES

The objectives for the chapters in Part one are as follows:

- □ To introduce the concept of the psychological importance of the face and mouth to the species and to the individual
- □ To explore and examine the psychophysiology of dental disease
- □ To document the objective need for dental care, that is, the incidence of dental disease by type as it varies with such factors as age, sex, race, psychology, and environment
- □ To examine the perceived need for dental care and how it relates to the demand for and utilization of dental care
- □ To identify the factors involved in the evolution of the provider in terms of career choice, selection, and education of dentists

Chapter 1

THE PSYCHOLOGICAL SIGNIFICANCE OF THE FACE AND MOUTH

It is now an accepted fact of life that the biology and pathology leading to oral disease or dysfunction arise from the same general principles that govern the biology of the rest of the body. At the same time, specialized biological functions and unique pathologies develop in association only with the oral cavity, as is true in the gastrointestinal system or eye.

Just as oral structures and functions involve both general and specialized human *biological* processes, they also involve general as well as specialized *psychosocial* phenomena. The mouth is important to everyone; however, it is apparently more important to some persons than to others. Some will allow the oral structures to become important to them because appearance, eating, or pain avoidance is important to them; no inconvenience or expense will deter persons so motivated. For others, appearance, eating, and even pain avoidance are not sufficient motivators toward good oral health; the perception of the significance of the oral cavities for these people may be trivial, nonexistent, or even strongly negative. Despite the simple and obvious validity of these observations, it has taken a long time for health care delivery systems in general, and dentistry specifically, to begin attending to more than the purely physical aspects of disease or dysfunction.

It is now recognized that the treatment of illness, any illness, is never only the treatment of diseased body parts—painful stomach, carious tooth, or bleeding gums. Successful diagnosis and treatment require "identifying the patient in the disease" and "the physician in the treatment." How the body works and how patients respond to this is now understood to be much more complicated than previously thought. The understanding involves such far-flung concerns as the cultural-ethnic background of the patient, family attitudes toward disease and "doctors," and the person's own health belief system. In other words, the physician has to find out what the patient is complaining about in broader contexts than objective signs represented by measurable pathology. Perhaps the patient is afraid of being deformed, of being hurt, or even of dying. The physician has to evaluate his or her own willingness or ability to respond to the patient's concerns as well as to the patient's body.

Why is this so? Why can't the physician, dentist, nurse, hygienist, social worker, or pharmacist simply attend to "what's wrong"—the broken part, the fever, the heightened glucose level, the pain, etc.? Why become involved in a morass of personal problems that may only complicate or confuse the health professional who is trying to find out what the "real problem" is and then address it with dispatch?

The answer is simple in theory, yet complicated in application. The simple part of the answer relates to our relatively new awareness that no disease process goes on in isolation from the rest of the patient's life—this is what is meant by "identifying the patient in the disease." A toothache is not simply a pure pain sensation; for the person involved the pain can have many meanings—dreaded treatment, disrupted appearance, and/or financial burdens. The complicated part of the answer relates to finding out which meaning is significant for a particular patient at a particular time and how the meaning attached to the disease symptom is likely to affect the patient's behavior before, during, and after treatment.

For example, a patient with a toothache must come to the dentist, sooner or later. However, the very act of deciding when to come is clearly a personal decision. The entire personal history of the patient as it affects the development of the present pain comes to bear. Why did the patient let it go so long? Was he or she influenced by family attitudes? Previous dental experience? Fear? Money? Who will the patient finally select as a dentist? Will the choice be the result of the recommendations of a neighbor? Walking in off the street? Will the patient choose someone in private practice? Someone in a dental school clinic? What kind of medication will the patient accept? Local anesthetic? Waking sedation? General anesthetic? What are the expectations of the patient? Exodontia only? Complex fixed-porcelain restorations? Endodontic therapy?

Not only patient-oriented but also dentist-oriented considerations are involved. Is the dentist available for emergencies? Does the dentist have personal preferences or biases for doing surgery as opposed to endodontics, etc.?

The patient's problem involves more than just objective pathology, and the dentist's response involves more than just clinical know-how. Thus health professionals find themselves attending to concerns (both patient and health professional oriented) that fall outside traditional clinical procedures. These concerns, taken together, have been labeled "psychosocial" factors in health and illness. For the patient, the term "psychosocial" refers to intra- and interpersonal forces that shape his or her development and maturation; such forces include consideration of the patient's social and cultural history and, most importantly, the patient's family relationships. A large portion of this book is devoted to demonstrating how the manner in which dental disease affects patients and the manner in which dentists provide care are both influenced by psychosocial factors. The mouth, oral structures, stomatognathic apparatus, etc. are known to have psychosocial as well as biological significance for persons. Although it seems more difficult to define with precision the psychosocial compared to the biological significance, the remainder of this chapter examines how the oral cavity becomes profoundly important to individuals.

OBJECTIVES

The objectives of this chapter are as follows:

1. To discuss the psychobiological basis of the significance of the orofacial area
2. To examine the different levels of psychobiological significance of the oral structures
3. To indicate the psychoanalytical interpretation of the importance of the oral cavity as an historical view

PSYCHOBIOLOGICAL BASIS OF THE SIGNIFICANCE OF THE OROFACIAL AREA

The basis of the importance of the face, mouth, and related structures can be traced biologically and psychologically. At the risk of being teleological, it may be said that the significance of the mouth and face may well result in part from the disproportionately large representation of the orofacial areas in the cerebral cortex. This is particularly so in the somatic sensory and motor systems, as shown in Fig. 1-1.

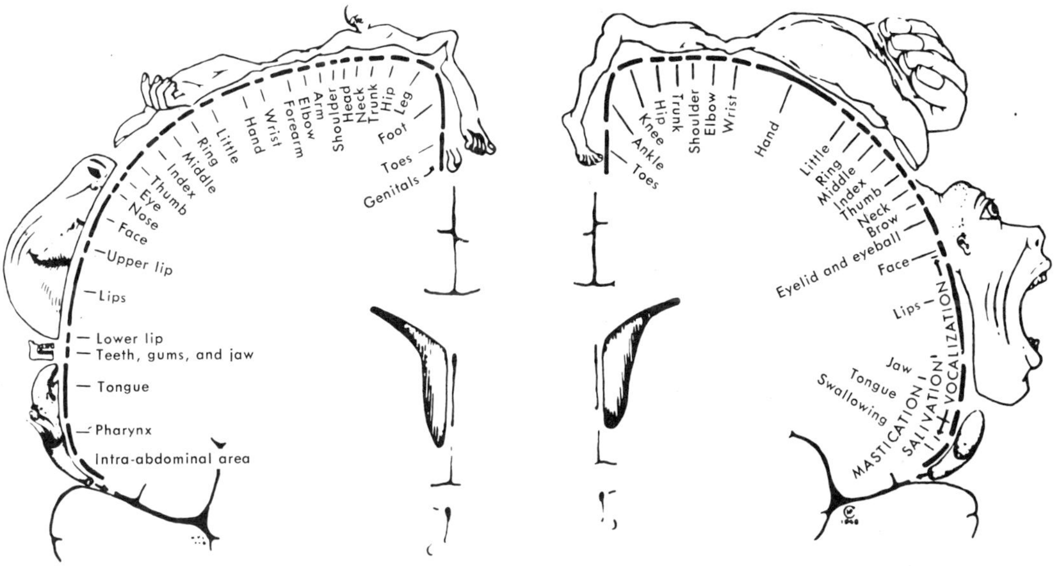

A B

Fig. 1-1. A, Sensory homunculus, drawn overlying a coronal section through the postcentral gyrus. **B,** Motor homunculus, drawn overlying a coronal section through the precentral gyrus. (From Penfield, W., and Rasmussen, T.: The cerebral cortex of man: a clinical study of localization of function, New York, 1950, Macmillan, Inc. Copyright 1950 by Macmillan, Inc.)

Other observations support the idea that there is a biological substrate for the psychological significance of the oral cavity. For example, within the hypothalamic pathways of the limbic system, there is a region associated with oral and aggressive behavior. Stimulation in this area elicits penile erection and aggressive behavior as well as biting and chewing activity. Fighting is frequently a preliminary to both feeding and mating.[16] Moreover this close relationship between oral and genital functions is phylogenetically related to the olfactory sense, which, of course, has played an important role in feeding and mating for more primitive species.

DIFFERENT LEVELS OF PSYCHOBIOLOGICAL SIGNIFICANCE OF ORAL STRUCTURES

The psychological significance of the face and mouth may be conveniently thought of in terms of the three different levels of needs identified by Maslow[17]: survival, socialization, and self-actualization.

Maslow suggests that until basic survival needs are met, persons can devote little energy or time to socialization, except as relationships with others are important to satisfying these needs. For example, needs relating to socialization such as love or self-esteem or one's perceived worth in the eyes of others must be postponed until basic oral needs relating to survival such as thirst, hunger, and sex are met.

The highest level of needs in Maslow's[17] hierarchy, self-actualization, is defined as relating to the need to fulfill one's potential: ". . . to become everything one is capable of becoming." Thus the ". . . musician must make music, the artist must paint, . . . a poet must write. . . . " The key word here is "must" for the mature personality *must* become what it can, but only after lower-order needs have been met.

Let us examine how the mouth and its surrounding structures may take on significance for individuals at each of these need levels.

Survival

The survival functions of the mouth begin at birth. The mouth is important in the taking in of food and water from the mother or surrogate, thus obtaining adequate nutrition for the organism.

At the same time, the mouth is one of the neonate's most important avenues for learning about the world. The newborn infant's first experiences with objects, spatial relations, and the discontinuity of self from external objects occurs via the mouth as a sense organ. Probably the infant's first prototypical experiences of pain and frustration are associated with hunger and the feeding experience, thus establishing the survival value of pain as a warning signal of impending danger to the body.

The teeth, together with the facial muscles, provide a major means for expressing the positive emotions of joy or pleasure and the negative emotions of fear and anger. The infant, for example, experiences pain associated with teething. Simultaneously the satisfaction is associated with hunger reduction and the entire nursing-eating experience. These emotions are signals that provide the organism with the actual means for the defensive or aggressive behavior necessary for survival.

With the development of speech, communication becomes a more efficient way to deal with others than acting out the experience. This development facilitates the cooperative behavior necessary for survival. Depending on the particular culture, mouth odors emitted or detected communicate information about personal habits, behavior, ethnicity, and physical health.[12]

For the adolescent and the adult the face and mouth also have a role in the initiation and repetition of sexual activity, a necessity for the survival of the species. The appearance of the face and mouth is important in the attraction between the sexes as well as in the expression of emotion, which facilitates sexual attraction.

The mouth is also significant as a source of highly gratifying and reinforcing sexual behaviors from kissing to oral-genital activity, although these behaviors may, for some, become sources of guilt, shame, or other conflict. The pleasure they provide encourages the repetition of sexual acts, thus increasing opportunities for reproduction.

Some interesting studies suggest a basic need for oral activity per se. For example, there is a report on the probability of an apparently innate diurnal, oral behavior cycle in humans that can be linked with the rapid eye movement (REM) sleep cycle.[5] By noting spontaneous oral activity such as the amount of smoking, drinking, and eating occurring within a given time period, as shown for one subject in Fig. 1-2, rhythmic cycles of oral activity averaging 96 minutes were described in waking patients. Interestingly the peaks of oral activity appeared to be directly related to the degree of alertness. Although some of the cyclic responses were undoubtedly related to physiological variables such as glucose level, one may infer from the authors that these oral activities may be the waking counterpart of REM sleep—increasing in frequency as do gastric secretions, muscle contractions, and penile erections when REM sleep is deprived.

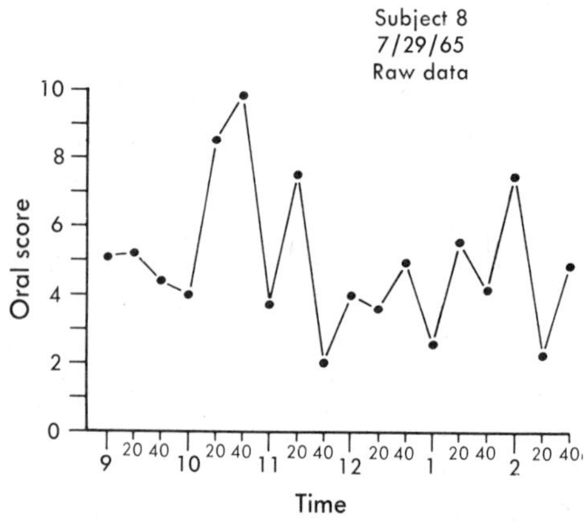

Fig. 1-2. Raw data of subject who showed "very noisy" cycles. The times listed in all the graphs refer to the 20-minute intervals beginning with the stated times. (From Friedman, S., and Fisher, C.: J. Am. Psychoanal. Assoc. **15**[2]:317, 1967.)

Socialization

The importance of the face and mouth in the socialization process begins with their role in perceptual development as the maturing infant differentiates "self" from others. As observed by Piaget, "the oral cavity with its tool tongue becomes the first organ of perception for the infant."[19] The child learns that although it can sense objects, that is, its own hand or foot or even the mother's breast, these sensed objects have an independent existence. By confrontation, then, with his or her own oral cavity, the child learns to perceive the different body parts as well as his or her separation from the rest of a world of external objects.[23]

Following differentiation of the world into self and others, the young child begins to recognize the importance of cooperative interaction with other individuals to attain goals and objectives. With the maturation of the facial muscles and the development of the organs involved in speech, the human organism is able to communicate using words and facial expressions. In contrast to lower animals, humans are able to effectively use these orally initiated symbols to express ideas. For example, we can orally express aggression, rather than being required to act it out by biting or attacking.

By virtue of its role as an organ of aggression, the mouth becomes not only a logical channel but also a susceptible target for symbolic expression. Harmful, nonmasticatory activities, often obviously aggressive in intent such as "gnashing the teeth in anger," are seen in bruxism (the clenching or gnashing of the teeth), with deleterious effects on the teeth, the temporomandibular joint, and related structures.

In addition to the previously mentioned nonmasticatory activities that are affected by social factors, the act of mastication is also influenced by the psychosocial context of eating behavior. In a study by Giddon et al.[7] comparing the ability of denture wearers and persons with natural dentition to differentiate the sweetness of solid food, it was found that the denture wearer took more than twice as long to render a judgment than a person with natural dentition: 15 seconds and 6 seconds, respectively. Using a psychophysical method to determine the differential threshold, as shown in Fig. 1-3, it can be seen that the discriminative ability of denture wearers was only half that of the patients with natural dentition. When the denture patient was restricted to 10 seconds, the maximum time that the natural dentition patient took to render a more accurate judgment, the discriminative ability as represented by the slope became zero, that is, the artificial denture patient was absolutely unable to distinguish among the cookies containing increasing levels of sucrose.

Generalizing to the situation in which eating behavior usually occurs, it is probable that the denture wearer can be placed in socially stressful situations. Like anyone else, the denture wearer does not like to look any more different than necessary; he or she will probably attempt to chew food at a rate faster than usual for denture wearers, thereby reducing the ability to perceive and enjoy the subtle differences in the flavor of solid foods. Some denture patients will also undoubtedly resent the inadequacies of dentistry to meet an important psychosocial need.

Part of the denture wearer's handicap results from the loss of adaptability and compensatory ability. Patients with natural dentition who are restrained by time or number of masticatory strokes compensate by increasing the forcefulness of each chewing stroke.[20] Unfortunately the denture wearer is at a decided disadvantage and does not even approach the chewing efficiency of the individual with natural teeth.[27] As noted earlier, the texture of the food and the associated sound will also be different and probably less satisfactory for the denture wearer. In addition to the satisfaction resulting from sound quality, the swallowing threshold is influenced by texture and feedback from the auditory system. Recall, for example, the changing

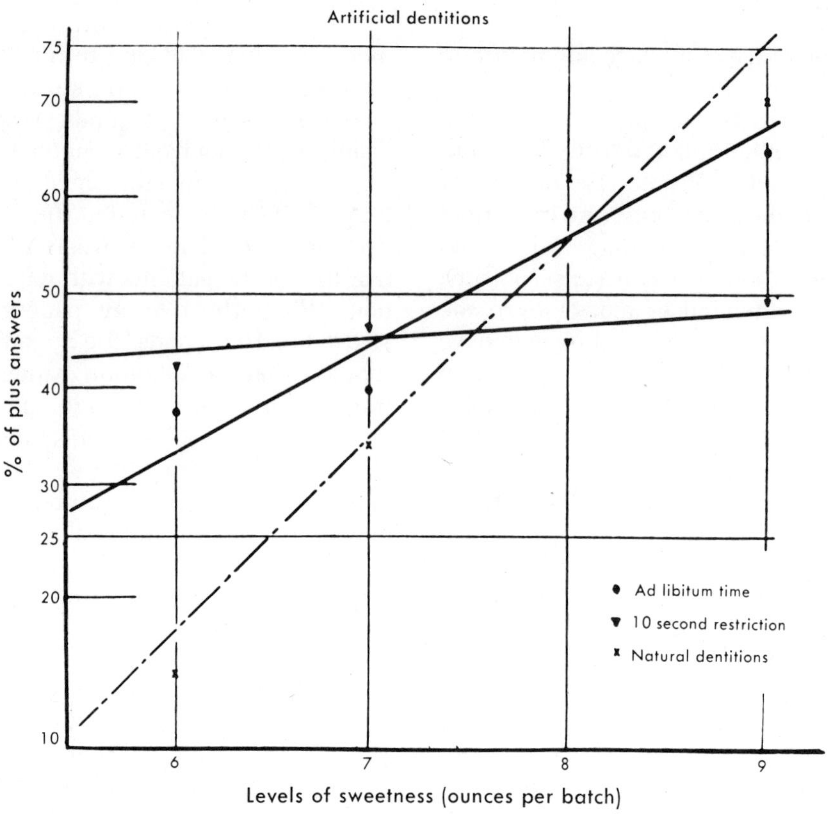

Fig. 1-3. Ability of denture wearers and natural dentition patients to discriminate sweetness. (From Giddon, D. B., Dreisbach, M. E., Pfaffman, C., and Manley, R. S.: J. Prosthet. Dent. **4**[2]:263, 1954.)

sound of carrots as one chews to the swallowing threshold.

Perhaps the most important socializing role of the face, with the mouth as the central feature, is in interpersonal communication. The face is intimately connected with both verbal and nonverbal communication processes.[15] The listener focuses on the speaker's face, and the speaker focuses on the face of the listener. These observations of the face in the communication process significantly augment the meaning of the speaker's words or the level of the listener's understanding or attention.

First impressions of individuals are formed from facial expressions, at least this is a very common belief. Many studies have, in fact, documented the importance of the face, and the mouth in particular, to perceived physical attractiveness and self-concept. Simply stated, the greater the physical attractiveness as perceived in the eyes of others, the greater the perceived self-esteem. Thus the importance that many patients attach to aesthetic restorations, orthodontics, and maxillofacial surgery is understandable in terms of self-esteem.

Although philosophers, artists, plastic surgeons, and orthodontists have long argued over the merits of one or more facial features and their various constellations, the first experimental study dates only as far back as 1921. In that simple research project, it was found that the mouth and face were high on the list of attributes that were used to distinguish the most attractive from the most "repulsive" women.[18] In a more recent, sophisticated, and less chauvinistic study, individual features of women students were rank ordered by approximately 100 men and women judges prior to ranking overall attractiveness. As expected, the median correlations with judg-

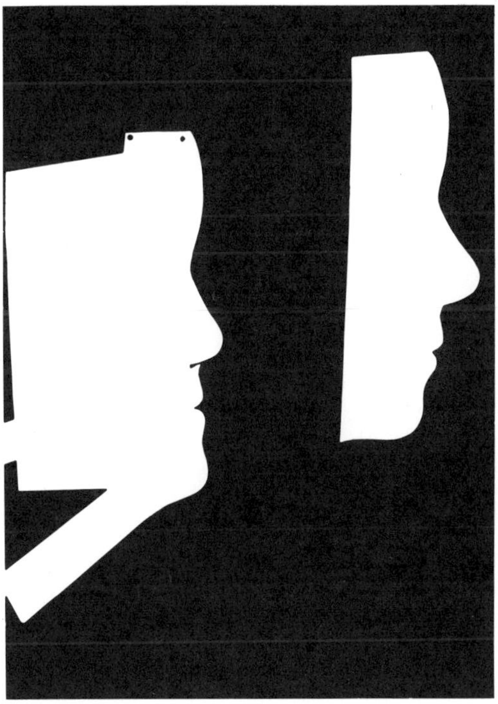

Fig. 1-4. Profile simulation device and fixed test profile. (From Giddon, D. B., Hershon, L. E., and Lennartsson, B.: Scand. J. Dent. Res. **82:**527, 1974.)

ment of overall attractiveness were highest for the eyes and smiles for both men and women judges.[9]

Such judgments undoubtedly are a complex function of sociocultural factors, influenced to some extent by the media of advertising, movies, television, and professional judgments of orthodontists and plastic surgeons as well as a function of the psychological characteristics of the judges.[26] With the help of a more sophisticated psychological methodology, it may be possible to determine the contribution each factor makes to these judgments.

It is no wonder that many patients attach such great significance to deformities or obvious defects of the mouth or related structures, since studies and common sense validate that physical attractiveness is extremely important to self-esteem. Each society seems to manifest preference for some ideal characteristic, and members who possess this societal norm for attractiveness are generally sought out.

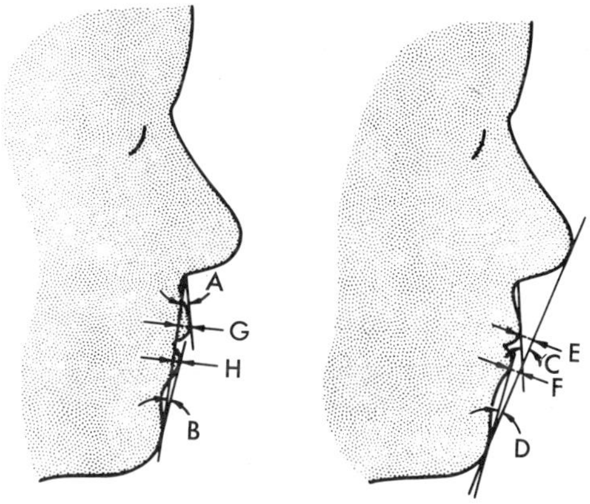

Fig. 1-5. Angular and linear profile measurements. (From Giddon, D. B., Hershon, L. E., and Lennartsson, B.: Scand. J. Dent. Res. **82:**527, 1974.)

Objective physical arrangement of features, however, is not the critical variable. Perception is the key; "beauty is in the eye of the beholder," to quote a trite cliché. For example, most people tend to err in the direction of what is thought to be socially accepted norms when asked to estimate their body dimensions such as hips, bust, and weight.[11] In a recent study subjects were asked to simulate their own profile for comparison with their actual profile. Using the simple device shown in Fig. 1-4, they underestimated the protrusiveness of their lips as determined by measurements made from their actual profiles, as shown in Fig. 1-5.[6]

Unfortunately it is very difficult to define beauty in our society. "Samuel Johnson contended that if we were more accustomed to deformity than beauty, the ideas now annexed to deformity would be attached to beauty. It is only because we are more accustomed to beauty that we approve it and admire it."[10] There is, however, the possibility that such preferences are innate or imprinted.[14] For example, some basic receptors and organizations of neurons within our central nervous system are responsive to or more easily excited by particular curves or configurations, and this may constitute part of the basis on which our aesthetic preferences are formed.[24]

Part of our socialization involves learning culturally determined appropriate distances for different kinds of communication.[1] The role that the face and the mouth play varies with these differing appropriate distances. Thus at "intimate distance" (up to 1½ feet), there is a mutual awareness through bodily contact of skin, muscle movements, temperature, and smell. Clear vision is limited to small areas of the face, and facial expressions are secondary to voice modulation. Within this distance, then, the facial area plays an important role. At "personal distance" (1½ to 4 feet), persons are still within arm's reach of each other, but physical contact, body odor, and heat perception are reduced. Vision of the whole body as well as of the face is important. At "social distance" (4 to 12 feet), where most interpersonal dealings are conducted, the whole body can be seen, and a louder voice is used. At "public distance" (greater than 12 feet), the voice must become louder, and observation of gross gestures and bodily stances becomes more important as a means of communication.[8]

The size of the space these intimate, personal, social, and public distances occupy varies considerably from culture to culture. For example, it would be improper in German society to intrude into one's social space, let alone personal space, without a specific invitation. However, the dentist must always work within the patient's intimate space, regardless of the culture. It is speculated that, for some patients, being at an intimate distance with a person with whom one is not intimate may be threatening. The loss of the accustomed cues of ordinary interpersonal relationships that occur at this distance requires the patient, in some cases, to make a significant adaptation.

Compared to the mouth, the contributions of the other parts of the orofacial apparatus to the socialization of the individual are less well recognized. For example, a group of investigators concluded that the unconscious display of the tongue is a universal sign of aversion to social encounter. The tongue is apparently used in this fashion by all races and by some primates, for example, orangutans and gorillas! The tongue is used to reflect intrapersonal states in other ways as well, some developing at a very early age. Toddlers, for example, tend to show their tongues when engrossed in difficult tasks such as climbing over obstacles and also when involved in awkward social situations such as being scolded for misbehavior. Similarly, adults show their tongues during tasks requiring intense concentration such as when making a tricky shot at pool, when backing into a small parking space, and during involvement in a socially threatening situation such as being interrupted in conversation. Gorillas and orangutans in close quarters were also found to exhibit a tongue display whenever engaged in complex tasks such as peeling bananas with their toes or in unpleasant situations such as being scolded for fighting.[21]

Another interpretation of these behaviors is that the tongue as well as other parts of the oral apparatus may be used to displace aggression or reduce tension. Common examples cited are the use of chewing gum and preferences for hard foods.

Thus the orofacial area is of great interest as a powerful source of nonverbal signals, especially in communication. We learn that the perception of another person's face leads to the belief that one can determine the degree of understanding in interpersonal encounters. As we shall see in Chapter 12, to know that one is understood both by thought and by affect is absolutely essential to a successful communication exchange.

Self-actualization

Having discussed the requirements of survival and socialization, we can turn to how the face and the mouth are used for satisfaction of the higher-order needs of self-actualization, or fulfillment. Once the basic survival and socialization needs are met, the mouth is available as a communication mechanism for the expression of profound thoughts, for enjoyment of supreme culinary delights, or for more exotic and erotic pleasures. All these activities can be directed toward personal growth and the enhancement of the quality of life. Some of these activities, although they were alluded to in the socialization process and are not necessary for survival, are essential to increased participation in the enjoyment of life's pleasures. When oral health is good, as a general rule, so is systemic health, and the significance of oral health as one component of a feeling of well-being cannot be overemphasized.

PSYCHOANALYTICAL INTERPRETATION OF THE IMPORTANCE OF THE ORAL CAVITY

Finally, no discussion of the psychological significance of the oral cavity would be complete without reference to the Freudian viewpoint. Here we will touch only on Freud and his followers' concept of the significance of the oral cavity; his theory of psychoanalysis will be discussed in Chapter 14.

Psychosexual development is believed by Freud to begin with the oral stage, characterized by the mouth being the prime source of sensual gratification for the infant from birth to 2 years of age.[4] There are two phases in the oral stage: The first is the passive oral receptive phase, relating to the intake of milk and other activities dependent on the mother. With the eruption of the teeth, beginning around age 6 months, the maturation of the nervous system, and activity directed toward mastery of the world, the infant moves to the second stage, the oral sadistic, or oral aggressive, stage.[2]

Additional significance attached to the oral stages may be of interest.[22a] For example, oral succorance combines both passive and dependent tendencies, the existence of which is inferred from oral habits such as prolonged sucking, compulsive eating and drinking, and perverse attachment to the nipple, breast, and thumb. When succorance behaviors predominate, aggressive tendencies are usually inhibited. In contrast, in oral-aggressive behaviors oral activity is combined with aggression as indicated by the presence of such habits as biting and chewing. Strong aggressive needs are expressed, and the world may be seen as being full of biting objects. Resentment of authority and the use of hostile words also occur. A third oral behavior constellation is that of oral rejection, which involves spitting-out behaviors, theoretically in disgust of oral activities and in fear of oral infection.

It must be remembered that these Freudian interpretations are just that, theoretical interpretations of what the person "really" means when engaging in nail-biting, sucking, or spitting. These interpretations are provided for the reader's interest. Great care must be exercised to resist the temptation by dentists to label patients as passive, aggressive, or rejecting solely on the basis of these oral behaviors.

SUMMARY

Clinically, dentists may hear patients lament bitterly about their dental misfortunes.[22] The most articulate representation of their unhappiness, however, is perhaps best left to the great writers of history.[28] As Don Quixote says, "I had rather have lost an arm, so it were not my sword arm; for a mouth without cheek-teeth is like a mill without a mill-stone, Sancho; and every tooth in a man's head is more valuable than a diamond."[3]

Considering the biopsychological importance of the oral cavity, it is no wonder that, compared to other parts of the body, pain and suffering relating to the oral cavity often appear far out of proportion to objective clinical signs. Stated more positively, the mouth and surrounding structures are essential to survival and socialization and contribute much toward appreciating and participating in those aspects of our society that enhance the quality of life.

REFERENCES

1. Abercrombie, M. L. J.: Face to face—proximity and distance, J. Psychosom. Res. **15:**395, 1971.
2. Abraham, K.: Selected papers of Karl Abraham, New York, 1960, Macmillan, Inc.
3. de Cervantes, M.: Don Quixote, New York, 1975, The New American Library, Inc.
4. Freud, S.: Cited in Brenner, C.: An elementary textbook of psychoanalysis, New York, 1955, International Universities Press.
5. Friedman, S., and Fisher, C.: On the presence of a rhythmic, diurnal, oral instinctual drive cycle in man: a preliminary report, J. Am. Psychoanal. Assoc. **15**(2):317, 1967.
6. Giddon, D. B., Hershon, L. E., and Lennartsson, B.: Discrepancy between objective and subjective profile measures, Scand. J. Dent. Res. **82:**527, 1974.
7. Giddon, D. B., Dreisbach, M. E., Pfaffman, C., and Manly, R. S.: Relative abilities of natural and artificial dentition patients for judging the sweetness of solid foods, J. Prosthet. Dent. **4**(2):263, 1954.
8. Hall, E. T.: The hidden dimension, New York, 1966, Doubleday & Co., Inc.
9. Hilzenrath, S.: The relation of judgments of attractiveness, Thesis, Brandeis University, Waltham, Mass., 1963.
10. Johnson, S.: Cited in MacGregor, F. C.: Transformation and identity: the face and plastic surgery, New York, 1974, Quadrangle/The New York Times Book Co.
11. Jourard, S. M., and Secord, P. F.: Body cathexis and the ideal female figure, J. Abnorm. Soc. Psychol. **50:**243, 1955.
12. Largey, G. P., and Watson, D. R.: The sociology of odors, Am. J. Sociol. **77**(6):1021, 1972.
13. Levy, D. M.: Experiments on the sucking reflex and social behavior of dogs, Am. J. Orthopsychiatry **4:**203, 1934.
14. Lorenz, K.: The companion in the bird's world, Auk **54:**245, 1937.
15. MacGregor, F. C.: Transformation and identity: the face and plastic surgery, New York, 1974, Quadrangle/The New York Times Book Co.
16. MacLean, P. D.: The brain's generation gap: some human implications, Zygon **8:**113, 1973.
17. Maslow, A. H.: Motivation and personality, ed. 2, New York, 1970, Harper & Row, Publishers.

17a. Penfield, W., and Rasmussen, T.: The cerebral cortex of man: a clinical study of localization of function, New York, 1950, Macmillan, Inc.

18. Perrin, F. A. C.: Physical attractiveness and repulsiveness, J. Exp. Psychol. **4:**203, 1921.
19. Piaget, J.: Cited in a paper by Pfeiffer, E. L., presented at the Sixth Annual Jean Piaget Conference, Philadelphia, June 12, 1976.
20. Rugh, J. D.: Variation in human masticatory behavior under temporal constraints, J. Comp. Physiol. Psychol. **50**(1):160, 1972.
21. Smith, J. W., Chase, J., and Lieblish, A. K.: Tongue showing: a facial display of humans and other primate species, Semiotica **11**(3):201, 1974.
22. Sosnow, I.: The emotional significance of the loss of teeth, Dent. Clin. North Am., p. 637, Nov., 1962.

22a. Spitz, R.: The first year of life, New York, 1965, International Universities Press.

23. Szczesniak, A. S., and Kahn, E. L.: Consumer awareness of and attitudes to food texture, J. Texture Stud. **2:**280, 1971.
24. Vitz, P.: Personal communication, 1976.
25. Watson, P.: Boss cows and sleepy, sexy sheep, Psychol. Today **9**(7):93, 1975.
26. Wiggins, J.: Men's preferences for different types of female figures, Med. Aspects Hum. Sexuality **5**(9):110, 1971.
27. Yurkstas, A. A., and Emerson, W. H.: Decreased masticatory function in denture patients, J. Prosthet. Dent. **14**(5):931, 1964.
28. Ziolkowski, T.: The telltale teeth: psychodontia to sociodontia, PMLA **91:**1, 1976.

Chapter 2

THE PSYCHOPHYSIOLOGY OF DENTAL DISEASE

The mouth and face may not only be a source of satisfaction or suffering, but can also be the target for the manifestations of life's adversities. There is, in fact, considerable evidence that, together with other biophysical host and environmental variables, social and psychological factors are important in the genesis of dental disease.

Since the mouth has the actual or prototypical functions of all body systems, the contribution of psychological and social factors to pathological changes in the oral cavity is to be expected. Portions of the respiratory and digestive systems and the musculoskeletal, cardiovascular, exocrine, and endocrine systems are all subject to the influences of the somatic and autonomic nervous systems.

To the extent that these systems are influenced by the central nervous system, they will be affected by variations in the psychological status of the individual. It follows, then, that noxious environmental events, acting through the senses and the central nervous system, have as much potential to produce malfunction or organ damage in the oral cavity as they do in other parts of the body.

Yet for many behavioral scientists and dentists, and even more for their patients, these ideas are somewhat surprising. Psychiatrists and psychologists are often amazed to discover that the mouth is more than a vestige of a Freudian psychosexual stage. One only need look into the mouth to study a disease that may be affected by psychosocial factors. Moreover, the disease may be easily quantified, for example, by the number and extent of carious lesions or inflamed gingival papilla.

The dentist can actually do much to increase patient concern with oral health and disease by emphasizing the impact of psychosocial factors. The patient of today readily accepts that psychological stress affects body organs. Why should the oral structures not be similarly affected, since they have blood vessels, nerves, and muscles like any other part of the body?

Understanding psychophysiological disorders provides the dentist with insight into the nature of patient complaints. Thus when a patient complains, that is, presents a symptom, the dentist is able to appreciate that the basis of the complaint may go beyond the observable organic pathological condition.

Indeed the typical psychophysiological disorder presents many more symptoms than signs. Symptoms are defined as the *patient's description* of the problem, for example, a report of a toothache; signs are defined as *objective, measurable* indices of pathology such as temperature and blood pressure. Unfortunately the dentist often dismisses the patient's complaint with an implicit or explicit diagnosis that the problem is "psychosomatic," that is, "it's all in your mind." In so doing, the dentist relegates the complaint to some poorly understood diagnostic category, and the disorder becomes more difficult to treat.

Understanding the psychological factors that affect disease does not require that one be a psychiatrist nor does it imply that dentists should stop cutting tooth structure and start "psychologizing" the decay. Rather, as we will see, this viewpoint encourages an integrated approach to the understanding of signs and symptoms and, as such, is an adjunct to dental diagnosis and treatment, not a substitute for it.

OBJECTIVES

The objectives of this chapter are as follows:

1. To explore the relationship between stress and disease (especially dental disease)
2. To determine the nature of psychophysiological disorders, including examining factors that determine the stressfulness of a situation for a given individual, the body's pathways of response to stress, and what organ system will be involved in responding to stress
3. To examine evidence relating psychological factors to disease

STRESS AND DISEASE

Concepts

In general, **disease** can be thought of as an unsuccessful attempt on the part of the body to deal or cope with environmental **stressors,** that is, disease is not the *result* of these environmental factors, but represents a failure to avoid, by appropriate preventive behavior, or to adapt to the adverse factors in the environment.[27] These stressors might include, at one extreme, the easily understood physical or biological stressors such as a pathogenic microorganism or the less well-understood psychosocial problems of interpersonal relationships such as marital conflict or moving to another community. Just as some individuals fail to avoid or to adapt to the presence of certain pathogens and become sick, others are not able to avoid or to adapt to pathogenic psychosocial situations.

Historical perspective

Since the Freudian revolution, diseases resulting primarily from the failure to adapt have been referred to as **psychosomatic,** or more recently, **psychophysiological.** Although both terms indicate acceptance of the reciprocal relationship between the mind and the body, the term "psychophysiological" reflects more recent knowledge about the mutual influences the mind and body have on each others' functioning.

Historically the medical models for understanding disease states, especially the germ theory of disease, have provided compelling explanations for organic pathological conditions. The inclusion of such seemingly vague considerations as psychological events or mental disturbance with the more observable etiological factors in illness was met, until relatively recently, with derision and denial on the part of the medical-dental establishment.

The label "psychosomatic disease" came to be applied to a particular group of diseases and their treatment. The psychosomatic diseases were so named because their primary etiological factors seem to be psychological. Typically the involved organ systems are connected to autonomic nervous system (ANS) activity. These diseases include peptic ulcer, ulcerative colitis, rheumatoid arthritis, essential hypertension, migraine, asthma, and certain allergic responses. Psychosomatic medicine became that specialty of medicine dealing with these diseases and their treatment.

The newer, somewhat broader term, **"psychophysiological disorder"** is now defined by the American Psychiatric Association in the following manner:

> . . . a group of disorders characterized by physical symptoms that are caused by emotional factors and involve a single organ system, usually with ANS innervation. The physiologic changes involved are those normally associated with certain emotional states, but in the psychophysiological disorder, these changes are more intense and sustained. In addition, the patient is

usually not aware of underlying emotional or stress relationships.*

The concept is that aberrations in mental functioning, somehow, may cause such strong and chronic physiological reactions that bodily breakdown can occur. The patient becomes ill for reasons that are, typically, not immediately obvious.

Disease as a response to psychosocial stressors

Psychosocially mediated disease can also be thought of as the result of the interaction of impinging psychosocial stimuli on the psychobiological program of the individual.[25] The individual's psychobiological program depends on genetic factors and early environmental influences. This sequence of events leading to disease or its precursors can be seen in Fig. 2-1.

In this theoretical conception, interacting variables can modify "causative" factors that might lead to disease. These interacting variables could be intrinsic or extrinsic factors, mental or physical, that promote or prevent disease. The sequence is not a one-way process, but constitutes a cybernetic system with continuous feedback.

*From American Psychiatric Association: Diagnostic and statistical manual of mental disorders (DSM-II), Washington, D.C., 1968, The Association.

The following analogy may assist the reader in understanding the relationship between stress, attempted adaptation, or coping behavior, and disease. Let us think of our human psychological and physiological responses to adverse environmental events as analogous to the response of an oyster to an irritating grain of sand. The oyster responds by making a pearl, whereas persons respond by changing cognitive and affective responses with the respective changes in physiological reactions.

Patterns of responding to stressors as a function of psychological or mental health status

"Normal/healthy" individuals. The normal human organism responds to physical and social stressors with different size "pearls," depending on the magnitude of the irritating environmental event. When the magnitude of the stressor is great as

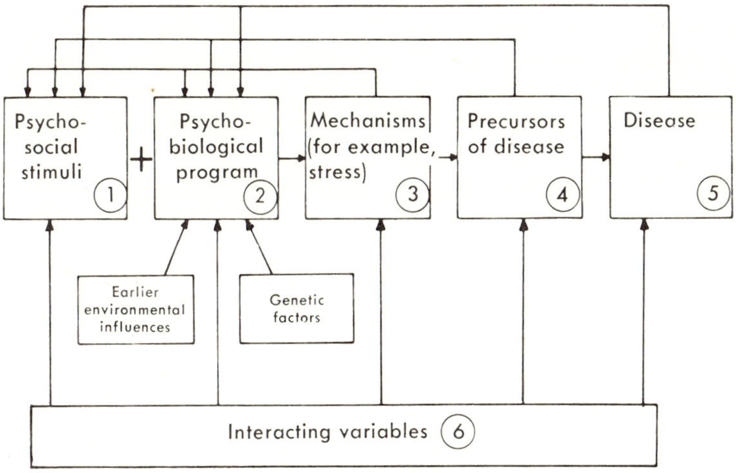

Fig. 2-1. A theoretical model for psychosocially mediated disease. The combined effect of psychosocial stimuli (1) and the psychobiological program (2) determines the psychological and physiological reactions, or mechanisms (3), for example, stress, of each individual. These may, under certain circumstances, lead to precursors of disease (4) and to disease itself (5). This sequence of events can be promoted or counteracted by interacting variables (6). The sequence is not a one-way process but constitutes part of a cybernetic system with continuous feedback. (From Kagan, A. R., and Levi, L.: In Reports from the lab for clinical stress research, Stockholm, 1971, Karolinska Sjukhuset.)

in the death of a close family member, so, too, is the psychophysiological response. It is, in fact, quite normal that a psychophysiological response to such real tragedy may last a long time. When the psychosocial or physical events comparable to the grain of sand are reduced in magnitude, so, too, are the psychophysiological responses.

Neurotic individuals. In neurotic individuals, the psychophysiological responses are out of proportion, that is, they are greatly exaggerated or greatly diminished in magnitude and/or duration in relation to the stressor. Thus the neurotic person may react with a large pearl even if the noxious environmental event is of smaller magnitude. A neurotic person's response may also be inappropriate when it persists beyond the duration of the increased environmental irritant or cause of stress. However, these reponses are really not so exaggerated when one considers that the response is actually proportional to the individual's exaggerated *perception* of the magnitude of the irritant. Such misperception is, in fact, the most characteristic neurotic response. When a person overreacts to society's demands, inappropriate attempts to adapt may become so excessive and/or numerous as to incapacitate the individual to the point of mental illness.

Although all of us have some neurotic tendencies, one may be diagnosed as having a neurosis when responses to emotional conflict become incapacitating and dominate one's mental life, leading to maladaptive behavior and discomfort.[20] For example, dentists with an obsession about cleanliness that results in compulsive hand-washing would obviously be engaging in counterproductive behavior for busy professionals. At the other extreme, dentists may compound their trouble if they only washed their hands after, rather than before, touching a patient. Some patients may believe they are being "put down" by such actions.

Psychotic individuals. A psychotic individual also attempts to adapt to environmental stressors. However, this person responds inappropriately either by thought processes (the schizophrenias) or emotional behavior (the affective psychoses) that are highly idiosyncratic, totally maladaptive, and often bizarre.

The difference between the neurotic and the psychotic is illustrated by the old adage that "the neurotic builds castles in the air and the psychotic lives in them," that is, the psychotic actually experiences a self-constructed world as real.

Sociopathic individuals. The sociopathic individual, who is characterized by his or her antisocial behavior, responds to physical-social irritation by moving against it. In other words, the sociopathic person may act out his or her response behaviorally, possibly by violent, destructive behavior. He or she may also react less antisocially by leaving the field of encounter, by running away, or by "copping out." Such a reaction, although appropriate in magnitude, is inappropriate in direction. The sociopathic individual appears to "not care" to an excessive degree about current behavior, personal relationships, or the effect of his or her behavior on others.

• • •

This general disease model is only a conceptual orientation. As such it is oversimplified, with many details omitted.

All individuals, whether psychologically healthy or ill, are subject to environmental changes that require continual adaptation. The objective presence or absence of the physical-social factors responsible for bodily adaptation are not so important for the occurrence of disease as the perceived or "felt" significance of an event. Adaptative efforts may be excessive because of distorted perception or motivational needs (Chapters 8 and 9). A person in relatively perfect mental health can respond to a real family tragedy with extensive behavior and/or neurohumoral manifestations that equals in magnitude the neurotic individual's response to something someone may have said.

Dental disease as an example of the stress-generated disease model

Dentistry offers an excellent model for the phenomenon of psychosocial stressors causing disease. Dental disease may result when the body fails to avoid, by appropriate preventive behavior, the accumulation of local irritants that can support pathogenic bacteria and/or when the host fails to adapt to noxious environmental events.

Acute necrotizing ulcerative gingivitis is an example of an infectious oral disease that fits the previously mentioned model. Patients with this disease demonstrate a significantly higher incidence of psychological disturbance than control patients.[16] Consistent with this "failure to avoid or adapt" model, the disease occurs when the individual fails to avoid the accumulation of local irritants and/or when the patient fails to adapt to noxious environmental events, for example, for neurotic reasons.

One can, in fact, postulate a threshold concept of tissue destruction such that, when any combination of adverse local and systemic factors reaches this threshold, the host tissue resistance to microorganisms is reduced, and tissue destruction is probable. If, for example, the "threshold" is arbitrarily set at 12 and local factors such as calculus and systemic factors such as nutritional deficiency or blood supply are each rated on a scale from 1 to 8, tissue destruction may result in a necrotic ulcer when, by some mathematical combination, these two factors reach 12. Similar to other diseases, both the probability of occurrence and the intensity of such dental diseases increase as a function of inadequate or inappropriate behavioral and/or neurohumoral adaptation to change in the physical-social environment.

NATURE OF PSYCHOPHYSIOLOGICAL DISORDERS

Given the preceding overview, we will now attempt to delineate the ways in which stress in general and psychosocial stressors in particular influence the structure and function of the oral cavity. This problem can be divided into three basic questions to be considered separately.

- What determines the stressfulness of a particular situation for a given individual?
- What are the physiological pathways involved in the body's response to stress?
- What determines which particular organ system will be affected?

What determines the stressfulness of a situation for a given individual?

Nature of the psychosocial stimuli (stressor). The first question may be simply rephrased to what environmental events—actual, imagined, or symbolic—trigger the central nervous system to start the chain of physiopathological events? To begin, let us define the term "stress" more precisely as a change in the external or internal environment of such intensity or duration that it requires more than the usual adaptative efforts to maintain homeostasis or life.[19] Included as stressors are changes such as intoxication, dehydration, bacterial toxins, or interhuman conflicts involving deprivation or frustration. In other words, the damaging agent can be mechanical, physicochemical, biological, or personal.

As Groen[19] indicates in the following quote:

> Human beings inflict damage on each other in many ways, one of them being the effects of social conflict. The types of interhuman conflicts are determined by the culture of the subgroup(s) to which the partners in the conflict belong. The ways in which they behave and thereby try to act out or solve their conflicts are not only individually but also culturally determined. Human cultures, particularly via their educational norms and goals, influence the personality structure of their members, the nature of the conflicts between them, the ways in which they respond to their conflicts, and

the types of the disease which occur as a result.*

Stress can thus be caused by social circumstances or cultural rules that frustrate or threaten to frustrate an individual by preventing him or her from developing or acting according to inborn, acquired, or gratifying behavior patterns.

Magnitude of the required adaptation. Although not always accessible to observation, some form of psychological obstruction usually precedes such varied psychophysiological disorders as gastrointestinal disturbance, asthma, back pain, cluster headaches, and even certain cancers. Events **(psychological antecedents)** that require such significant personal readjustment include changes in family constellation, sexual activity, marital status, occupation, economic status, residence, group and peer relationships, education, religion, recreation, and health. Recently, in fact, Rahe et al. established the relative stressfulness of readjustment to changes in these different life events. In several studies from different cultural subgroups, the number of times a relatively serious life event occurred prior to the disease was found to correlate with the onset and frequency of illness.[34] The occurrence of each of these events usually requires some adaptive or coping behavior that, if unsuccessful, may result in disease. Those events that evoke in an individual feelings of *resentment, frustration, depression, anxiety,* and/or *helplessness,* in that order, have greater potential for disease than events that may evoke other kinds of feelings.[29]

Regardless, then, of whether the stress is associated with physical or psychosocial factors, *what is most important in the onset of disease is the amount of real or perceived change to which the individual must adapt to maintain a relatively steady state*. Tables 2-1 and 2-2 indicate the relative stressfulness of different life events for samples of American and Swedish young and old individuals.

Such a perspective makes it easier to understand that disease of any kind, or even accidents, may be related to stress. Looking at it another way, the world may be divided into the following three groups: those who adapt well to stress, those who do not, and those in the middle. It is most likely that poor adaptors make up the group who are more illness or accident prone than the general population. These are patients with the thickest or heaveist hospital record folders. One study showed that 75% of the illnesses or accidents, that is, time lost from work for any reason, were accounted for by only 25% of the group studied.[22]

As indicated earlier from the data on readjustment, *stress does not have to be negative to cause disease or accidents.* Changes in positive or pleasant direction require coping. For example, although getting married is generally considered a positive event, it requires adaptation. Similarly, unpleasantness or adversity is not restricted to excessive stimulation; deprivation of stimulation may also be stressful, as shown in Fig. 2-2. For example, understimulation such as is involved in parental deprivation, often seen in urban slums of developing countries, can seriously increase the risk of disease.

Some of the psychosocial stimuli related to stressfulness in this model follow:

1. Deprivation or excess of parental care related to
   a. Antagonism to child or mutual antagonism of parents
   b. Favoritism, particularly in relation to sustenance, play, and advice
2. Social and economic deprivation or excess related to
   a. Group membership at school or work and during leisure (friends, gangs, or clubs)
   b. Interpersonal relationships (family, friends, co-workers)

*From Groen, J. J.: In Levi, L., ed.: Society, stress and disease, vol. I. The psychosocial environment and psychosomatic disease, London, 1971, Oxford University Press.

Table 2-1 □ SRRQ item mean scores and rank orderings* for young Americans and young Swedes†

Item	American		Swedish	
	Rank	Score	Score	Rank
Death of spouse	1	914	956	1
Divorce	2	640	652	3
Marital separation	3	536	594	5
Death of close family member	4	507	549	7
Marriage	5	500	500	10
Detention in jail‡	6	484	752	2
Major personal injury or illness‡	7	404	630	4
Retirement from work	8	398	462	12
Being fired from work‡	9	365	504	9
Marital reconciliation§	10	351	444	14
Sexual difficulties‡	11	348	534	8
Death of a close friend‡	12	334	490	11
Major change in health of family‡	13	316	556	6
Pregnancy‡	14	298	460	13
Major change in financial state	15	294	330	18
Major change in arguments with wife	16	292	280	22
Addition of new family member‡	17	285	416	16
Major business adjustment‡	18	282	426	15
Changing to different line of work‡	19	261	379	17
Mortgage foreclosure	20	236	254	26
Start or end of formal schooling	21	219	233	28
Major change in work responsibilities‡	22	212	329	19
Son or daughter leaving home§	23	200	308	21
In-law troubles	24	194	258	25
Mortgage or loan over $10,000§	25	171	268	23
Wife starting or ending work‡	26	156	239	27
Trouble with boss‡	27	154	260	24
Outstanding personal achievement	28	136	164	35
Major change in living conditions‡	29	135	314	20
Changing to a new school‡	30	126	207	29
Major change in working conditions‡	31	120	202	30
Major revision of personal habits§	32	114	201	31
Major change in social activities‡	33	102	190	32
Major change in recreation‡	34	100	164	34
Mortgage or loan less than $10,000§	35	97	132	38
Change in residence†	36	92	172	33
Major change in church activities‖	37	88	152	36
Major change in family get-togethers‖	38	74	108	40
Major change in sleeping habits‡	39	66	119	39
Major change in eating habits‖	40	64	99	41
Vacation§	41	51	88	42
Christmas	42	36	57	43
Minor violations of the law‡	43	26	142	37

*Items listed according to the younger American sample rank ordering.
†From Rahe, R. H., Lundbergh, U., Bennett, L., and Theorell, T.: J. Psychosom. Res. **15**:241, 1971.
‖$p \leq 0.05$.
§$p \leq 0.01$.
‡$p \leq 0.001$.

Table 2-2 □ SRRQ item mean scores and rank orderings* for older Americans and older Swedes†

Item	American		Swedish	
	Rank	Score	Score	Rank
Death of spouse	1	636	694	1
Divorce	2	558	556	4
Marital separation	4	494		
Death of close family member‡	5	396	572	3
Marriage	3	500	500	7
Detention in jail§	6	378	552	5
Major personal injury or illness	7	374		
Retirement from work	9	331	408	11
Being fired from work	10	326	622	2
Marital reconciliation	8	362		
Sexual difficulties	13	296	354	18
Death of a close friend‡	26	182	394	13
Major change in health of family‡	12	305	508	6
Pregnancy	17	258		
Major change in financial state§	11	320	389	14
Major change in arguments with wife‖	18	248	313	22
Addition of new family member‡	14.5	290	400	12
Major business adjustment	16	288	273	25
Changing to different line of work§	14.5	290	409	10
Mortgage foreclosure‡	21	213	458	8
Start or end of formal schooling	28	161		
Major change in work responsibilities‡	19	230	372	16
Son or daughter leaving home‡	25	191	327	20
In-law troubles‡	23.5	198	314	21
Mortgage or loan over $10,000‡	22	210	346	19
Wife starting or ending work‡	27	174	257	27.5
Trouble with boss‡	29	156	422	9
Outstanding personal achievement‡	20	220	366	17
Major change in living conditions‡	23.5	198	388	15
Changing to a new school	37	112		
Major change in working conditions‡	30	146	304	23
Major revision of personal habits‡	34	126	272	26
Major change in social activities§	32.5	130	190	34
Major change in recreation‡	32.5	130	236	29
Mortgage or loan less than $10,000‡	39.5	104	257	27.5
Change in residence‡	31	134	297	24
Major change in church activities‡	35	118	218	31
Major change in family get-togethers‡	36	114	220	30
Major change in sleeping habits‡	38	110	212	32
Major change in eating habits‡	39.5	104	202	33
Vacation‡	41	94	181	35
Christmas	42	73		
Minor violations of the law	43	65		

*Items listed according to the older American sample rank ordering.
†From Rahe, R. H., Lundbergh, U., Bennett, L., and Theorell, T.: J. Psychosom. Res. **15:**241, 1971.
‖$p \leq 0.05$.
§$p \leq 0.01$.
‡$p \leq 0.001$.

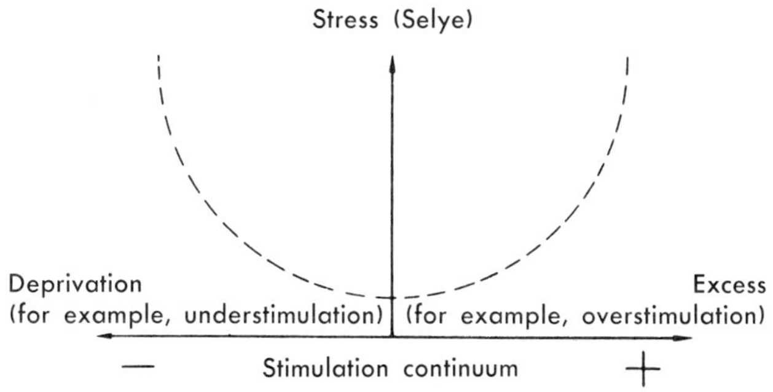

Fig. 2-2. Theoretical model of the relation between physiological stress as defined by Selye and various levels of stimulation. According to this hypothesis, deprivation of stimuli as well as excess is accompanied by an increase in "stress (Selye)." (Redrawn from Levi, L.: Stress and distress in response to psychosocial stimuli: laboratory and real life studies on sympathoadrenomedually and related reactions, Oxford, England, 1972, Pergamon Press Ltd.)

c. Communication (family, friends, or strangers)
d. Environmental change
e. Privilege, status, and self-esteem
f. Degree of affluence
g. Self-concept and security
3. Freedom of action
4. Limitations imposed by health status

As discussed earlier, the greater the magnitude, duration, frequency, unpredictability, and/or suddenness of these psychosocial stimuli, the greater the physiological consequences.

Variables affecting the individual's ability to adapt to stress. The bodily response to stress can be either increased or decreased by the following intervening variables*:

I. Psychosocial factors—combinations of noxious psychosocial environmental stimuli
II. Physicosocial factors—physical environmental stimuli such as heat, cold, noise, chemical hazards, altitude, malnutrition, and overcrowding, alone or in combination
III. Constitutional factors
  A. Genetic
  B. Acquired
IV. Lack of "protective" intervening variables
  A. Mental processes
    1. Habituation
    2. Adaptation
    3. Availability of acceptable substitute activities
    4. Increasing tolerance of ambiguity
    5. Learning by imprinting or conditioning
  B. Psychosocial factors
    1. Belonging to a group
    2. Availability of acceptable substitute activities
    3. Availability of someone to talk with about own troubles
    4. Education
  C. Physicosocial factors
    1. Nutrition
    2. Clothing
    3. Housing
  D. Constitutional factors
    1. Genetic
    2. Acquired

Perhaps the most important class of protective intervening variables are the psychosocial factors, particularly those relating to interpersonal resources. For example, Foa[8] identifies six resource classes (Fig. 2-3) that are potentially but not actually available to everyone. The social implications of "resource deprivation" for the question of "what is stressful" are well known. It has been demonstrated that re-

*Adapted from Kagan, A. R., and Levi, L.: In Reports from the lab for clinical stress research, Stockholm, 1971, Karolinska Sjukhuset.

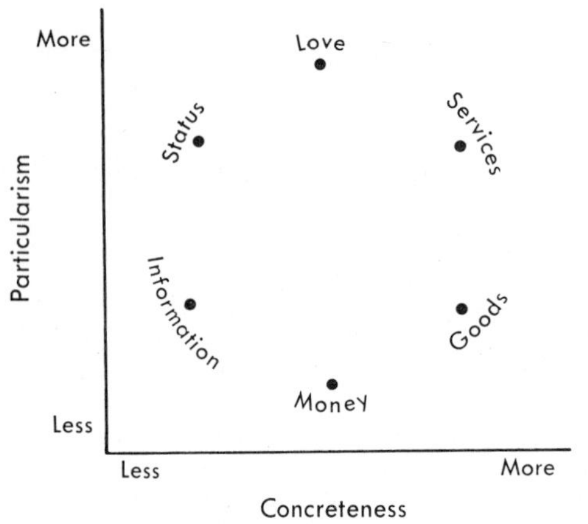

Fig. 2-3. Six resource classes. (From Foa, U. G.: Science **171**[3969]:345-351, 1971. Copyright 1971 by the American Association for the Advancement of Science.)

source deprivation, particularly at an early age, impairs social functioning. Thus impoverishment of experience during the early months can retard the development of intelligence, and hence coping skills, as per the following quote:

> When a needed resource is not readily available through access to appropriate institutional channels, the deprived individual may be forced to take longer and more devious routes to achieve what he needs, and his or her behavior may appear peculiar to the outsider. A good example is provided by the following behavior patterns which have been ascribed to some American Blacks: (1) preference for conspicuous consumption items like flashy cars and clothes, rather than purchasing more "solid" items; (2) demanding integrated facilities where there is separation, and separate ones where there is integration; and (3) enrolling in Black studies programs which do not provide training for specific future jobs. There seems to be little in common among these behaviors except that none of them appears oriented toward long-range goals. A meaningful picture emerges, however, when they are seen as different paths to achieve status, the resource of which Black people have been most deprived. Conspicuous consumption goods are exchangeable with status. Refusal of social contact, by insisting on separate facilities, means taking away status from those who originally rejected them; thus the real issue is not integration versus separation, but who is taking away status from whom. The information gained in Black studies may not be useful on the job, but it is a means to a needed increase in self pride.*

Foa goes on to say that when an individual is denied the most needed resource, he or she tends to give or receive the resource that is nearest the order to the preferred one. When the only resource available is on the side of the circle opposite the preferred one, the intensity of response may be proportional to the distance between the preferred and the available resource; and/or the need satisfaction will be inversely related to the distance. Thus a person who needs to be loved and can obtain only money will never be satisfied no matter how rich he or she becomes. In the same manner, an individual who has been insulted (deprived of status) and can retaliate only by destroying goods belonging to the insulter, will inflict a great deal of material damage and still be left with a grudge.

Such an analysis explains in part the exchange involved in U.S. welfare institutions that often required clients to lose status for the money they receive. This transaction deprives clients of a resource that is already scarce for them, thus further reducing their chances of autonomous performance as resource exchangers in society. Similarly, the decrease in aggression and destruction of property during riots may be attributed to the acquisition of more status among deprived minorities or to their increased ability to reciprocate in kind by taking away status from the privileged majority, rather than "burning their shops."

Conclusion. In summary, everyone has his or her own peculiar set of physical or social events that create stress; the magnitude of the event and consequent response is much more related to the individual's subjective *perception* of the event than the objective characteristics of the event as

*From Foa, U. G.: Science **171**(3969):345-351, 1971. Copyright 1971 by the American Association for the Advancement of Science.

observed by others. Consider, for example, the interpretation of the two letters of the alphabet: A and E. Although we all recognize them as communication symbols, in a variety of shapes, distorted or otherwise, it is really not that simple. Perception of these letters as such depends on two basic components, the structural and the functional. Structural factors include the physical stimuli and neural events contributing to the basic sensation level without meaning. Functional factors include affect, past experience, and learning that contribute to the interpretation of sensation or perception.

In this example, the stimulation of the retina by black lines on white paper, specifically four horizontal, two diagonal, and one vertical line, is without meaning until the functional factors of learning establish the configuration of those lines as the letters A and E. With learning and experience they can become symbols for use in written communication, the most familiar to students being examination grades.

Although everyone objectively sees these lines as A and E, these letters can produce at least two very different subjective perceptions and consequent physical responses. If, for example, the names Mr. Dworkin and Mr. Ference were put before the letters A and E respectively, there is little difference in responses emanating from these individuals. If, however, these line symbols are subsequently identified as examination grades (with A being the highest), Mr. Dworkin and Mr. Ference would have very different reactions to those same objective stimuli. Mr. Dworkin would react with a subjective response of pleasure and associated physiological changes, whereas Mr. Ference would experience disappointment or frustration and consequent physiological manifestations. Everyone else would have intermediate psychophysiological responses, depending on their individual identification with Mr. Dworkin or Mr. Ference. This all-important matter of perception is discussed in detail in Chapter 9.

What are the physiological pathways involved in the body's response to stress?

The example just given logically leads to our second question: Once the nervous system has been triggered by whatever is stressful for a given individual, two physiological pathways are involved—the relatively voluntary somatic motor system and the more involuntary neuroendocrine system, which may result in organ malfunction or damage.

Volitional pathways. The following are examples of overt behavioral reactions that coopt the voluntary pathways and that have been associated with actual dental disease. This category includes most of the semiautomatic *habits* associated with dental disorders.

Oral hygiene. The deleterious effects of poor oral hygiene on both hard and soft tissues of the oral cavity are well established. The role of psychosocial factors in health behavior such as oral hygiene has been extensively reviewed elsewhere.[35] The failure to engage in preventive health behavior such as oral hygiene or other known preventive measures is but another example of the contribution of social factors to disease. More detail is offered in the subsequent discussion of factors of psychosocial factors affecting demand and utilization of health care resources.

Oral habits. Typical examples of habits that may be harmful to oral tissues are those that utilize the masticatory apparatus for nonmasticatory activities, for example, bruxism and teeth clenching have been correlated by some authors with latent aggression[40] and depression.[32] Gum chewing similarly has been reported to be responsible for temporomandibular joint disturbances,[7] whereas sucking of the gingiva, tongue-thrusting, thumb-sucking, and tics involving the lips or face are socially inappropriate as well as potentially deleterious.

Other potentially harmful habits include the introduction of noxious vapors, liquids, and air currents that affect tissue moisture or temperature. Perhaps the most insidious is smoking, which, according to several researchers,[16] is related unquestionably to acute necrotizing ulcerative gingivitis and probably to other oral diseases. Smoking is also inversely related to many psychosocial variables associated with mental health.[31] What is not known, however, is whether smoking is itself of direct etiological significance or whether it is a symptom of some underlying psychological disturbance that has a more important role in the pathogenesis of these diseases. This qualification, however, does not minimize the direct local irritating effect of nicotine and tars on the tissue and, probably, less directly, their role in the formation of calculus. Mouth breathing with a more complex psychological or physical etiology may also affect the integrity of the oral tissues.

Coffee drinking is another habit that may act locally, as a result of thermal or chemical properties, and systemically, as a result of caffeine content. Coffee drinking is more frequent among smokers[31] and has also been shown in one of our unpublished studies to be greater among patients with acute necrotizing ulcerative gingivitis than among patients with normal gingivae.[9]

Another habit of psychological significance is the consumption of alcohol. Alcohol may act on the gingiva locally as an irritant and systemically via the neurohumoral system and other metabolic pathways.

Dietary factors. Diet as the more volitional aspect of nutrition can also influence the gingival tissue at both the local and the systemic levels. There is much in the literature relating psychiatric disorders to appetite levels. For example, loss of appetite (anorexia nervosa) or ravenous increase in appetite (bulimia) have been related to psychosocial stress. Taste preferences can also affect oral health. Tastes varying from the craving for sweets to the preference for hot spicy foods have been attributed to psychosocial factors such as cultural practices, need for oral gratification or stimulation, and personality type.[36] Failure to voluntarily avoid the previously mentioned irritants or to effectively remove them by proper oral hygiene will greatly increase the chances of initiating or aggravating oral disease.

Nonvolitional pathways. Knowledge about the internal (nonvolitional) pathways that lead to pathology, commonly referred to as the psychosomatic hypothesis, stems largely from the works of Pavlov, Cannon, Freud, and Selye. There is now little question of the role of the neuroendocrine systems in the pathogenesis of psychosomatic or psychophysiological reactions in general. Psychosomatic disease in the sense used here refers only to those diseases in which the alteration in the function of the neuroendocrine pathway results in observable organic disease. This is in contrast to "hysteria" or conversion symptoms involving the voluntary somatic nervous system in which no organic basis can be found for apparent paralysis or sensory loss.

These neuroendocrine pathways may be divided into the sympathetico–adrenal medullary system, presumably involved in reaction to more short-term acute stress, and the pituitary–adrenal cortical system and probably the parasympathetic branch of the autonomic nervous system, which are involved in response to more prolonged or chronic stress. Although the reader should refer to a text of endocrinology, physiology, or physiological psychology for details of these pathways, a brief overview of the role and function of some of the hormones in the nonvolitional pathway is offered here.

Hormones associated with response to stress. Hormones regulate body processes principally by their influence on (1) morphogenesis, or the building of the structure of the body; (2) the integration of body functions together with the nervous system; and (3) the maintenance of the internal environment, or homeostasis, compatible with life.

The hormones themselves are regulated by a complex interaction of neurons, hormones, and chemical regulators that vary in response to the physiological state of the organism. Thus some hormones are controlled by trophic hormones or other hormones from the anterior pituitary or master gland. A second group of hormones is governed by a physicochemical feedback, or the amount of presence of substances that they control in the bloodstream. A third group of hormones is primarily controlled or regulated by the nervous system itself.

The release of trophic hormones from the anterior portion of the pituitary is controlled by the hypothalamus. The most important trophic hormones are adrenocorticotropic hormone (ACTH), which controls the secretions of the adrenal cortex such as cortisone; thyroid-stimulating hormone (TSH), which controls the secretion of the thyroid gland; follicle-stimulating hormone (FSH), which controls the development of the follicle to ovulation and the testes to sperm production; luteinizing hormone (LH), which controls estrogen and ultimately progesterone secretion and ovulation in the female and acts on interstitial cell stimulating hormone (ICSH) to stimulate the interstitial cells of the testes to produce hormones responsible for the secondary sex characteristics in the male. Prolactin, or luteotropic hormone (LTH), initiates the maintenance of lactation and possibly maternal behavior. In addition, somatotropic, or growth, hormone (STH) has recently been shown to be responsive to physical and psychological stress in addition to being essential for normal growth.

An example of a second group of hormones that are governed by the amount of the substance they control in the bloodstream is insulin, which is determined by the level of circulating blood glucose. Insulin is involved in controlling the utilization of glucose by cells. Similarly, the secretion of parathyroid hormone (PTH) varies inversely with the amount of calcium in the bloodstream.

An example of hormones that are regulated primarily by neurogenic mechanisms is adrenaline, or epinephrine, which may also be involved in the regulation of ACTH. Epinephrine is secreted by the adrenal medulla, which is on the outer portion of the adrenal gland located over each kidney. Histologically, the medulla resembles nervous tissue and modified ganglion cells and thus is similar to the postganglionic nerve endings of the sympathetic branch of the autonomic nervous system, which secretes norepinephrine.

Epinephrine is associated with the acute response to stress causing increases in heart rate, blood pressure, pupillary dilation, and blood sugar level and, conversely, a reduction in digestive activity. All these reactions are consistent with the "fight-or-flight" reaction described by Cannon.[39]

The outer portion of the adrenal gland, or adrenal cortex, is regulated by ACTH and is responsible for more than 30 secretions necessary for life. Principal among these are the glucocorticoids, especially 17-hydroxycorticosteroids, which influence carbohydrate metabolism, wound healing, allergic response, and inflammation.

In the presence of iodine the thyroid gland produces and secretes a hormone called **thyroxin.** *This is another most important hormone that is sensitive to psychosocial stimuli.* It increases the metabolic rate and the turnover of carbohydrates, fats, and cholesterol. Hyperthyroidism, also called Graves' disease, is associated with increased metabolic and heart rates, etc. and may be precipitated by an "acute emotional crisis." On the other hand, hypothyroidism is associated with an overall reduction in metabolic rate, manifested by lowered oxygen consumption, body heat, and heart rate. If not corrected in early childhood, mental retardation or cretinism may result.

Role of the autonomic nervous system in response to stress. Of at least equal importance in the neuroendocrine translation of psychosocial stress into organic pathology is the more acutely responding autonomic nervous system (ANS), which is composed of sympathetic and parasympathetic branches. In general, the control of the sympathetic nervous system is more diffuse, affecting larger regions of the body, whereas the parasympathetic innervation is more specific to particular organs.

The sympathetic nervous system consists of a chain of 22 ganglia that connect with all of the spinal nerves after they emerge from the spinal cord (in the thorax and lumbar region), although not necessarily on a one-to-one basis. There is one synapse between the target organ and the ganglia located within the head and abdominal cavity. In contrast, the parasympathetic system follows cranial nerves III, VII, IX, X, and XI and sacral nerves II, III, and IV of the spinal nerves and synapse very close to the organs they innervate.[39]

The autonomic nervous system (ANS) in general functions to maintain, along with the hormones, the internal environment necessary for life. It helps regulate the energy exchange that permits the voluntary somatic neuromotor system to engage in overt behaviors essential to coping with change in the external environment. All the changes take place at a relative reflex level in the lower brain stem, or medulla, in centers that contain groups of ANS neurons involved in the regulation of specific bodily functions. The center for temperature regulation, for example, involves respiration, vasodilation, sweating, etc.

The hypothalamus, in turn, is responsible for organizing these centers into response patterns that are associated with specific activities such as mating, hunger, sleep, and rage. The relation of these behaviors to such emotions as anger, fear, and love is coordinated within the limbic system. When to apply the repertoire of "emotional" responses is then determined by the highest level of the nervous system, the cerebral cortex, where learning experience and reality appraisal operate to determine the appropriateness of behavior. If the stimulus is exciting enough, however, whether pleasant or unpleasant, cerebral control decreases in favor of lower level dominance by the limbic system. For example, animals that have had the cortex removed exhibit a "sham rage" response similar to what humans might do when subjected to strong emotion-producing situations.[43]

What determines which particular organ system will be affected?

Why then does a particular organ system, including the oral cavity, become a target of the pathophysiological process? This question has produced a number of theories in response. The major theoretical issues have centered on whether physiological or psychological specificity is responsible for organ specificity. Explanations of the mouth as the target organ vary from the psychoanalytical to a genetic basis for organ weakness.

Some workers were convinced that certain diseases were associated with specific conflicts such as ulcers being related to dependency or asthma to fear of separation.[1] Others believed that disease was related to certain personality-specific coping styles,[6] that is, ulcers and passive-dependent patterns. Another view, supported by experimental evidence, attributed some diseases, for example, hives and urticaria,[18] to specific attitudes.

Early conditioning experiences offered further promise as an explanation. Experience with stress such as a problem with feeding at a critical period in infant development could predispose the adult to revert to undifferentiated, total patterns of physiological responding when confronted with any stress in later life. Thus the child may be reinforced by a grandmother who responds supportively to the occasional gastric upset such as pain or diarrhea—the result in later life being gastrointestinal response to stress-producing situations. The common pathophysiological concept for all these theories is that persistence of these emotionally arousing situations produces a breakdown in a particular organ system.

A comprehensive synthesis of the various approaches has been made by Wolff, who said the following:

> The stress accruing from the situation is based in large part on the way the affected sub-

ject perceives it: perception depends upon a multiplicity of factors including the genetic equipment, basic individual needs and longings, earlier conditioning influences, and a host of life experiences and cultural pressures. No one of these can be singled out for exclusive emphasis. The common denominator of stress disorders is *reaction* to circumstances of threatening significance to the organism.*

As noted earlier, *everyone,* however, *does not perceive or respond to the same noxious stimuli in the same way.*

> The particular adaptation pattern evoked by a noxious agent is the resultant of past life experiences which condition individuals to react in specific ways. Hence, "etiology" in disease becomes a function, not merely of the precipitating incident and setting, but also a function of the past of the individual. . . . An individual may have been a potential "nose reactor" or "colon reactor" all his life without ever actually having called upon a particular protective pattern for sustained periods because he did not need to. A given protective pattern may remain inconspicuous during long periods of relative security, and then with stress, become evident as a disorder involving the gut, the heart and vascular system, the nasorespiratory apparatus, and skin or general metabolism.*

These conclusions were based on clinical observations of the affected organ systems of individuals in states of tranquility and during stressful interviews. Changes indicative of inappropriate adaptive response were observed in the gastric and colonic mucosa. Other examples are blanching of nasal mucosa with fear, increased blood pressure in hypertensive subjects, increased sebum production in patients with acne vulgaris, and increased response to local irritation and histamine in allergic patients. More generalized metabolic effects such as alterations in blood clotting and in carbohydrate metabolism were also observed.

The thesis of organ specificity has also been supported by the experimental observations that individuals respond with an idiosyncratic pattern of autonomic responses regardless of the stress imposed.[26] Further support for this concept was obtained by finding that the particular organ or system to which body complaints were referred exhibited greater reactivity to standardized stressors than other body areas. Specifically, it was observed that cardiac patients responded to stress with increased heart activity, headache-prone patients with increased electromyographic responses of the neck muscles,[30] hypertensive patients with elevations in blood pressure, and rheumatoid arthritis patients with higher levels of muscle activity.[33]

*From Wolff, H. G., STRESS AND DISEASE, 1953. Courtesy of Charles C Thomas, Publisher, Springfield, Illinois.

EVIDENCE RELATING PSYCHOSOCIAL FACTORS TO DISEASE

Even disease processes involving known specific pathogens may be influenced by psychosocial variables.

History of tuberculosis—an example

The history of tuberculosis might serve as an example of how the psychophysiological viewpoint became an integral part of medical theory and practice. Even at the time of Koch, reports indicated differential familial susceptibility to tuberculosis. The tubercle bacillus was apparently more pathogenic for some families than others. As many of the sources of tuberculosis were eliminated via vaccine, sanitation, raising of nutritional standards, etc., the concept of bacillus specificity of the disease was questioned. More than just the pathogen has to be considered in order to adequately comprehend the changes in reported epidemiology of the disease. Tuberculosis is now considered a disease of multiple etiology, with equal weight given the person and the bacillus. Critical covariables include the individual nature of the stress response, general hormonal imbalance, and the psychological disposition of the individual toward handling long-time dependency needs. The relationship between the virulence of the organisms and the resistance of the host thus constitute a complex interaction of physiological states, psychological history, and current life situation.

Studies relating psychosocial variables to oral pathology

More relevant to the mouth are case studies[17] demonstrating that daily counts of beta hemolytic streptococci in the pharynx are increased during times of frustration. There are also experimental reports of increased dental caries in stressed animals and interference with cementogenesis in rats subjected to stress.[22]

The possible role of the pituitary-adrenocortical axis in mediating the effects of a neurogenic stress on the oral cavity has also been investigated. Auditory stress has been shown to increase the weight of the adrenal glands in one experiment,[11] and in another study mice subjected to noxious auditory stress were more likely to develop a vesicular stomatitis in response to herpes virus inoculation than were nonstressed mice.[24]

Oral ulcerations have also been produced by restraint "stress" in rats.[44] A similar technique has been used to produce cleft palates in the offspring of stressed female mice.[37]

Examples of pathology produced by more direct manipulation of neurohumoral pathways are the production of ulcerative oral lesions in dogs in response to direct central nervous system irritation[4] and a greater frequency of destruction of the interdental papilla following incidental inflammation in cortisone-treated animals.

There is also little question of the association of psychological status and qualitative or quantitative alternations in saliva.[3,10,15] The literature is replete with studies relating physical and chemical characteristics of saliva to dental disease.

Salivary functions may also directly reflect activity of the physiological pathways involved in the mediation of stress. For example, activity of the adrenal cortex is reflected in the elevation of steroid levels in saliva in response to parenteral injections of ACTH.[38] Similarly, the level of a cholinesterase-like substance in saliva is affected by autonomically active agents and psychological stress.[12]

Other measures of autonomic nervous activity have been investigated in various disease states, particularly those presumed to have a psychological factor in their etiology.[42] Let us look at how a dental disease, gingivitis, was studied by evaluating the ANS. Using the method of Wenger et al., several autonomic measures were compared in normal subjects and in patients with gingival disease.[14] The results for two studies are shown in Table 2-3. Nine of the 15 variables show an apparent trend toward dominance of the sympathetic nervous system in the gingivitis groups. Four of these were significantly different: combined autonomic balance ($\bar{A}$) score, salivary output, sublingual temperature, and heart period. Dermal latency (capillary response to tactile irritation), however, was also significantly different, but in the opposite, or parasympathetic, direction. These differences in autonomic activity were apparently not a result of differences in anxiety level, as measured by two psychological tests.

In addition to implications for the pathogenesis of gingivitis, several interesting findings emerged from these studies. For example, two of the significant variables reflect differences in oral physiology such as a lower salivary output and a higher sublingual temperature for the gingivitis group.

This same autonomic battery of tests was given to a series of patients with acute necrotizing ulcerative gingivitis (ANUG) during the acute phase of the disease and to unaffected control groups at the same time. The tests were repeated 6 weeks later for both ANUG and control groups. Similar differences in the direction of sympathetic dominance were found for the ANUG group during the acute phase, which diminished on retesting during clinical recovery 4 to 6 weeks later. An interesting exception was the response of the cutaneous blood vessels to local irritation

Table 2-3 □ Mean resting autonomic measures: combined data from first and second studies*

Test	Units of measure	Normal (N = 35)	Gingivitis (N = 14)	t ratio
Salivary output	ml	2.6	1.9	2.12 (S)†‡
Sublingual temperature	° F	98.6	99.0	1.82 (S)†
Palmar conductance	μmho	8.62	9.71	0.68 (S)
Volar conductance	μmho	5.85	6.32	0.78 (S)
Log conductance change	Log μmho	0.501	0.479	0.31 (S)
Diastolic blood pressure	mm Hg	71.6	72.6	0.28 (S)
Heart period	milliminutes/10 cycles	156.1	146.6	1.91 (S)§
$\bar{A}$ score		73.2	67.4	2.32 (S)‡
Systolic blood pressure	mm Hg	117.2	122.1	1.35 (S)
Pulse pressure	mm Hg	45.4	50.2	1.37 (?S)
First finger temperature	° C	32.0	32.8	0.75
Second finger temperature	° C	33.1	33.2	0.10
Second − first finger temperature	° C	1.1	0.4	0.77
Dermal latency	sec	15.3	11.3	1.68§
Dermal persistence	min	30.5	33.5	0.68
Pupillary diameter	mm	5.4	5.1	0.81 (S)
Respirations per minute	cpm	17.7	16.9	0.96

*From Giddon, D. B.: J. Dent. Res. **45**(6):1627, 1966.
†$p < 0.01$
‡(S) indicates difference in direction of relative sympathetic dominance for gingivitis patients.
§$p < 0.05$

(dermal latency). In contrast to the relatively parasympathetic cutaneous vascular reaction noted previously for simple gingivitis, the cutaneous response to the ANUG group indicated sympathetic dominance that was consistent with a necrotic lesion of ischemic origin, as in ANUG.

These studies implicating autonomic regulation of the vascular system as a principal pathway in the pathogenesis of gingival disease prompted further investigation of the vascular bed of the affected tissues. A photoelectric method was developed for continuous measurement of the vascular reaction of a single human gingival papilla (Fig. 2-4).

The volume pulse recorded from a normal interdental papilla simultaneously with the cutaneous volume pulse and several other physiological variables is shown in Fig. 2-5. Both physical and psychological stimuli such as anticipation of distress reduced the amplitude of the volume pulse of the gingiva as well as of the finger. The similarity of the gingival and digital cutaneous vascular responses, occurring

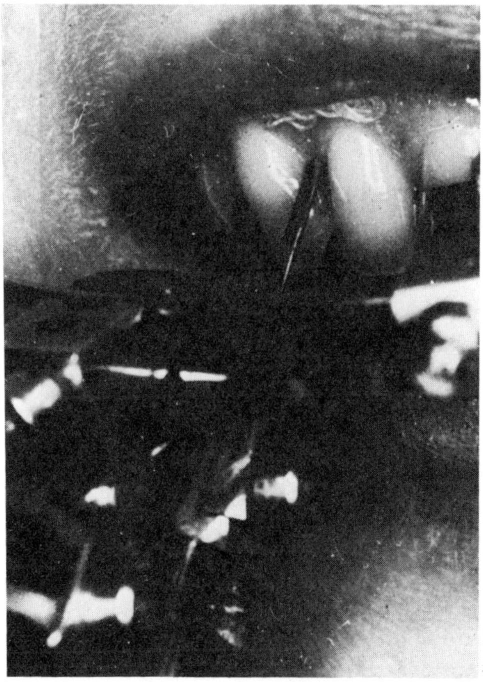

Fig. 2-4. Photoelectric probe for monitoring vascular responses of a single gingival papilla. (From Giddon, D. B.: J. Dent. Res. **45**[6]:1627, 1966.)

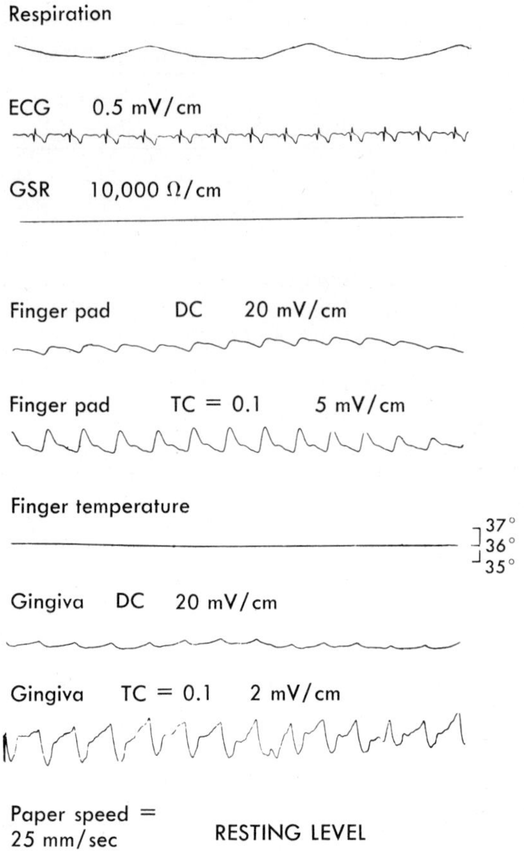

Fig. 2-5. Polygraph recording of gingival and digital volume pulses and other physiological variables. (From Giddon, D. B.: J. Dent. Res. **45**[6]:1627, 1966.)

simultaneously with other variables, to both the anticipation of stress and the actual cold presser stimulation is shown in Fig. 2-6. This method was subsequently used to demonstrate differences between ANUG and control groups in gingival and digital vascular responses.[5,13]

The observation that the *oral tissues are acutely responsive to anticipation of stress as well as the actual stress is, of course, most important for the diagnosis and treatment of oral disease*. Even variations in response to expectations of local anesthetics become more understandable in view of the acute sensitivities of the oral tissues to psychological factors.[46]

SUMMARY

Although there is considerable clinical evidence relating psychological stress to disease, there has been little experimentally controlled hard data definitely establishing the specific physiological connections. Some of the difficulty is, of course, related to the understandable ethical question of producing a disease in human beings who are subjected to experimental stress. The case must of necessity be made with animals. Only recently, for example, the importance of the psychological variable of control in the regulation of somatic stress was demonstrated in rats. Those animals that received ulcer-producing levels of shock but that could turn the shock off by escaping or moving a switch developed fewer ulcerations than their matched controls that had no means of turning off the shock.[41]

One approach to determine the possible contributions of psychosocial factors rela-

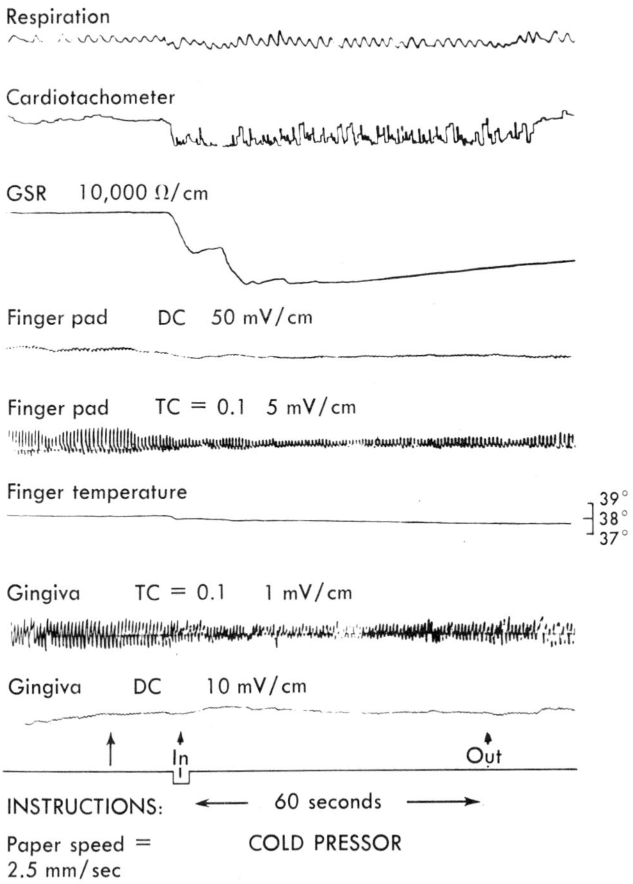

Fig. 2-6. Comparison of gingival and digital vascular response to cold pressor stimulation with other physiological variables. Note apparent vasoconstriction of gingival and finger pad immediately prior to the stimulus and during the 60-second stimulus period and then subsequent recovery. (From Giddon, D. B.: J. Dent. Res. **45**[6]:1627, 1966.)

tive to other biological or physical variables is through the science of epidemiology, the study of the distribution or occurrence of disease and its possible determinants. These epidemiological studies have attempted to look at the relationship between disease in general and a number of variables as potential stressors. In Chapter 3, we will examine the relationships of dental disease to the magnitude of each of these variables—physical, biological, geographical, and the component personal, socioeconomic, and cultural factors.

REFERENCES

1. Alexander, F.: Psychosomatic medicine—its principles and applications, New York, 1950, W. W. Norton & Co., Inc.
2. American Psychiatric Association: Diagnostic and statistical manual of mental disorders (DSM-II), Washington, D.C., 1968, The Association.
3. Barber, T. X., and Chauncey, H. H.: Effect of hypnotic and non-hypnotic suggestions on parotid gland response to gustatory stimuli, Psychosom. Med. **26**:374, 1964.
4. Chauncey, H. H., and Quintarelli, C.: Preliminary investigation on the relationship between the central nervous system and the oral cavity, Oral Surg. **12**:1257, 1959.
5. Clark, R. E., and Giddon, D. B.: Body geometry of patients having had recurrent attacks of acute necrotizing ulcerative gingivitis, Arch. Oral Biol. **16**:205, 1971.
6. Dunbar, H. F.: Mind and body: psychosomatic medicine, New York, 1947, Random House, Inc.
7. Elman, E.: Gum chewing and the temporomandibular joint, J. Am. Dent. Assoc. **71**:1416, 1965.
8. Foa, U. G.: Interpersonal and economic resources, Science **171**(3969):345, 1971.
9. Giddon, D. B.: Unpublished data.

10. Giddon, D. B.: The relation of a cholinesterase-like substance in parotid saliva to psychological stress, Doctoral Dissertation, University of Michigan, Ann Arbor, Mich., Dissert. Abstr. **24:**2115, 1963.
10a. Giddon, D. B.: Psychophysiology of the oral cavity, J. Dent. Res. **45**(6):1627, 1966.
11. Giddon, D. B., and Goldhaber, P.: Effect of auditory stress upon healing of experimental periodontal lesions, J. Dent. Res. **39:**746, 1960.
12. Giddon, D. B., and Lisanti, V. F.: Cholinesterase-like substance in the parotid saliva of normal and psychiatric patients, Lancet **1:**725, 1962.
13. Giddon, D. B., Clark, R. E., and Varni, J. G.: Apparent digital vasomotor hypotonicity in the remission stage of acute necrotizing ulcerative gingivitis, J. Dent. Res. **48:**431, 1969.
14. Giddon, D. B., Tanzer, D. W., and Gustafson, L. A.: Marginal gingivitis and resting autonomic activity, Int. Assoc. Dent. Res. Abstr. **41**(170):77, 1963.
15. Gilchrist, J. C., and Furchgott, E.: Salivary pH as a psychophysiological variable, Psychol. Bull. **48:** 193, 1951.
16. Goldhaber, P., and Giddon, D. B.: Present concepts concerning the etiology and treatment of acute necrotizing ulcerative gingivitis, Int. Dent. J. **14:**468, 1964.
17. Gottschalk, L. A., and Kaplan, S.: A quantitative method of estimating variations in intensity of a psychological conflict of state, Arch. Neurol. Psychiatr. **79:**688, 1958.
18. Grace, W. J., and Graham, D. T.: The specificity of the relation between attitudes and disease, Psychosom. Med. **14:**243, 1952.
19. Groen, J. J.: Social change and psychosomatic disease. In Levi, L., ed.: Society, stress, and disease, vol. 1. The psychosocial environment and psychosomatic disease, London, 1971, Oxford University Press.
20. Hines, F. R., and Pfeiffer, E.: Behavioral science, a selective view, Boston, 1972, Little, Brown & Co.
21. Hinkle, L., Jr.: The concept of "stress" in the biological and social sciences, Sci. Med. Man. **1:** 31, 1973.
22. Hollomand, R.: Anxiety and the oral cavity in experimental animals, Int. Assoc. Dent. Res. Abstr. **40**(227):60, 1962.
23. Hunt, J. M.: Intelligence and experience, New York, 1961, The Ronald Press Co.
24. Jensen, M. M., and Rasmussen, A. F.: Stress and susceptibility to viral infections, II. Sound stress and susceptibility to vesicular stomatitis virus, J. Immunol. **90:**21, 1963.
25. Kagan, A. R., and Levi, L.: Health and environment—psychosocial stimuli: a review. In Reports from the lab for clinical stress research, Stockholm, 1971, Karolinska Sjukhuset.
26. Lacey, J. I., and Lacey, B. C.: Verification and extension of the principle of autonomic response—stereotype, Am. J. Psychol. **71:**50, 1958.
27. Levi, L., ed.: Society, stress, and disease, vol. 1. The psychosocial environment and psychosomatic disease, London, 1971, Oxford University Press.
28. Levi, L.: Stress and distress in response to psychosocial stimuli: laboratory and real life studies on sympathoadrenomedually and related reactions, Oxford, England, 1972, Pergamon Press Ltd.
29. Luborsky, L., Docherty, J., and Penick, S.: Onset conditions for psychosomatic symptoms, Psychosom. Med. **35:**187, 1973.
30. Malmo, R. B., and Shagass, C.: Physiologic study of symptom mechanisms in psychiatric patients under stress, Psychosom. Med. **11:**25, 1949.
31. Matarazzo, J. D., and Saslow, G.: Psychological and related characteristics of smokers and nonsmokers, Psychol. Bull. **57:**493, 1960.
32. Molin, C., and Levi, L.: A psycho-odontologic investigation of patients with bruxism, Acta Odontol. Scand. **24**(3):373, 1966.
33. Moos, R. H., and Engle, B. T.: Psychophysiological reactions in hypertensive and arthritic patients, J. Psychosom. Res. **6:**227, 1962.
34. Rahe, R. H., McKean, J. D., Jr., and Arthur, R. J.: A longitudinal study of life-change and illness patterns, J. Psychosom. Res. **10**(4):355, 1967.
34a. Rahe, R. H., Lundberg, U., Bennett, L., and Theorell, T.: The social readjustment rating scale: a comparative study of Swedes and Americans, J. Psychosom. Res. **15:**241, 1971.
35. Rayner, J. F., and Cohen, L. K.: School dental health education. In Richards, N. D., and Cohen, L. K., eds.: Social sciences and dentistry: a critical bibliography, Leiden, 1971, A. W. Sijthoff, International Publishing Co. BV.
36. Richards, N. D., and Barmes, D.: Social factors in dental epidemiology. In Richards, N. D., and Cohen, L. K., eds.: Social sciences and dentistry: a critical bibliography, Leiden, 1971, A. W. Sijthoff, International Publishing Co. BV.
37. Rosenzweig, S., and Blaustein, F. M.: Cleft palate in CD-1 mice from restraint and deprivation of food and water, J. Dent. Res. **50**(2):503, 1971.
38. Shannon, I. L., Prigmore, J. R., Brooks, R. A., and Feller, R. P.: The 17 hydroxycorticosteroids of parotid fluid, serum and urine following intramuscular administration of repository corticotrophin, Clin. Endocrinol. Metabol. **19:**1477, 1959.
39. Sternbach, R. A.: Principles of psychophysiology, an introductory text and readings, New York, 1966, Academic Press, Inc.
40. Vernallis, F. F.: Teeth grinding: some relationships to anxiety, hostility and hyperactivity, J. Clin. Psychol. **11:**389, 1955.
41. Weiss, J.: Psychological factors in stress and disease, Sci. Am. **226:**(6):104, 1972.

42. Wenger, M. A., Clemens, T. L., and Cullen, T. D.: Autonomic functions in patients with gastrointestinal and dermatological disorders, Psychosom. Med. **24:**267, 1962.
43. Wenger, M. A., Jones, F. N., and Jones, M. H.: Physiological psychology, New York, 1956, Holt, Rinehart & Winston, Inc.
44. Whittaker, D. K., and Wilson, T. R.: The effect of age and strain differences on the incidence of restraint-induced oral and gastric ulcers in 3 strains of rats, J. Dent. Res. **51:**519, 1972.
45. Wolff, H. G.: Stress and disease, Springfield, Ill., 1953, Charles C Thomas, Publisher.
46. Zelechowski, K., Giddon, D. B., and Clark, R. E.: Gingival vascular response to anticipated and actual punctate stimulation, J. Dent. Res. **48:**419, 1969.

Chapter 3

THE OBJECTIVE NEED FOR DENTAL CARE

A description of observable dental disease in relation to socioeconomic and environmental factors

It is difficult for the dental student and even the relatively isolated individual dentist concerned with a clinical practice to fully appreciate the extent to which dental disease affects humanity. It is probably even more difficult to comprehend how information is gathered about the distribution of caries, periodontal disease, and, often, oral pathologic conditions. Finally, once the information is gathered it must be analyzed according to some rational plan. Certain analyses come readily to mind: Does age have anything to do with the prevalence of caries and/or periodontal disease. How about sex differences—do men and women suffer dental disease at the same rate? But other factors that contribute to the pattern of dental disease may not be so readily apparent. It turns out, for example, that ethnicity, culture, and psychosocial factors affect the distribution of caries, periodontal disease, malocclusion, and oral malignant disease.

OBJECTIVES

Chapter 3 is intended to provide an estimation of the magnitude of clinically determined dental disease, based in part on examination of a representative sample of the population by the U.S. Public Health Service as part of the National Health Survey.[32] The failure to seek dental treatment for a variety of reasons has resulted in a staggering amount of untreated oral disease among the American public.

From this epidemiological information, inferences can be made about the objective need for dental care in the United States. Unfortunately, these data are not up-to-date because dental disease is not a legally reportable disease such as tuberculosis or syphilis.

Other important sources of information include the periodic publication of the American Dental Association entitled "Bureau of economic research and statistics survey of needs for dental care" among American patients,[12] and the World Health Organization survey data, which are based on a classification of dental disease within the International Classification of Diseases.[64]

In descriptive epidemiology the terms "experience," "incidence," and "prevalence" are used to describe different aspects of the disease. **Experience** refers to the cumulative effect of the disease, past and present. **Incidence** refers to the number of new cases of a disease over a period of time. **Prevalence** refers to the proportion of the population affected by a disease at any point or period in time.[16] These terms will be used in relating some of the major dental diseases to psychosocial and environmental variables.

In addition to the distribution of disease,

the epidemiological approach is also used to describe the distribution of possible determinants of the disease. These determinants have been traditionally divided into host, agent, and environmental factors. **Host factors** include age, sex, heredity, national or ethnic group, diet as the volitional aspect of nutrition, and certain intrinsic psychological factors. **Agent factors** are physical and biological factors that affect the disease process. For example, the agent for caries, microbial in nature, may be involved in the actual production of decalcification and consequent loss of tooth structure. **Environmental factors** can be either external or internal. Among the external factors are the composition of water, diet, and sociopolitical elements. Internal environmental factors include motivation to engage in preventive health behavior such as oral hygiene practices.[16]

The objectives of this chapter are to acquaint the reader with the prevalence of and host and environmental factors associated with the following conditions:

1. Dental caries
2. Periodontal disease
3. Malocclusion
4. Cleft lip and cleft palate
5. Oral cancer

DENTAL CARIES

Prevalence

Approximately 95% of all Americans experience dental caries, which is the most prevalent of all chronic diseases.[28,30] A recent survey of a probability sample of the adult population of the United States projected that 20 million people have no natural teeth.[32] Among the 90 million others, there were an estimated 855.4 million missing teeth and 127.4 million teeth with unfilled carious lesions. Stated as an average these were 1.4 decayed (D), 9.4 missing (M), and 7.0 filled (F) teeth for a total of 17.9 DMF teeth per person.[37]

The magnitude of each component of the total number of D + M + F teeth reflects a different aspect of the disease or therapeutic process. The number of D teeth indicates the need for treatment, whereas the number of F teeth reflects the treatment received. Thus the sum of D and F teeth or surfaces is the measure of the caries experience of an individual. Because the number of M teeth could be the result of deep decay or periodontal disease, the ratio of F/D teeth and F/F + D teeth provides an even better indication of the care received relative to need.[31]

Despite certain limitations, the DMF count is the most commonly used index for caries survey in a population and is valuable for measuring the variations in dental experience between different groups of people. These variations can then be related to environmental or social factors and behavioral practices. DMF counts, for example, have been shown to vary with numerous social factors such as diet, fluoride content of the drinking water, oral hygiene, and frequency of visits to the dentist.[49]

Host factors

Age. Although the number of DMF teeth increases with age, the D component of the DMF total decreases with age as a result of the decreasing availability of vulnerable surfaces, whereas the M component increases.[32]

Sex. There is no consistent finding of greater prevalence of dental caries among either females or males, as shown in Fig. 3-1.

Race and ethnic background. Although there is considerable evidence for genetic factors in caries susceptibility of animals and humans, the causes of racial or ethnic differences are difficult to determine. In addition to genetic racial factors, there may be considerable variations in life-style, including dietary habits and health behaviors. For example, both Chinese and black populations have a lower caries incidence than whites living in the United States,[16] whereas Chinese children in Malaysia[64] and French Polynesia[6] had a greater incidence of caries than other racial-ethnic groups.

In the United States, the DMF index is higher in white than in black adults (18.7

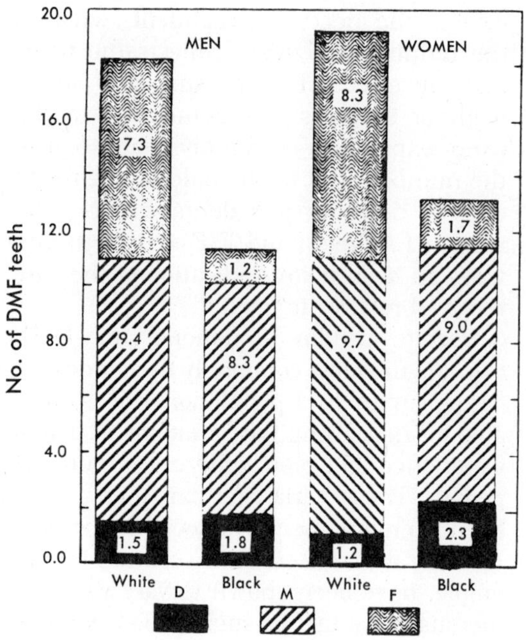

Fig. 3-1. Mean number of decayed, missing, and filled (DMF) teeth among dentulous men and women by ethnic group: United States 1960-1962. (From Kelly, J. E., Van Kirk, L. E., and Garst, C. C.: Decayed, missing, and filled teeth in adults—United States—1960-1962. Vital and health statistics, Series 11, No. 23, Public Health Service Pub. No. 1000, Washington, D.C., February, 1967, U.S. Government Printing Office.)

vs 12.2), primarily as a result of the higher number of F teeth in white adults. On the other hand, there is a higher need for fillings and extractions among black patients.

Psychological factors (psychosomatic or emotional influences). Recent reviews of the social and psychological factors in dental disease suggest that some individuals have a personal style of coping with stressful situations that results in increased caries.[49,57,61] For example, acute caries was observed in 24% of adult subjects within a month after the onset of stress. This short latency period suggests that changes in oral hygiene or diet alone could not have accounted for the lesions.[61] Other investigators, however, have found no consistent relationship between anxiety or stress and the DMF score in humans.[14,17,46] In animals it has been demonstrated that stress associated with physical restraint or intermittent electric shocks significantly increased caries susceptibility in young rats placed on cariogenic diets.[21,61]

In an attempt to elucidate possible mechanisms by which stress can influence the oral disease process, a number of investigators have focused on the indirect effects of sociopsychological stress by examining some of the variables that are known to directly affect the carious process. Studies of saliva and the salivary gland indicate that there are qualitative and quantitative alterations of the saliva during stress.[4,22,25] With activation of the sympathetic branch of the autonomic nervous system, as would occur under acute stress, the saliva would be expected to become more viscous with less volume and more acid, that is, have a lower pH. Prolonged or chronic stress, presumably by activation of the pituitary-adrenocortical axis and the parasympathetic nervous system, would most likely increase the salivary volume and pH.

Perhaps the most important intervening variable in dental disease is the formation of plaque on the tooth surface. The control of plaque, in turn, seems to depend most on the number of physiochemical and psychological factors. In physiochemical terms, plaque forms by the adsorption of bacteria to salivary glycoprotein on the tooth surface.[19] Eating and oral hygiene habits, however, also have a profound influence on the rate and fate of plaque formation. Although several authors have confirmed that toothbrushing is effective in reducing periodontal disease by reducing plaque,[41,62] the evidence for the effectiveness of toothbrushing for the prevention of caries is inconclusive.[19] Prevention and the concern of the dentist with regard to preventive dentistry will be discussed in Chapter 18.

Environmental factors

Although caries susceptibility is in large part genetically determined,[11] environmental factors appear to be more important, at least for those who are susceptible. There is, for example, a greater similarity of caries experience among members of the same household than would be expected for a random group of individuals stratified by age, sex, race, and social class. In general the data from the national health surveys and other studies indicate that the higher the socioeconomic status, the lower the DMF index.[37]

On the other hand, differences in income and education do not explain the wide differences in DMF teeth observed in different races. For example, the higher DMF index for both white men and women compared to their black counterparts suggests that higher levels of education and affluence do not always correlate with a lower DMF index level. In fact, when worldwide comparisons are made between areas of lower socioeconomic development and nations with improved socioeconomic status, there is a marked increase in the prevalence of dental caries in the more affluent areas. This increase has been attributed to the increased consumption of fermentable carbohydrate foods and the lack of oral hygiene.

PERIODONTAL DISEASE

Prevalence

Progressive destruction of the periodontal or supportive structures of the teeth, or periodontal disease, is the major cause of tooth loss in patients over age 40 years.[16] As measured by the Russell Periodontal Index, periodontal disease increases with age.[35] It was estimated that 39% of the children from age 6 to 11 years had periodontal diseases[34]; this rate increased to 68% for youth from age 12 to 17 years.[55] Periodontal disease in children, however, does not appear to be as closely associated with poor oral hygiene (Simplified Oral Hygiene Index) as has been reported for adults.[34]

Age. As noted earlier, the amount of periodontal disease increases almost linearly with age.[35]

Sex. There is little difference between the periodontal indices of men and women,[35] although white males required slightly more extractions as a result of periodontal disease than did women of similar age.[16] Although there is a definite increase in gingivitis during pregnancy, even in the absence of increased oral debris,[1] there is still some question about the relative importance of increased hormone levels or decreased oral hygiene in gingivitis.

Race. Both prevalence and severity of periodontal disease are substantially less for white than for black Americans, much of this being primarily a function of socioeconomic differences between the two groups.[35]

Psychological factors. Behavioral and emotional factors have been associated with the occurrence of periodontal disease in several studies.[3,3a,26,43] Psychiatric illness, independent of oral hygiene or bruxism, appears to predispose patients to the development of periodontal disease.[7,8] For example, severity of periodontal disease appears to be related to the degree of anxiety a person experiences.[49] Other experimenters noted a positive relationship between Periodontal Index (PI) scores and stress. Schizophrenia and anxiety as measured by the Minnesota Multiphasic Personality Inventory (MMPI) also have been found to correlate with periodontal disease.[14]

In military populations, dental emergencies including periodontal conditions increase in combat, with stress and poor oral hygiene linked to increased gingival and periodontal problems.[9] As mentioned earlier, acute necrotizing ulcerative gingivitis (ANUG) is a well-known example of a stress-related disease. In several studies psychological stress such as that occurring during examination periods and interpersonal disagreements has been found to be associated with ANUG.[23,24,27]

Although hypertension has been directly related to the extent of periodontal disease, this relationship is confounded by the fact that persons with higher blood pressure also tend to have poorer oral hygiene habits and greater psychological problems than those with lower blood pressure.[33]

Environmental factors

Oral hygiene. The role of psychosocial factors in oral hygiene practice has been extensively reviewed by Rayner and Cohen.[48] The deleterious effects of poor hygiene on both hard and soft tissues of the oral cavity have been discussed previously.

Use of noxious substances. The effects on the oral tissues of noxious substances such as tobacco, coffee, and alcohol have been previously discussed. As with tobacco, how many of the changes observed in oral health are the result of the action of social drugs or the result of a particular life-style associated with the use of drugs or stimulants is not known.

When compared with other psychiatric patients of similar age groups, alcoholic patients in particular were observed to have a greater dental need. Both alcoholics as a group and other psychiatric patients showed severe oral neglect; the alcoholics as a group, however, had significantly more missing and nonrestorable teeth.[15,38]

MALOCCLUSION

Prevalence

Overall it has been estimated that 60% of American children have orthodontic conditions severe enough to warrent treatment; for 25% of these, the condition is deforming or crippling.[28]

Using the Treatment Priority Index (TPI), it is estimated from the National Health Survey that 24.4% of children were classified as having normal occlusion, 39.0% had only minor manifestations (0 to 3 on the TPI scale), and 22.4% had definite malocclusion for which the treatment was elective. Of the remaining children, 8.7% had a severe handicap (7 to 9 on the TPI scale), and for an additional 5.5% treatment was mandatory.[36]

Host factors

The average TPI score for all children from age 6 to 11 years in the United States was 3.3, with no difference between the sexes.[36] In the United States there seems to be little difference in the prevalence of malocclusion between the white, Indian,[18] and black races,[36] whereas in eastern Europe, children with broader skulls were found to be less likely to need orthodontic treatment.[20]

Environmental factors

Although popular and dental opinion have long held that malocclusion is caused by oral habits such as finger-sucking, mouth-breathing, and tongue-thrusting, there is little conclusive evidence in support of this. Thumb-sucking, however, is a common habit for approximately 60% of all children from age 6 to 11 years.[36]

CLEFT LIP AND CLEFT PALATE

Prevalence

The most frequently occurring birth defects are the cleft lip and cleft palate; the incidence in the United States is estimated to be between 0.6 to 1.8 per 1000 live births. The incidence in locations outside the United States was within the range of 0.6 to 1.9 per 1000 live births, with the exception of Japan, which reported a high rate of 2.68, probably associated with World War II.[44] These anomalies were familiar to ancient medicine, being noted in archeological findings from Corinth dated as long ago as the fourth century BC.[58] Even busts of Demosthenes appeared to show a harelip, undoubtedly associated with his famous speech impediment.[10]

The occurrence of these anomalies has been shrouded in mysticism and superstition. The most common folk explanations include cleft lip as evidence of sexual irregularities. Accordingly it was thought that when persons act like animals, they may expect their offspring to be like animals—hence the name "harelip."[13] Old wives' tales have thus added to the belief that psychological stress during pregnancy can result in congenital malformations.[50]

Host factors

Although considerable research exists, there is still no clear-cut evidence as to the precise contribution of genetic factors.

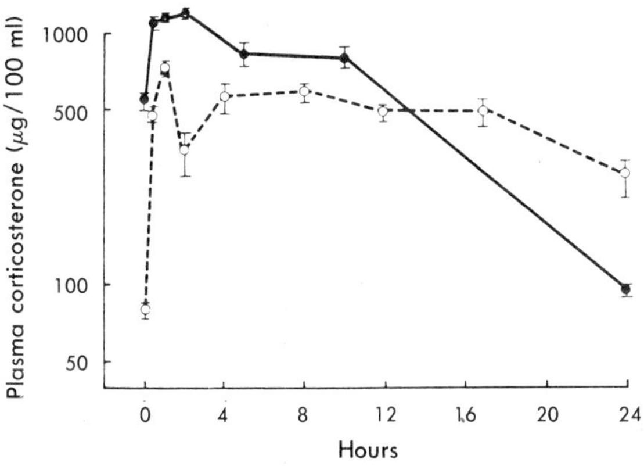

Fig. 3-2. Plasma corticosterone levels following subcutaneous injection of 2.5 mg (100 mg/kg) of corticosterone on day 14 of pregnancy (• —— •) or during the 24 hours of restraint begun on day 14 of pregnancy (○ ---- ○). Vertical bars indicate standard error (SE). (From Barlow, S., McElhattan, P., and Sullivan, F.: Teratology **12:**97, 1975.)

Most of the relevant discussion about this condition, therefore, appears as related to environmental factors, mostly with respect to the mother or the parents.

Environmental factors

Environmental factors act in at least two ways: by altering genetic material and/or by facilitating the expression of genetically determined abnormalities predisposing the formation of clefts. Factors that have been positively associated with the birth of children with oral clefts are older parents, lower socioeconomic status, threatened abortion, pelvic X-ray examination prior to pregnancy, emotional factors, and low birth weight. The consumption of tobacco and alcohol by mothers of children with clefts may be more of an indicator of underlying emotional turbulence than a cause of cleft palate.[56]

The consumption of certain types of drugs such as teratogens, for example, tranquilizers, may be stress related; moreover, the drug itself or a related compound, for example, cortisone, may be a major component in the pathway connecting stress with developmental disorders such as cleft palate. It has, in fact, been shown that corticoids act directly on the fetal palatal shelf tissues to induce cleft palate.[59]

Although the etiology of cleft lip and palate for animals is not necessarily the same as in humans, there is considerable evidence from animal studies that stress and cortisone increase the incidence of cleft palate.[5,51] The application of an experimental stress is generally associated with an increase in the weight of the adrenal glands and a consequent rise in corticosteroid level. Stressors that have been shown to induce a higher incidence of cleft palate in mice are restraint,[51] avoidance conditioning,[50] deprivation of food and/or water,[51] and disruption of regular dark and light cycles.[52] The observation that restraint causes a rise in plasma corticosterone level similar to that seen after the injection of teratogenic doses of corticosterone supports the conclusion that the teratogenic action of restraint is mediated via the release of endogenous corticosterone (Fig. 3-2).[5]

ORAL CANCER

Prevalence

Although oral cancer is encountered only infrequently by the dentist, its seriousness and the importance of early detection give it a greater significance. Cancer of the mouth accounted for 3% of all cancers diagnosed in the United States. In 1965 there were 7568 deaths from cancers occurring in sites commonly under super-

Table 3-1 □ Rate of malignant neoplasms of the buccal cavity and pharynx by race (United States, 1959-1961)*

Race	Death rates		
	Men	Women	Both sexes
All races	5.4	1.6	3.5
White	5.5	1.6	3.5
Black	4.1	1.3	2.7
Indian	1.1	0.4	0.7
Chinese	16.2	3.6	10.9
Japanese	1.6	0.7	1.1
Others	4.3	1.0	2.9

*From Public Health Service, National Center for Health Statistics: Factors, facts of life and death, Washington, D.C., 1967, U. S. Government Printing Office.

vision by dentists, including 6501 deaths from neoplasms of the buccal cavity. The crude death rate in 1965 was 3.4 per 100,000 persons.[47]

Host factors

Age and sex. Oral cancer seldom occurs in persons under 40 years of age, with the risk increasing steadily with age after 40 years of age. The risk is three times greater for men than women for both whites and blacks.[2]

Race and ethnic background. Geographical variations in cancer mortality are difficult to separate from racial factors. Primitive cultures appear to have lower rates of all types of cancer. In the United States, the death rate as a result of oral cancer is low among Japanese Americans and American Indians; however, it is high among the Chinese population living here and elsewhere.[2] Other groups having relatively high risk of oral cancer were Irish men and immigrants from Canada and Germany.[29]

Area and community. An association exists between urbanization and cancer mortality as well as any number of other chronic diseases. Although these differences may be explained by variation in the accuracy of case reporting in urban and rural areas, the data do indicate a pronounced increase in risk of urban residents in the United States for cancer of the lung, oral cavity, and esophagus.[40]

Psychological factors. The belief that psychological factors may be involved in the etiology and pathogenesis of cancer derives from the ancient theory of body humors. Clinical impressions have long suggested a relationship between the experience of major emotional loss and the first noted symptoms of cancer. Based on limited data, certain types of personality organization seem to predispose to a shortening of the length of time between appearance of the neoplasm and death. As with other diseases, personality and coping styles appear to be related to the type and location of the cancer.[39]

Environmental factors

Environmental agents most certainly have a role in the etiology of oral cancer. Among those who smoke and drink heavily, the probability of developing cancer of the mouth is approximately 1 in 35. For people who neither smoke nor drink, the probability is only 1 in 350. Probably two thirds of oral cancer could thus be prevented by reduced alcohol and tobacco consumption. Moreover, it has been demonstrated that alcohol and tobacco act synergistically to increase the risk beyond that of either one acting alone.[54]

Pipe and cigar smoking in particular appear to increase the probability of oral cancer more than cigarette smoking. Similarly, tobacco chewing, although infrequent today, has also been linked to buccal cancer. In areas such as India, where reverse smoking, or smoking with the lit end of the cigarette in the mouth, is practiced, oral cancer is among the most common forms of cancer. Inveterate betel nut chewing is another pernicious habit practiced in Southeast Asia that results in abrasion of the teeth and atrophy of the periodontal tissues and is highly associated with cancer of the buccal mucosa.[45]

SUMMARY

An overview of the magnitude of dental disease and associated psychosocial factors has been presented. No attempt has been made to be inclusive; rather, the reader is referred to textbooks on epidemiology and/or dental public health for detailed findings.[16] Our intent has been primarily to identify the major factors that contribute to the initiation and maintenance of oral health problems that dentists will encounter.

REFERENCES

1. Adams, D., Carney, J. S., and Dicks, D. A.: Pregnancy gingivitis: a survey of 100 antenatal patients, J. Dent. Res. **54**(1):106, 1974.
2. Bailar, J. D., King, H., and Mason, M. J.: Cancer rates and risks, Public Health Service Pub. No. 1148, Washington, D.C., 1964, U.S. Government Printing Office.
3. Baker, E. G., Crook, G. H., and Schwabacher, E. D.: Personality correlates of periodontal disease, J. Dent. Res. **40:**396, 1961.

3a. Baker, E. G., and Schwabacher, E. D.: Psychological considerations in periodontology, Dent. Clin. North Am. pp. 651-658, Nov., 1962.

4. Barber, T. X., and Chauncey, H. H.: Effect of hypnotic and non-hypnotic suggestions on parotid gland response to gustatory stimuli, Psychosom. Med. **26:**374, 1964.
5. Barlow, S., McElhatton, P., and Sullivan, F.: The relation between maternal restraint and food deprivation, plasma corticosterone and induction of cleft palate in the offspring of mice, Teratology **12:**97, 1975.
6. Baume, L. J.: Caries prevalence and caries intensity among 12,344 school children of French Polynesia, Arch. Oral Biol. **14:**181, 1969.
7. Belting, C. M., and Gupta, O. P.: Incidence of periodontal disease among persons with neuropsychiatric disorders, J. Dent. Res. **39:**744, 1960.
8. Belting, C. M., and Gupta, O. P.: The influence of psychiatric disturbance on the severity of periodontal disease, J. Periodontol. **32:**216, 1961.
9. Bernier, J. L., and Sumnicht, R. W.: The emergence of preventive dental practice in the U.S. Army, Milit. Med. **131:**520, 1966.
10. Bien, S. M.: Why Demosthenes mouthed pebbles, Lancet **2:**1152, 1967.
11. Bordoni, N., Doño, R., Manfredi, C., and Allegrotti, I.: Prevalence of dental caries in twins, J. Dent. Child. **40:**440, 1973.
12. Bureau of economic research and statistics survey of needs for dental care, 1965, J. Am. Dent. Assoc. **73:**1128, 1966.
13. Crocker, E., and Crocker, C.: Some implications of superstitions and folk beliefs for counselling parents of children with cleft lip and cleft palate, Cleft Palate J. **7:**124, 1970.
14. Davis, C., and Jenkins, C. D.: Mental stress and oral disease, J. Dent. Res. **41:**1045, 1962.
15. Dunkley, R. P., and Carson, R. M.: Dental requirements of the hospitalized alcoholic patient, J. Am. Dent. Assoc. **76:**800, 1968.
16. Dunning, J. M.: Principles of dental public health, ed. 2, Cambridge, 1970, Harvard University Press.
17. Feldman, H.: Caries susceptibility, anxiety, and stress, J. Am. Soc. Psychosom. Dent. Med. **15:**28, 1968.
18. Foster, L. W.: Dental conditions in White and Indian children in northern Wisconsin, J. Am. Dent. Assoc. **29:**2251, 1942.
19. Frandsen, A., ed.: Oral hygiene, a symposium at Malmo, Sweden, 1971, Copenhagen, 1972, Munksgaard, International Booksellers & Publishers, Ltd.
20. Gardiner, H. J.: Malocclusion in Europe, Br. J. Orthodont. **1**(3):69.
21. Gerstein, H. A.: The effects of prolonged psychic stress on the albino rat, Thesis, University of Nebraska, 1960.
22. Giddon, D. B.: The relation of a cholinesterase-like substance in parotid saliva to psychological stress, Doctoral Dissertation, University of Michigan, Ann Arbor, Mich., Dissert. Abs. **24:**2115, 1963.
23. Giddon, D. B., Goldhaber, P., and Dunning, J. M.: Prevalence of reported cases of acute necrotizing ulcerative gingivitis in a university population, J. Periodontol. **34:**366, 1963.
24. Giddon, D. B., Zackin, S. J., and Goldhaber, P.: Acute necrotizing ulcerative gingivitis in college students, J. Am. Dent. Assoc. **68:**381, 1964.
25. Gilchrist, J. C., and Furchgott, E.: Salivary pH as a psychophysiological variable, Psychol. Bull. **48:**193, 1951.
26. Goldberg, H., Ambinder, W. J., Cooper, L., and Abrams, A. L.: Emotional status of patients with gingivitis, NY State Dent. J. **22:**308, 1956.
27. Goldhaber, P., and Giddon, D. B.: Present concepts concerning the etiology and treatment of acute necrotizing ulcerative gingivitis, Int. Dent. J. **14:**468, 1964.
28. Green, J. C.: Dental health needs of the nation, J. Am. Dent. Assoc. **84:**1073, 1972.
29. Haenszel, W.: Cancer mortality among the foreign-born in the United States, J. Natl. Cancer Inst. **26:**37, 1961.
30. Hollinshead, B. S.: The survey of dentistry: The final report—commission on the survey of dentistry in the United States, Washington, D.C., 1961, American Council on Education.
31. Jackson, D.: Measuring restorative dental care in communities, Br. Dent. J. **134:**385, 1973.
32. Johnson, E. S., Kelly, J. E., and Van Kirk, L. E.: Selected dental findings in adults by age, race and

sex—United States—1960-1962. Vital and health statistics, Series 11, No. 7, DHEW Pub. No. (HRA) 74-1274, Washington, D.C., August, 1973, U.S. Government Printing Office.
33. Kelly, J. E., and Engel, A.: Selected examination findings related to periodontal disease among adults—United States—1960-1962. Vital and health statistics, Series 11, No. 33, DHEW Pub. No. (HRA) 75-1293, Washington, D.C., September, 1974, U.S. Government Printing Office.
34. Kelly, J. E., and Sanchez, M. J.: Periodontal disease and oral hygiene among children—United States. Vital and health statistics, Series 11, No. 117, DHEW Pub. No. (HSM) 72-1060, Washington, D.C., June, 1972, U.S. Government Printing Office.
35. Kelly, J. E., and Van Kirk, L. E.: Periodontal disease in adults—United States—1960-1962. Vital and health statistics, Series 11, No. 12, Public Health Service Pub. No. 1000, Washington, D.C., November, 1965, U.S. Government Printing Office.
36. Kelly, J. E., Sanchez, M., and Van Kirk, L. E.: An assessment of the occlusion of the teeth of children 6-11 years—United States. Vital and health statistics, Series 11, No. 130, DHEW Pub. No. (HRA) 74-1612, Washington, D.C., November, 1973, U.S. Government Printing Office.
37. Kelly, J. E., Van Kirk, L. E., and Garst, C. C.: Decayed, missing and filled teeth in adults—United States—1960-1962. Vital and health statistics, Series 11, No. 23, Public Health Service Pub. No. 1000, Washington, D.C., February, 1967, U.S. Government Printing Office.
38. King, W. H., and Tucker, K.: Dental problems of alcoholic and non-alcoholic psychiatric patients, Q. J. Stud. Alcohol **34:**1208, 1973.
39. LeShan, L. L.: Psychological states as factors in the development of malignant disease: a critical review, J. Natl. Cancer Inst. **22:**1, 1959.
40. Levin, J. L., Haenszel, W., Carrol, B. E., Gerhardt, P. R., Handy, V. H., and Ingraham, S. C.: Cancer incidence in urban and rural areas of New York State, J. Natl. Cancer Inst. **24:**1243, 1960.
41. Löe, H., Theilade, E., and Jensen, S. B.: Experimental gingivitis in man, J. Periodontol. **36:**177, 1965.
42. Masi, M. B.: The pattern of dental disease in the South Pacific area of the Pacific Basin, Int. Dent. J. **23**(4):573, 1973.
43. Miller, S., Thaller, J. L., and Soberman, A.: The use of MMPI as a diagnostic aide in periodontal disease—a preliminary report, J. Periodontol. **27:** 44, 1956.
44. Moller, P.: Dentofacial deformities: malocclusion. In Pelton, W. J., Dunbar, J. B., McMillan, R. S., Moller, P., and Wolff, A. E.: The epidemiology of oral health, Cambridge, Mass., 1969, Harvard University Press.
45. Paymaster, J. C.: Cancer of the buccal mucosa: a clinical study of 650 cases in an Indian hospital, Cancer **9:**431, 1956.
46. Phipps, G. T., and Marcuse, F. L.: Anxiety and dental caries, J. Dent. Res. **36:**362, 1957.
47. Public Health Service, National Center for Health Statistics: Factors, facts of life and death, Washington, D.C., 1967, U.S. Government Printing Office.
48. Rayner, J. F., and Cohen, L. K.: School dental health education. In Richards, N. D., and Cohen, L. K., eds.: Social sciences and dentistry: a critical bibliography, Leiden, 1971, A. W. Sijthoff, International Publishing Co. BV.
49. Richards, N. D., and Barmes, D.: Social factors in dental epidemiology. In Richards, N. D., and Cohen, L. K., eds.: Social sciences and dentistry—a critical bibliography, Leiden, 1971, A. W. Sijthoff, International Publishing Co. BV.
50. Rosenzweig, S.: Psychological stress in cleft palate etiology, J. Dent. Res. **45**(6):1585, 1966.
51. Rosenzweig, S., and Blaustein, F.: Cleft palate in A/J mice resulting from restraint and deprivation of food and water, Teratology **3:**47, 1970.
52. Rosenzweig, S., Clark, R. E., Giddon, D. B., Blaustein, F. M., and Steinert, R.: Cleft palate incidence increased by disruption of regular dark-light cycles in CD-1 mice, Int. Assoc. Dent. Res. **47:**78, 1969.
53. Rothman, K. J.: Diseases of the mouth. In Clark, D. W., and MacMahon, B., eds.: Preventive medicine, Boston, 1967, Little, Brown & Co.
54. Rothman, K. J., and Keller, A. Z.: The effect of joint exposure to alcohol and cancer of the mouth and pharynx, J. Chronic Dis. **25:**711, 1972.
55. Sanchez, M. J.: Periodontal disease among youths 12-17 years—United States. Vital and health statistics, Series 11, No. 141, DHEW Pub. No. (HRA) 74-1623, Washington, D.C., June, 1974, U.S. Government Printing Office.
56. Saxen, I.: Cleft lip and palate in Finland: parental histories, course of pregnancy and selected environmental factors, Int. J. Epidemiol. **3**(3): 263, 1974.
57. Schwabacher, E. D.: Interpersonal factors in rampant dental caries, J. Am. Soc. Psychosom. Dent. Med. **4:**108, 1957; **5:**2, 1958; **5:**97, 1958; **6:**20, 1959.
58. Skoog, T.: A head from ancient Corinth, Scand. J. Plast. Reconstr. Surg. **3:**49, 1969.
59. Spain, K. M., Kisieleski, W., and Wood, N.: Cleft palate induction: quantitative studies on ^{3}H corticoids in A/Jax mouse tissue after maternal injections of ^{3}H cortisol, J. Dent. Res. **54**(5): 1069, 1975.
60. Steinman, R. R.: The effect of stress on the incidence of dental caries, J. South. Calif. Dent. Assoc. **28:**367, 1960.
61. Sutton, P. R. N.: The early onset of acute dental

caries in adults following mental stress, NY State Dent. J. **31:**450, 1965.
62. Theilade, E., Wright, W. H., Jensen, S. B., and Löe, H.: Experimental gingivitis in men. II. A longitudinal clinical bacteriological investigation, J. Periodont. Res. **1:**1, 1966.
63. World Health Organization: Application of the international classification of diseases to dentistry and stomatology, (ICD-DA) 1973, Geneva, The Organization.
64. Yassin, I., and Low, T.: Caries prevalence in different racial groups of school children in West Malaysia, Community Dent. Oral Epidemiol. **3:** 179, 1975.

Chapter 4

THE PERCEIVED NEED FOR DENTAL CARE

How it relates to the demand for and utilization of dental care

As shown in Chapter 3, almost everyone needs dental care as objectively determined by clinical examination. Additionally, the need for preventive care in dentistry places the potential users of dental services at nearly 100% of the population. However, not all individuals in need of care seek it. The next question thus becomes "Who of those persons with dental disease seeks care"? In other words, what forces motivate or deter the person with dental disease (need) in seeking the dentist's help and/or utilizing health care resources (demand)? The decision to seek care is primarily a voluntary choice based on the individual's *perception of his or her need relative to the perceived availability, acceptability, and accessibility of resources for providing care.*

In this discussion, **objective need** indicates those persons with disease or deficiency as recognized by the dentist, whereas **demand** implies the seeking of care by the patient. **Utilization** of dental resources occurs when the patient actually receives dental care. *The principal variable intervening between objective need and demand is the perceived or subjective need.* **Perceived need** is defined as the patient's subjective experience that dental care is required. The relationship and sequence of these different factors are shown in Fig. 4-1.

The general subject of perception will be discussed extensively in Chapter 8. In Fig. 4-1 note the importance of variables such as age, sex, and socioeconomic status that predispose an individual to acquire knowledge and beliefs influencing the perception of two important areas: an individual's needs and the possibility for meeting those needs. It is the patient-consumer's perception of a subjective need—not the objective need as determined by the dentist—and of the availability, accessibility, and acceptability of resources for providing needed care that determines the utilization of therapeutic and/or preventive dental care services. This fact has important implications for the dentist's understanding of patient attitudes and behavior. It also has significant impact on planning any health care delivery system.

OBJECTIVES

The objectives of this chapter are as follows:

1. To review the discrepancy between the objective and the perceived need for dental care
2. To discuss factors related to the patient's perceived need for dental care
3. To explore factors decreasing the demand for dental care
4. To discuss the utilization of dental services

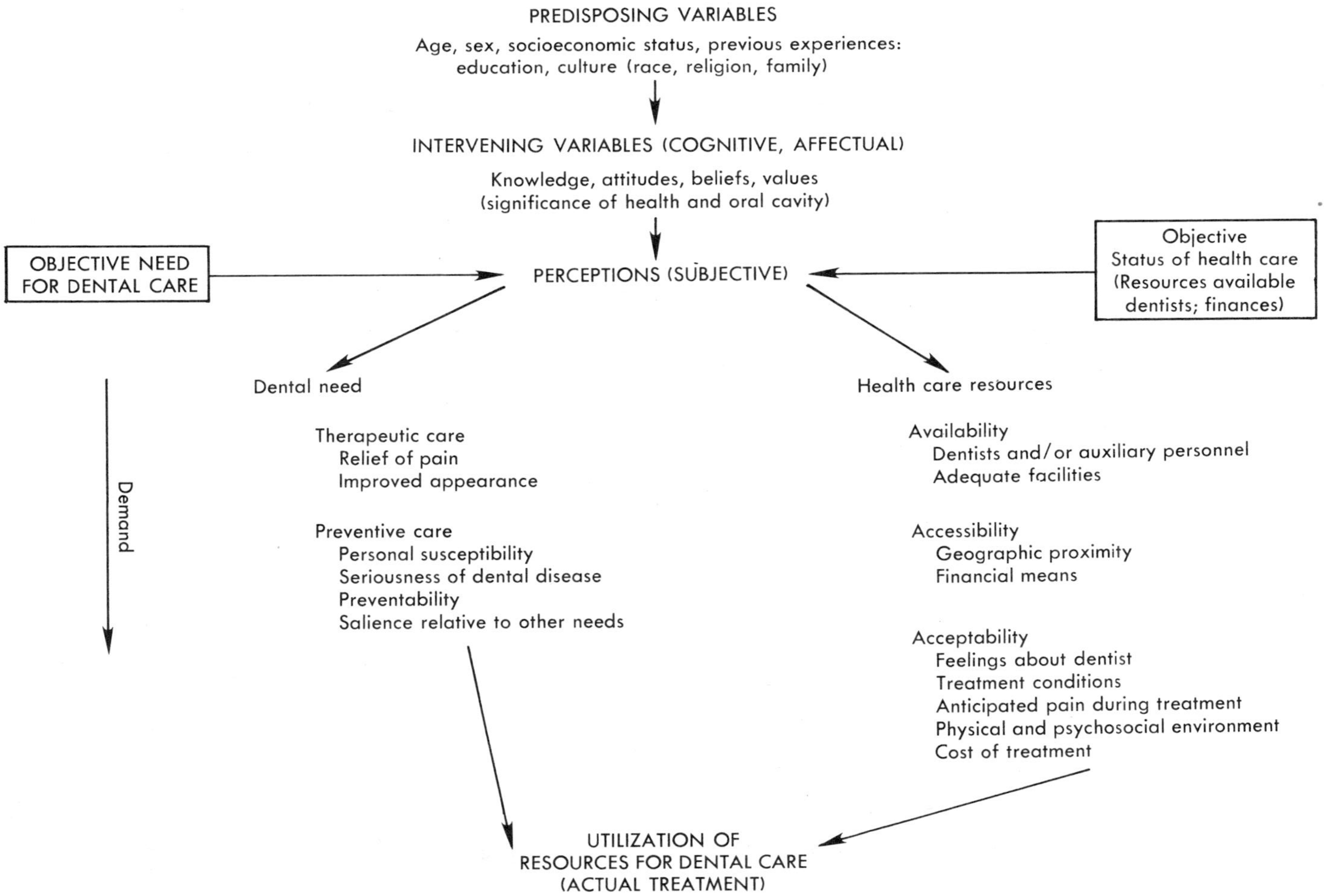

Fig. 4-1. Variables affecting demand and utilization of dental care resources. (From Giddon, D. B., Silberman, S. L., Prasad, L., and Bikofsky, C. G.: In Ward, H. O., ed., *A Preventive Point of View,* in press. Courtesy of Charles C Thomas, Publisher, Springfield, Illinois.)

DISCREPANCY BETWEEN OBJECTIVE AND PERCEIVED NEED FOR DENTAL CARE

Several studies document the discrepancy between the objective and the perceived need for dental care.[15,17] Using random population samples from several English towns, we found little relation between individuals' self-assessment of dental need and actual need as determined by clinical examination. Although dental care utilization was, as expected, correlated with social status, the patients obviously used different criteria than the dentist in determining need for dental treatment. For example, few adults were aware they had periodontal disease.

For dental caries, the relationship between objective and perceived need can be expressed quantitatively using a combination of bioassay and psychophysical methods.[15] The proportion of subjects with favorable self-assessments (good vs bad teeth or "I do not need treatment" vs "I need treatment") for each increment of the total of decayed (D), missing (M), or filled (F) teeth is determined. A mathematically determined line best fitting these points is then calculated, from which a 50% point for DMF teeth or for component D, M, or F teeth is determined. Using this method, Giddon et al.[17] demonstrated that men and women differ quantitatively in the relationship between self-assessment and objective need for treatment, as shown in Fig. 4-2. Women, as a group, are less aware of objective need than men, but, as shown in repeated surveys of dental practice, they utilize dental services more often than men.[1] This approach to quantification of the relation of perceived to objective need can also be extended to comparison of other groups of varying demographic or sociopsychological characteristics.[17]

Another way of expressing the relationship between objective need and actual utilization behavior can be seen by comparing the proportion of patients with a given dental condition to those with a given condition who made dental visits (Table 4-1).[29]

Note the great discrepancy between the frequency of the objective clinical situation and the percentage of utilization. Addition-

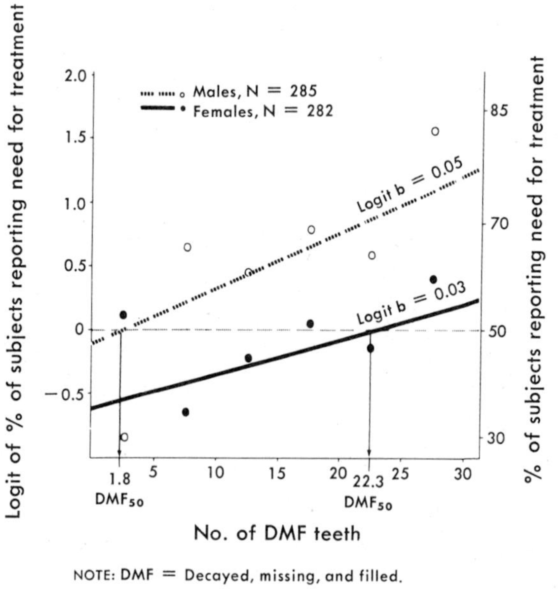

Fig. 4-2. Weighted least squares determination of relation of DMF teeth to reported need for treatment. (From Giddon, D. B., Mosier, M., Colton, T., and Bulman, J. S.: Public Health Rep. **91**(6): 508, 1976.)

Table 4-1 □ Distribution of dental conditions and the proportion of persons with conditions who made dental visits*

Condition	Proportion (%) with condition†	Proportion (%) with condition who made a visit†
Toothache	20 (9330)	75 (1401)
Sore or bleeding gums	8 (9302)	45 (698)
Loss of permanent tooth	5 (9321)	61 (451)
Pain in tooth when drinking hot or cold liquid	14 (9302)	54 (1256)
Tartar or stains on teeth	25 (9255)	57 (2363)
Crooked teeth	7(9311)	32 (698)

*From Newman, J. D., and Anderson, O. W.: Patterns of dental service utilization in the United States: a nationwide social survey, Research Series 30, Chicago, 1972, Center for Health Administration Studies. The University of Chicago Press.
†Number in parentheses is actual number with condition.

Table 4-2 □ The most important reason for taking care of teeth and gingiva*

Most important reason	Boys	Girls	Both
No. who answered question	1083	1126	2209
To help your appearance	37%	37%	37%
To prevent other illnesses	3%	3%	3%
To avoid later expensive treatment	10%	8%	9%
To avoid future pain and trouble	19%	16%	18%
To keep your teeth as long as possible	31%	35%	33%

*From Linn, E. L.: J. Am. Dent. Assoc. **92**:946, 1976. Copyright by the American Dental Association. Reprinted by permission.

Table 4-3 □ Dental conditions worried about most*

Dental condition	Boys	Girls	Both
No. who answered the question	1196	1159	2355
Broken or lost permanent teeth	44%	26%	35%
Discolored teeth	15%	25%	20%
Sore or bleeding gingiva	7%	7%	7%
Poorly aligned teeth	11%	16%	14%
Tooth decay	24%	26%	25%

*From Linn, E. L.: J. Am. Dent. Assoc. **92**:946, 1976. Copyright by the American Dental Association. Reprinted by permission.

al data on the reasons for visiting dentists, particularly individuals' perceived need for maintaining or improving their appearance, can be seen in Tables 4-2 and 4-3.[23]

FACTORS RELATED TO PATIENT'S PERCEIVED NEED FOR DENTAL CARE

Relief from pain

The complex role of pain perception is well recognized by the dental profession. Pain of dental origin, which is discussed in Chapter 17, is a prime factor in the patient's perceived need for dental care. On the other hand, many patients are deterred by the fear of pain incurred in the course of treatment.

Attractiveness

Although considerable data exist on the importance of physical attractiveness to such vital dimensions of mental health as self-esteem, self-concept, and behavior,[32,39] there is little agreement on what is physically attractive and how it relates to the patient's perceived need for dental care. As noted previously,[23,29] specifically in Tables 4-1 to 4-3, a large portion of the demand for dental care of all types results from the patient's concern with appearance.

Even with the apparent cultural shift in current Western society to minimize physical assets as essential to social acceptance, experimenters have repeatedly shown that most persons are highly motivated to obtain and maintain physical beauty. This concern for physical attractiveness begins in early childhood[12,39] and continues through dating and mating behavior.[6,25,39-41] Such interest is reflected in the increasing number of cosmetic surgical procedures for men and women of all ages and for many parts of the body, whether ordinarily visible or visible only in intimate relationships.

Similarly, there has been increasing interest in those dental procedures that maintain or enhance the attractiveness of the orofacial area: aesthetic restorations of the anterior teeth; orthodontics for adults as well as for children, including surgical corrections; and endodontics and periodontics to conserve natural teeth.

Using orthodontics as one example, let us examine the factors contributing to the demand for specialized care, that is, who becomes the orthodontic patient? Objective evaluation by the orthodontist and subjective assessment by the potential patient do not necessarily agree.[13] The decision to treat or not to treat is based on some as yet unknown combination of the subjective judgments of patients, parents, and physicians.

Even with objective measurements of angulation, length, etc. of interdental and profile relationships, there is no reliable index that incorporates these easily available objective findings contained in the Treatment Priority Index (TPI) with the subjective preferences of patients and physicians.[7,18] Although orthodontists admit that approximately 80% of their patients seek orthodontic treatment for cosmetic purposes, there is still a considerable difference of opinion between physician and patient as to aesthetic preferences.[32] Thus objective classification and subjective clinical judgment of malocclusion and facial harmony by the dentist continue to be the main factors in determining whether to treat orthodontic patients—regardless of the perceptions of the patient and family. Consequently, the patients with only marginal clinical malocclusion who should be treated because of psychological handicaps related to their self-image may not receive treatment if the objective measurements do not fall within certain standards. Conversely, treatment of a patient with aesthetically pleasing bimaxillary protrusion uncomplicated by posterior malocclusion may properly be deferred or may not be sought if the patient is unconcerned.

The contribution of psychological factors cannot be overestimated and may, in fact, be significantly more handicapping than the functional impairments associated with malocclusion.[8,9] As noted in Chapter 1, the importance of the mouth and face to personality development and psychosocial interaction has long been recognized[16,37] and undoubtedly contributes to the motivation to seek orthodontic care.

Other factors leading to orthodontic treatment include parental socioeconomic and ethnic background and experience with orthodontists. The mother, in particular, is a most important determinant of the demand for orthodontic care.[4,5] Her motivation appears to depend on her perceptions of the need for correction of a dentofacial anomaly: her perception of the correction of her child's dentofacial deformity as possibly resolving her own problems of self-concept; her achievement orientation, possibly seeing orthodontic treatment as a symbol of status or belonging; and/or her attempted resolution of other family problems by displacement onto the child's orthodontic problem.[4] Similarly, among adolescents the desire for orthodontic treatment was related (in addition to improved facial aesthetics and importance of self-perception) to pressure from parents, peers, and friends.[22]

Health beliefs and perceptions about preventive behavior

Four perceptual factors have evolved as being crucial to the decision to seek preventive dental care.[19] In most proposed relationships between health beliefs, perceptions, and behavior, it is assumed that all dental visits are to some extent preventive, that is, preventing new disease as well as further deterioration resulting from any existing disease process. Visits for preventive purposes only are those in which little or no therapeutic intervention is provided, for example, the 6-month checkup. The four perceptions that have been identified as pertaining to the decision to seek preventive dental care are as follows:

1. **Susceptibility.** Dental disease can happen to oneself.
2. **Seriousness.** Consequences of disease might be clinically severe or interfere with other considerations deemed important by the individual.

3. **Preventability.** Adoption of a certain behavior will prevent the disease.
4. **Salience.** Doing something about the disease is more important than doing other things.

Perceived susceptibility. Perceived susceptibility in relation to dental disease has been measured or inferred from other data such as individual evaluation of teeth,[35,38] or perceived likelihood of occurrence of the worst problem[19] or of decay.[20] In general the more one perceives that the disease can occur, the greater the number of preventive trips to the dentist.[19]

Perceived seriousness. The perception of seriousness in relation to dental disease can include several different dimensions: clinical severity, interference with important activities, and impact on one's appearance. In general there is no consistent relationship between perceiving the seriousness of dental disease and visiting the dentist for preventive care, that is, most people do not believe that preventing dental disease is a serious enough problem to allocate resources or to change behavior that might be directed elsewhere.[14,19] However, there are some very specific exceptions, particularly involving those dental services related to appearance such as orthodontics.

Perceived preventability. There is an undoubtedly widely held belief (50% of those studied) that daily toothbrushing and flossing and regular visits to the dentist are beneficial.[10,19] Even though there is some question of the oral health benefit of some preventive health behaviors, the prevalence of these health beliefs[30] accounts for the relatively high proportion of persons engaging in toothbrushing and visits to the dentist.

Perceived salience. Although some investigators found that money spent on teeth or time talking about dental health was perceived as worthwhile,[3] the frequency of preventive dental visits was still more related to socioeconomic level[19] than to other variables. In other words, after meeting needs perceived as relatively more important or salient than dental needs, the potential patient will seek dental care if he or she can afford it.

FACTORS DECREASING THE DEMAND FOR DENTAL CARE

Several factors reduce the number of patients in need of dental treatment who actually seek care. Stated succinctly, dentistry for many individuals is economically and psychologically painful.

In addition to the obvious economic barrier for some persons, few would disagree that a major factor preventing persons from utilizing dental service is fear. Some patients are so fearful that they avoid necessary care and, indeed, suffer a fear so out of proportion to the situation that it can be classified as a phobia.[21] Estimates vary as to the number of patients who do not demand care out of fear alone. In one study of 51% of the persons who did not visit a dentist regularly, 9% reported fear as the reason.[14] Based on this and other studies, the number of persons who avoid the dentist out of fear is estimated to be between 10 and 12 million.[11,19]

The reason for this fear is difficult to determine. Fears are acquired by a process of conditioning and association. Experience with patients, however, indicates that fear sometimes exists even in the absence of any actual negative experience with the dentist, for example, a family member might have had an unpleasant experience.[34] Similarly, in a survey of the dental experiences of 1375 adults in Sweden, 10% of those questioned considered a visit to the dentist so painful that they were unable to follow through with dental care. Interestingly, women reported more severe discomfort than men, even though they visited the dentist more frequently.[24]

This extraordinary fear of dental treatment, even among those who actually visit the dentist, is closely linked to dental pain experience out of proportion to the actual stimulus (Chapters 1 and 17). A partial explanation for this reaction is the great psychobiological significance attached to the oral cavity, which, in turn, may be a reflection of the disproportionate representation in the cerebral cortex[36] (Chapter 1). These differences also result in part from past experience and family history. Thus each patient who enters the dental treatment situation has an individual set of psychosocial factors that will affect his or her perception of the pain experience.

UTILIZATION OF DENTAL SERVICES

Finally, let us examine how these factors influence actual utilization of dental services. Research on utilization of dental services has historically focused on descriptive and demographic factors.[31] Almost no information has been available for nations other than the United States, England, and Scandinavia. Surveys made by the American Dental Association, the Health Information Foundation, and the National Opinion Research Center constitute the major sources of information in the United States.

Most studies of the actual utilization of dental health services have attempted to examine the roles of the following variables as they affect visits to the dentist for therapeutic or preventive purposes[31]:

1. **Predisposing factors.** This includes age, sex, marital status, social class, family size, education, race, and related cultural/ethnic group.
2. **Enabling characteristics.** This includes financial resources such as income, health insurance, etc. and community factors related to geographical accessibility and availability.

Predisposing factors

U.S. Public Health Service data related to utilization of dental services indicate that age and sex affect patterns of use (Figs. 4-3 and 4-4). Although visits to a physician are not age related, dental visits peak between the ages of 10 and 20 years and decline over time.

As shown in Fig. 4-4, the highest utilization of dental services is by women, whether working or at home. Women visit the dentist 1.6 times per year, whereas

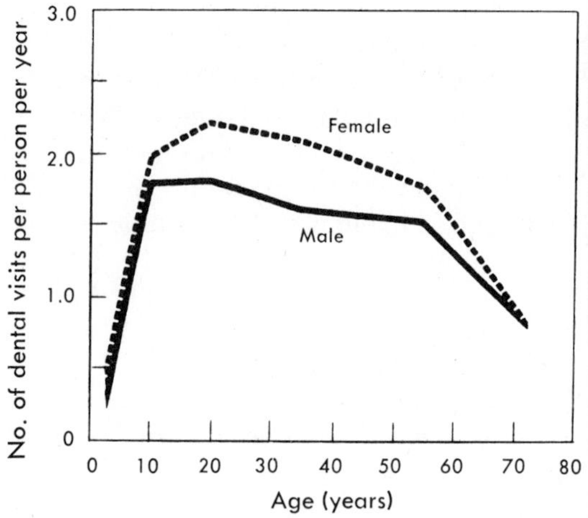

Fig. 4-3. Number of dental visits per person per year by sex and age: United States, 1963-1964. (From Alderman, A. J.: Volume of dental visits—United States, July, 1963–June, 1964. Vital and health statistics, Series 10, No. 23, Public Health Service Pub. No. 1000, National Center for Health Statistics, Washington, D.C., 1965, U.S. Government Printing Office.)

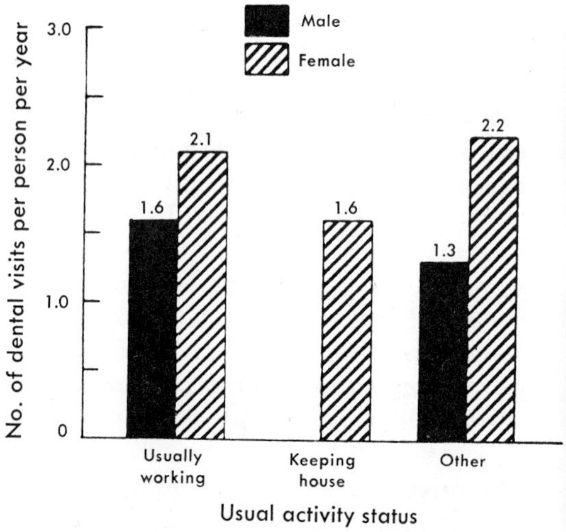

Fig. 4-4. Number of dental visits per person per year (aged 17+ years) by sex and usual activity status: United States, 1963-1964. (From Alderman, A. J.: Volume of dental visits—United States, July, 1963–June, 1964. Vital and health statistics, Series 10, No. 23, Public Health Service Pub. No. 1000, National Center for Health Statistics, Washington, D.C., 1965, U.S. Government Printing Office.)

men do so only 1.4 times per year.[29] Although there has actually been a gradual change from the time when almost two out of every three patients visiting a dentist were women, the latest U.S. Public Health Service report (1973) still indicates that the majority of U.S. patients are women.[26] These data can be contrasted with those of other countries, for example, Israel, where factors of age and sex are not related to dental service utilization.[33]

Enabling characteristics

Income or financial resources such as health insurance for dental services are obviously important determinants of the utilization of dental services. Comparison of utilization patterns in the United States with utilization in countries where the financial barriers have been reduced lends import to the argument that financial resources are the most important, but not the only, variable.

For example, in a National Opinion Research Center (NORC) comparison of the United States and Sweden (which provides national health insurance), the overall utilization rates were slightly higher in Sweden: 43% as compared to 39%. In both countries, however, high social class, smaller families, urban location, and female sex were associated with greater utilization of dental services for prevention or symptomatic relief of dental disease.[2]

In England and Wales relatively few statistics are available on utilization prior to the introduction of the National Health Service in 1948. After its introduction, however, utilization increased from 18% to 41% from 1949 to 1968; this rate is still not greater than that of the United States.

Based on surveys by the American Dental Association and NORC, the percentage of the population receiving dental care in the United States has been steadily increasing. In 1949 only 40% of the population had been to the dentist at least once a year.[28] This increased to 46% by 1969.[26] In 1973 the percentage of persons visiting the dentist had increased to 48.9%[26]; however, it was estimated that only 15% to 20% of the population receives regular care.[19] Data from a NORC survey of 1965 indicated that 33% of all dental visits were primarily preventive; the remaining visits were for relief of symptoms. As expected, the higher the level of income and education, the greater the utilization of dental services for preventive purposes.[30]

REFERENCES

1. Alderman, A. J.: Volume of dental visits—United States, July, 1963–June, 1964. Vital health and statistics, Series 10, No. 23, Public Health Service Pub. No. 1000, Washington, D.C., 1965, U.S. Government Printing Office.

1a. American Dental Association Bureau of Economic Research Statistics: A motivational study of dental care, J. Am. Dent. Assoc. **56:**437, 1958.

2. Anderson, R., Smedby, B., and Anderson, O. W.: Medical care use in Sweden and the United States, Research Series 27, Center for Health Administrative Studies, Chicago, 1970, The University of Chicago Press.

3. Antonovsky, A., and Kats, R.: The model dental patient: an empirical study of preventive health behavior, Soc. Sci. Med. **4:**367, 1970.

4. Baldwin, D. C.: Psychological factors motivating orthodontic treatment J. Mass. Dent. Soc. **14:** 235, 1965. (Abstract.)

5. Baldwin, D. C., and Barnes, M. L.: Patterns of motivation in families seeking orthodontic treatment, Int. Assoc. Dent. Res. **44:**142, 1966.

6. Brislin, R. W., and Lewis, S. A.: Dating and physical attractiveness: a replication, Psychol. Rep. **22:**976, 1968.

7. Carlos, J. P.: Indices of malocclusion: characteristics and uses. Paper presented at National Institute of Dental Research Workshop on Psychosocial Aspects of Craniofacial Malformation, Hilton Head Island, S.C., Oct. 15-17, 1974.

8. Cohen, L. K., and Horowitz, H. S.: Is child's oral self-image important? Public Health Rep. **84**(3): 245, 1969.

9. Cohen, L., and Horowitz, H. S.: Occlusal relations in children born and raised in an optimally fluoridated community. III. Social-psychological findings, Angle Orthod. **40:**159, 1970.

10. Cohen, L. K., O'Shea, R. M., and Putnam, W. J.: Toothbrushing: public opinion and dental research, J. Oral Ther. Pharmacol. **4:**229, 1967.

11. Crockett, B.: Dental survey: Southeastern State College, J. Okla. Dent. Assoc. **51:**25, 1963.

12. Dion, K. K., and Berscheid, E.: Physical attractiveness and evaluations of children's transgressions, Sociometry **37**(1):1, 1974.

13. Draker, H. L.: Judgments of peers in assessing

the orthodontic handicap, J. Public Health Dent. **30:**134, 1970.
14. Friedson, E., and Feldman, J.: The public looks at dental care, J. Am. Dent. Assoc. **57**(3):325, 1958.
15. Giddon, D. B., and Nornoo, D.: Development of quantitative index of perceived relative to objective need for dental treatment, J. Dent. Res. **53** (special issue):209, 1974.
16. Giddon, D. B., Hershon, L. E., and Lennartsson, B.: Discrepancy between objective and subjective profile measures, Scand. J. Dent. Res. **82:** 527, 1974.
17. Giddon, D. B., Mosier, M., Colton, T., and Bulman, J. S.: Quantitative relationships between perceived and objective need for health care: dentistry as a model system, Public Health Rep. **91**(6):508, 1976.
17a. Giddon, D. B., Silberman, S. L., Prasad, L., and Bikofsky, C. G.: A behavioral science analysis of preventive dentistry. In Ward, H. O., ed.: A preventive point of view, Springfield, Ill., Charles C Thomas, Publisher. (In press.)
18. Katz, R.: Associations between eight orthodontic indices and two oral diseases: periodontal disease and dental caries. Paper presented at National Institute of Dental Research Workshop on Psychosocial Aspects of Craniofacial Malformation, Hilton Head Island, S.C., Oct. 15-17, 1974.
19. Kegeles, S.: Why people seek dental care: a review of present knowledge, Am. J. Public Health **51**(9):1306, 1963.
20. Kirscht, J. P., Haefner, D. P., Kegeles, S., and Rosenstock, I. M.: A national study of health beliefs, J. Health Soc. Behav. **7:**248, 1966.
21. Lautch, H.: Dental phobia, Br. J. Psychiatry **119** (541):151, 1971.
22. Lewitt, D. W., and Virolainen, K.: Conformity and independence in adolescents' motivation for orthodontic treatment, Child Dev. **39:**1189, 1968.
23. Linn, E. L.: Teenagers' attitude, knowledge, and behaviors related to oral health, J. Am. Dent. Assoc. **92:**946, 1976.
24. Molin, C., and Seeman, K.: Disproportionate dental anxiety: clinical and nosological considerations, Acta Odontol. Scand. **28**(2):197, 1970.
25. Murstein, B. I.: Physical attractiveness and marital choice, J. Pers. Soc. Psychol. **22:**8, 1972.
26. National Center for Health Statistics: Profile of American health, 1973, Public Health Rep. **89**(6):502, 1974.
27. National Center for Health Statistics, U.S. Public Health Service: Dental visits: volume and interval since last visit: United States, 1969, Washington, D.C., 1972, U.S. Government Printing Office.
28. National Opinion Research Center: Public attitudes and practices in the field of dental care, Chicago, 1960, The Center.
29. Newman, J. D., and Anderson, O. W.: Patterns of dental service utilization in the United States: a nationwide social survey, Research Series 30, Chicago, 1972, Center for Health Administration Studies, The University of Chicago Press.
30. O'Shea, R. M., and Gray, S. B.: Dental patients' attitudes and behavior concerning prevention, Public Health Rep. **83:**405, 1968.
31. Richards, N. D.: Utilization of dental services. In Richards, N. D., and Cohen, L. K., eds.: Social sciences and dentistry: a critical bibliography, Leiden, 1971, A. W. Sijthoff, International Publishing Co. BV.
32. Rosenberg, M.: Malocclusion and craniofacial malformation: self-concept implications. Paper presented at State of the Art Workshop, National Institute of Dental Research, Hilton Head Island, S.C., 1974.
33. Schwarz, E.: A socio-dental study of a kibbutz community, Doctoral Dissertation, Hebrew University, Jerusalem, 1974.
34. Shoben, E. J., and Borland, L.: An empirical study of the etiology of dental fears, J. Clin. Psychol. **10:**171, 1954.
35. Shuval, J. T.: Social and psychological factors in dental health in Israel. In O'Shea, R., and Cohen, L., eds.: Toward a sociology of dentistry, Milbank Memorial Fund Q. **49**(3):95, 1971.
36. Sternbach, R. A.: Pain: a psychophysiological analysis. New York, 1968, Academic Press, Inc.
37. Story, R.: Psychological issues in orthodontic practice, Am. J. Orthod. **52:**584, 1966.
38. Tash, R., O'Shea, R., and Cohen, L.: Testing a preventive-symptomatic theory of dental health behavior, Am. J. Public Health **59**(3):514, 1969.
39. Walster, E.: Psychosocial aspects of craniofacial malformations. Paper presented at the National Institute of Dental Research Workshop on Psychosocial Aspects of Craniofacial Malformation, Hilton Head Island, S.C., Oct. 15-17, 1974.
40. Walster, E., Berscheid, E., and Walster, G. W.: New directions in equity research, J. Pers. Soc. Psychol. **25:**151, 1973.
41. Walster, E., Aronson, V., Abrahams, D., and Rottman, L.: Importance of physical attractiveness in dating behavior, J. Pers. Soc. Psychol. **4:**508, 1966.

Chapter 5

EVOLUTION OF THE PROVIDER

The evolution of the providers of dental care begins with the first inclination to study dentistry, whether in childhood, in adolescence, or during the college years. Age, sex, socioeconomic level, education, sociocultural background, and geographical origin all interact in the selection and attainment of dentistry as a life's work. These factors, in turn, affect the potential provider's knowledge, attitudes, beliefs, values, and interests, all of which influence perceptions of one's own abilities, personality, and assessment of the profession. These perceptions ultimately determine whether or not an individual will decide to become a member of the profession.

OBJECTIVES

The objectives of this chapter are as follows:

1. To discuss characteristics of students interested in becoming dentists
2. To explore how dental students are selected
3. To discuss the education of the dentist
4. To explore some prospects for the future of dental education

CHARACTERISTICS OF STUDENTS INTERESTED IN BECOMING DENTISTS

Among college-bound students planning to enter a profession, many more express a desire to become physicians, engineers, lawyers, chemists, or architects than to become dentists.[24] However, certain common characteristics are found among students interested in dentistry.

Factors correlated with a preference for dentistry

The academic interests of students entering or planning to enter dentistry are generally matched with a desire to be independent, to work with people, and to use one's hands in one's profession. This combination of intellectual and manual pursuits, in particular, distinguishes predental students from other preprofessionals.

Most students who express an interest in dentistry come from a middle-class background. Thus the income level is usually great enough to undertake the high cost of dental education. The mean level of the father's education is, similarly, average or above average.[24]

A trend toward interest in dentistry exists among fathers of students interested in dentistry. The interest of fathers in dentistry as a career for their children apparently stems from their aspiration for their children's upward social mobility. In many cases the fathers of prospective dental students themselves have been upwardly mobile. Students with this background often perceive dentistry as a career offering high satisfaction and status with relatively easy access.[22]

Predental students also show psychosocial characteristics in common. On personality tests such as the Edwards Personal

Preference Inventory, predental students display similarities to medical students. They generally rank high on endurance and deference and low on dominance and change. On the California Personality Inventory, prospective dental students have been shown to be conventional, conforming, conservative, and concerned about seeming proper and right in the opinion of others.[12] Such interests reflect to some degree the predental student's academic ability and role orientation. Predental students were found to score highest in mechanical, technical, and scientific aptitude and lowest in physical science aptitude.[25]

Prospective dental students' perception of dentistry as a career

Other important factors influencing predental students' desires to become dentists are their occupational values and perceptions of what dentistry has to offer. In agreement with lay opinions, most students perceive dentistry as a career offering prestige and financial success.[22] These perceptions are supported by many studies of the prestige and status ascribed by the public to dentistry relative to other professions.[3,5,14]

Public opinion of dentistry as a career affects prospective students' perception of the profession. In one study, six specific criteria were identified as those by which the public judges dentists: the quality of the dentist's treatment, the dentist's manner in relating to patients, the fees charged, the dentist's ability and concern in minimizing pain, the dentist's personal cleanliness, and the kind of dental equipment used.[14] The aspect of dentistry that the public often mentions as positive factors for *continuing* dental treatment is a dentist who takes personal interest in the patient and has a pleasing personality. But the most important quality responsible for the patient's confidence in his or her dentist is the dentist's ability to minimize pain. Thus it is obvious that the public expects more from the dentist than simple mechanical delivery of health care and that the public's opinions of the dentist are based on many more personal factors than technical ability.

Surveys conducted between 1947 and 1973 have revealed a steady increase in the public's ranking of the dentist's image relative to other professions. In a 1947 National Opinion Research Center (NORC) survey, dentists were rated sixth behind physicians, professors, bankers, clergymen, and lawyers.[12a] A 1961 study polling American high school students revealed that dentists were rated in the middle third of nine professions; eight variables were used, including honesty, prestige, and value to the community.[18] By 1963, the NORC survey revealed that dentists had risen in public esteem above bankers and clergymen.[12a]

In a more recent opinion poll (1971) of predominantly white middle-class Americans, the dentist was rated third behind physicians and clergymen.[21] The pervasiveness of particular occupational stereotypes throughout various segments of American society is surprisingly great. Members of the "general public" appear to have definite and consistent images of various occupational groups at any given point in time.

The dentist who is accorded high prestige takes a personal interest in a patient's dental problems and volunteers information about care of the teeth. Additional reasons for the increased prestige accorded dentists are related to improvements in methods of care such as use of the high-speed drill, taking x-ray films of teeth, and administration of anesthesia to reduce pain.[13]

Even though the dentist is generally held in high esteem by the public, a great number of patients, estimated at approximately 12 million, do not visit the dentist because of fear.[6] Those patients who had lost confidence in their dentist reported experiences of rough or painful treatment and lack of concern by the dentist about the pain to which the patient was subjected. It is also possible that some patients may believe the risk of incurring dental disease as a result of lack of care may not be as serious as the risk of receiving an anesthetic in the dental office.

In a recent survey of attitudes toward the use of expanded-duty auxiliary personnel in the health profession, it seems that the general public is willing to accept their performance of many tasks normally performed by the physician or dentist.[9a] We have noticed in our surveys, however, comments such as "We don't care who does it since we don't like any of you," which are unfortunate for the dentist.

Part of the lack of public empathy with dentistry or dentists is a result of the general insensitivity of the dental profession to the feelings of the public as well as of auxiliary personnel and other peers. This is documented to some extent by the surveys in which it was found that the dentist perceives his or her public rating as higher than it actually is.[4] The mass media also does its part to place dentistry in an unfriendly light, promoting images such as the television stereotypes of the dentist as a buffoon or as a nonhero, lost in a world of teeth. The dentist bears some of the responsibility for this stereotyping by his or her conspicuous absence from newspaper lists of members of citizens' committees and community projects.[10]

Some of the difficulty may also result from an "identity crisis" related in part to a discrepancy between the perceived role and the actual status of the dentist.[4] Although many dental schools are expanding their programs to include dentistry more as a part of comprehensive health care, including emergency first aid and mass casualty care, the public still views dentists in a narrow, traditional role.[9,19] Regardless of the roles that dentists may assume in providing a wider range of health care duties, the status ascribed to them by the public still remains below that ascribed to physicians.

Generally, however, the public respects dentists for their technical skill and professional concern for patients. Depending on the prospective student's individual experience, it is likely that his or her perceptions of dentistry as a career are affected by public opinion.

The prospective student forms other attitudes toward dentistry from personal experiences as a patient. Depending on the quality and quantity of these experiences, the patient may or may not seek to become involved in the dental treatment situation. So, too, prospective dental students will be more favorably inclined to dentistry as a career if they have had favorable experiences as dental patients.

In a study by Mann and Parkin,[16] the most frequently mentioned reasons for entering the dental profession were autonomy, freedom to choose working hours, working with one's hands, and working with people. Perhaps surprisingly, mention of the desire to help others was low in priority.[15]

The actual study of dentistry is perceived by prospective dental students as well defined, practical, and straightforward. Before the student enters dental school, there is little interest in, or even awareness of, the theoretical and artistic aspects of dentistry. Thus dentistry is perceived by prospective dentists as a well-ordered, high-status occupation, providing straightforward, practical knowledge and the security of a well-defined career.

SELECTION OF DENTAL STUDENTS

The second step in the evolution of the dentist is the selection of students with a biotechnical aptitude for dentistry from the pool of applicants who generally possess the characteristics described earlier. The spaces currently available (1975) in dental schools each year are 5617. According to U.S. government projections,[2] this number is not adequate to meet the growing demands for dental care.

The number of places available in dental school is, in part, determined by the amount and kind of financial support for dental training programs, which, in turn, depend on government and professional estimates of manpower need. Except for temporary setbacks as a result of economic recession, the demand for dental care is rising faster than the supply of dentists.

The selection of these potential providers must be made from a pool of 14,842 applicants.[2] In the United States selection is based on admissions committees' judgments of the applicants' aptitudes, achievements, and psychosocial characteristics.

Some attempts to reduce the discrepancy between supply and demand for dental care providers include changes in the organization of dental manpower training. Special emphasis is now being placed on training and utilization of highly skilled dental auxiliary personnel to assist dentists in meeting the increased demand for dental care. Assuming this trend continues, the dentist will be expected to become a manager of dental health care delivery teams as well as a clinically competent dental health care provider. Working with auxiliary personnel as well as with other members of the health team, for example, in group practice, requires characteristics other than those attributed to the usual dental applicant and/or practitioner.[3]

Coupling this information with personality studies that describe dental students as conforming, conventional, nonintellectual, and inflexible, with a tendency toward authoritarianism,[3] we have an interesting paradox. Even though the evolving role of the dentist includes the functions of team member and manager, in addition to necessary technical skills, today's dental student, with a desire for autonomy and a tendency toward authoritarianism, may not be prepared to work harmoniously with other members of the health team. Authoritarian and related characteristics have, of course, always been a barrier to successful physician-patient relationships.

DENTAL EDUCATION

Changes in attitude associated with a dental education program

There is some indication that the dental educational system may have a negative influence on the socialization of the dental student toward identifying with patient-centered needs, whether objective or perceived. One study[17] indicated increasing conservatism; less acceptance of chronically ill, aged, and handicapped patients; and greater interest in obtaining monetary rewards[23] as the student proceeds from the preclinical years through the third and fourth year of the educational program.

Many aspects of the dental education program contribute to these attitudes. In general, dental schools offer few electives for study. Additionally, schools do not select or orient faculty members to become role models for socially responsible or responsive behavior. Little emphasis is placed on values or ethics in course work or in clinics, except as a pragmatic advantage. Although the educational system pays lip service to concern for total patient care, there has been little or no curriculum time devoted to the development of management skills, including such skills as interpersonal communication, management of pain and anxiety, and/or assessment of patients' or coworkers' psychosocial needs. The result is that students tend to decrease in social sensitivity as they proceed through dental school.[7]

Although social sensitivity was not directly measured, the deleterious effect of regimentation on students in dental schools may be exemplified in a study of the effect of alphabetical sectioning, which is maintained throughout many large dental schools over most of their 4-year programs. Although there were no differences in the average academic standing among alphabetized sections during the first year they were formed, the mean academic scores of the students in the sections increasingly became significantly different from each other with each successive year. Moreover, the students within each section became more like each other academically (and, perhaps, in other ways) and less like students from the other sections.[8]

On the positive side, there are many "socially sensitive" students in dental schools today. In fact, curricula have been developed within some dental schools that provide opportunities to develop and enhance social and interpersonal awareness. Such programs also provide students with opportunities to learn the skills necessary to deal with factors of our social system that may affect the delivery of health care.

Years of observations with many students have shown us that dental students are really no different from medical students, art students, and college undergraduates. The traditional dental and medical school learning environment has so constricted students that they can easily slide into the mold of the conservative educational process.[3] As schools stop trying to teach social sensitivity and behavioral change by the lecture method and begin to listen to the students, students also begin to listen to themselves and become aware of their own feelings, goals, and interests. In working with proper faculty role models, they become conscious of and concerned for the well-being of other individuals. Such sensitivity is the basic requisite for involvement in one's own personal environment and for investment in one's own personal effectiveness.[7]

Recommendations for dental education in relation to the organization of dental practice

It is important to look at the possible contribution of behavioral science principles to the planning and implementation of improved health care delivery. If our dental schools are to have an impact on changing the health care delivery system, there must be a closer relationship between the dental education program and what is required in actual practice. Presently, less than ideal examples of health care delivery systems exist within most dental educational institutions. Good examples of health care delivery systems and more faculty role models who exhibit patient-oriented care in a humane teaching environment are needed. The use of expanded-function auxiliary personnel is also necessary to give students the opportunity to work effectively with other health professionals in delivering dental care as well as to expand and refine their interpersonal and management skills. Furthermore, students will learn to identify with modes of delivering care that are presently well accepted and growing in the medical field. It is thus essential that dental schools provide the training necessary for the establishment and management of group practice that effectively utilizes auxiliary personnel.

SOME PROSPECTS FOR THE FUTURE OF DENTAL EDUCATION

We would like to offer some predictions for the future of dental educational programs that will benefit the providers, that is, the dentists. We expect the educational process to become more related to the practice of dentistry, which, we will assume, will become more related to what society needs. With some form of national health insurance, there should be a greater congruence between need and demand for health care. The present situation is one in which the perceptions of practitioners and government are at variance. The federal government has been basing its planning and actions on the need for care that, as indicated earlier, almost everyone has. Consequently, the great problem of government planners is the lack and/or the maldistribution of dentists in various areas of the country. On the other hand, the private practitioner continues to respond to the *demand* for care, that is, the 50% of our general population in *need* of and actually seeking dental services. Obviously, there are great geographical variations, depending on the particular economic climate of the region. Although we must be aware of such differences in perceptions and resulting action, we cannot continue to allow them to unduly influence our educational programs, nor should we be disproportionately influenced by the parochial concerns of state boards, professional organizations, or even the albatross of tradition. Educational programs must be developed that prepare our graduates to best serve society's needs. The examining boards should, in turn, evaluate whether or not this is being accomplished.

One proposal is to convene representatives of examiners and educators (to do what logically should have been done years ago before we decided to have expanded duties, auxiliary personnel, increased enrollment, etc.) to determine what functions or duties are required for the practice of dentistry. This group would include representatives of different boards of dental examiners, the American Dental Association, the American Association of Dental Schools, and consumer and dental education groups. They would be asked to determine precisely what functions and duties are required for maintaining and improving dental health as part of comprehensive health care.

With the aid of computers, the following stage would involve deciding what personnel are required to perform these tasks and functions or how these tasks and functions should be properly divided among dentists, dental specialists, hygienists, dental assistants, laboratory technicians, receptionists, or any other kind of auxiliary personnel that the computer-assisted task analysts might evolve.

The next stage would be to develop appropriate educational programs for each individual group of providers. The programs would be appropriate to the special tasks and functions each group would perform with respect to the entire dental field. This responsibility should fall primarily with the educators, in concert with the boards of dental examiners and the Council on Dental Education of the American Dental Association. Based on the requirements of these educational programs, a continuing responsibility of dental educators would be to develop criteria for admission to these programs.

Once having decided what functions or duties are required for the practice of dentistry, what personnel are necessary, and what kind of educational programs are appropriate for each group, the final stage would be to evaluate whether or not the criteria have been met before allowing anyone to practice dentistry. Responsibility for the tasks would be shared by the appropriate licensing agencies and the educational institutions. Intermediate evaluation of student achievement, for example, would continue within the educational institutions. Educational programs would be periodically reviewed by process of an external evaluation group, presently the Commission on Accreditation.

Hopefully, such recommendations will result in major changes in the organization of dental education programs so that they become more related to dental practice as a delivery system for oral health care. Some schools have already replaced the traditional block system of clinical education with a modular system, or group practice. For example, the clinical educational program may be organized into a system of modules with a team of students (under the faculty supervision of a general practice resident) who would be responsible for the comprehensive dental care of a group of patients. This model is similar to the present practice of hospital medicine, where faculty members have the responsibility for the care of the patient, even though the services are actually provided by the students. Under such a system, if patient care is not completed by dental students in a given time period, the faculty leader would complete the treatment.

Let us assume that in addition to the clinical skills the dental student is learning, the future dentist will also perform higher order functions such as decision making, judgment, and executive management. Auxiliary personnel will also be trained to perform certain clinical services under the supervision of dentists. The implications for the students' education, then, are that dental students would obtain more training and experience in diagnosis and problem solving, treatment planning, pain control, and related medical and surgical subjects. Courses in the specialty areas of endodontics, periodontics, and surgery, which have been heretofore minimized in the predoctoral program, would be increased. In the past, this minimization has often been related to the specialists' unwillingness to relinquish expertise in these areas to the predoctoral student, rather than to a lack of student ability. Additionally, more courses will be offered in the areas of management, interpersonal skills, genetic counseling, medical sociology, etc.

Conversely, the students would receive less training in some of the more reversible mechanical procedures of restorative dentistry, which could be assumed by trained auxiliary personnel. Thus the student would be trained both in the clinical skills necessary to provide care and in the ability to manage a more complex organization to deliver care.

Relative to the basic medical sciences, a reordering of those basic science areas important for the practice of dentistry will probably occur. There will be fewer actual laboratory experiences and more audiovisual simulation. For those basic medical sciences that are essential, the learning process will become more efficient. Some changes currently under discussion would include placing certain basic science courses as well as the humanities and the social/behavioral science courses earlier in the student's predoctoral years in college or even in high school.

It is possible that some of the hallowed subjects such as organic chemistry may be deemphasized in the college years. The American Association of Medical Colleges, for example, recently found from a survey that organic chemistry, although still considered important for mastery of the medical school curricula, was seen as relatively unimportant for the actual practice of medicine.[1] Thus more time will become available for greater emphasis on quantitative methods, information science, and relevant behavioral sciences directed toward the development of problem-solving skills and the ability to cope with change.

An example of an integrated and more relevant curriculum might be to build on the course content of anatomy and physiology relevant to the speech and hearing apparatus for later courses in communication sciences: ordered communications essential to management and good interpersonal relations and disordered communications associated with psychopathology and ineffective interpersonal relations.

Similarly, the clinical portion of the curriculum might be more self-paced within the group practice modules. Rather than the simple system of requirements that still exists in many dental schools, students will be expected to maintain a certain level of proficiency, which will vary according to the individual student. At the same time, students could be given experience in peer review and other aspects of quality assurance while in dental school. Positive attitudes toward third-party payment and continuing education might become an integral part of their professional life. There could be greater emphasis on prevention, not only of dental disease, but also of environmental threats to the dentist's health —currently mercury, anesthetic gases, etc. If less emphasis were placed on removable dentures, etc., curriculum time could be available for adult orthodontics and other problems of growth and development such as craniofacial anomalies and geriatrics. Applied behavioral science could be expanded to include the psychological significance of the orofacial areas to self-concept, self-esteem, motivation for seeking dental care, stress, and oral disease. Most importantly, the dental student could have increased opportunities to gain an appreciation of the mouth and related structures to the "quality of life."

After demonstrating proficiency in all the necessary clinical disciplines in the group practice setting, the student would be free to pursue advanced clinical training, research, or community activities. Based on a reevaluation of the need for specialists and the government's interest in reducing specialty programs, there will probably be more of what is now reserved for postgraduate specialty training included in the predoctoral curriculum. The graduate might then become some type of a "supergeneralist."

With increased control of caries and resultant longer tooth life, an expanded role for the specialties of endodontics, periodontics, orthodontics, and prosthodontics and, of course, an increased emphasis on community preventive programs will occur. The graduating student of the future will know more of what is now reserved for the specialties of the orthodontist and the oral surgeon—particularly in the areas of pain control. Consequently, the orthodontist and oral surgeon will probably become more involved with transplantation, implantation, and reconstructive surgery—areas presently assumed by some of our medically qualified colleagues. In other words, future educational programs will follow the changes in responsibility of the dentist; for example, at present 80% of a dentist's time is spent repairing the ravages of carious lesions, but by the year 2000 only an estimated 30% will be spent on this problem. In contrast to the present distribution of dental education time, the student will spend significantly less time in the restorative areas of dental practice and more time in preventively oriented specialty training.

In summary, dentistry of the future will require, in addition to bioclinical competence, an even greater attention to the social, psychological, and personal aspects of dentistry. Such developments must be reflected in the recruitment and selection of dental students as well as in the education and preparation of the dentist. Certainly dentistry now requires an individual with characteristics very different from those who previously chose and were selected and trained for dentistry. The dentist of the present and the future must cooperate with other individuals as part of a total health team.

REFERENCES

1. Angel, J.: Personal communication, 1976.
2. Council on Dental Education: Dental education supplement 7 to annual report 1974-1975, Chicago, 1975, American Dental Association.
3. Counsell, L. A.: The intraprofessional image of dentistry, J. Public Health Dent. **28:**35, 1968.
4. Engle, D.: Social status of the dentist, N.M. Dent. J. **20:**42, 1969.
5. Fusillo, A. E., and Metz, A. S.: Social science research on the dental student. In Richards, N. D., and Cohen, L. K.: Social sciences and dentistry: a critical bibliography, Leiden, 1971, A. W. Sijthoff, International Publishing Co. BV.
6. Gale, E. N., and Ayer, W. A.: Treatment of dental phobias, J. Am. Dent. Assoc. **73:**1304, 1969.
7. Giddon, D. B.: Irrelevance of dental education to future health delivery systems. Paper presented at Student-Faculty Conference on Preventive Dentistry, New York University, New York, March 17, 1970.
8. Giddon, D. B., Brown, M. W., and McCabe, G. D.: The influence of alphabetically assigned sections upon the academic performances of dental students, Int. Assoc. Dent. Res. **47:**186, 1969.
9. Giddon, D. B., Fischer, T. E., Dressler, D. P., and Hozid, J. L.: Disaster preparedness training for dental students, J. Dent. Educ. **35:**40, 1971.

9a. Gilmore, N. D., Stevens, C., Pierce, V., and Giddon, D. B.: Consumer and provider attitudes toward dentists and expanded auxiliary functions, J. Am. Dent. Assoc. **3:**614, 1976.

10. Goodman, S. E.: The crack in the dental image, Dent. Manag. **5:**35, 1965.
11. Hein, J.: Future professional responsibilities of dental academicians, J. Dent. Educ. **40**(12):775, 1976.
12. Heist, P. A.: Personality characteristics of dental students, Educ. Record **41:**240, 1960.

12a. Hodge, R. W., Siegel, P. M., and Rossi, P. H.: Occupational prestige in the United States, 1925-1963, Am. J. Sociol. **70**(3):286, 1964.

13. Kriesberg, L.: The bases of occupational prestige: the case of dentists, Am. Sociol. Rev. **27:**238, 1962.
14. Kriesberg, L., and Treiman, B. R.: The public's views on dentistry as a profession, J. Dent. Educ. **25:**247, 1961.
15. Linn, E. L.: Work objectives and skills associated with high school students interested in dentistry, J. Can. Dent. Assoc. **34:**321, 1968.
16. Mann, W. R., and Parkin, G.: The dental school applicant, J. Dent. Educ. **24:**16, 1960.
17. Moosbruker, J. B., and Giddon, D. B.: Effect of experience with aged, chronically ill, and handicapped patients on student attitudes, J. Dent. Educ. **30:**278, 1966.
18. Nelson, H. A., and McDonagh, E. C.: Perception of statuses and images of selected professions, Soc. Sci. Res. **46:**3, 1961.
19. O'Shea, R. M., and Fusillo, A. E.: The dentist's role and parents' expectations, HSMHA Health Rep. **86:**915, 1971.
20. Richards, N. D.: Utilization of dental services. In Richards, N. D., and Cohen, L. K., ed.: Social sciences and dentistry: a critical bibliography, Leiden, 1971, A. W. Sijthoff, International Publishing Co. BV.
21. Rotter, J. B., and Stein, D. K.: Public attitudes to-

wards trustworthiness, competence, and altruism of twenty selected occupations, J. Appl. Soc. Psychol. **1:**334, 1971.

22. Sherlock, B., and Cohen, A.: The strategy of occupational choice: recruitment to dentistry, Soc. Forces **44:**303, 1966.
23. Steinberg, D. N.: Changes in attitudes of dental students, J. Dent. Educ. **37:**36, 1973.
24. Wertz, C. E.: Career choice patterns, Soc. Educ. **40:**348, 1967.
25. Witteman, J. K., Schimpfhauser, F. T., and Crownley, A.: Dentistry, medicine, pharmacy: treatment interests, ability and socio-economic index of three stable career groups, J. Dent. Res. **54**(3):548, 1975.

Part two

LEARNING THE LINES

Principles of interpersonal behavior

Now that the stage has been set, and the characters, including the dentist and the patient, have been cast, it is time to learn the lines.

In this drama, the lines consist of basic principles that the dentist must understand to be in full character. He or she can then more effectively deliver the lines in the upcoming drama, when dentist and patient meet. As in any drama, the main character must be very familiar with the lines; in fact, the character must practice them until they come naturally. To maximize learning of the basic principles in Part two, the student must agree to learn the lines by practicing them. After having learned the lines, the drama will begin: dentist and patient will meet and begin to interact.

OBJECTIVES

The objectives for the chapters in Part two are as follows:

- To examine the process of drawing up a psychological contract
- To explore the concept of learning style
- To investigate the importance of understanding human motivation
- To explore the ways in which perception shapes our behavior
- To look at individual and group approaches to problem solving
- To understand conflict and ways to manage it
- To practice communication skills and how they relate to giving and receiving help
- To examine how interpersonal influence is related to the change process

In summary, the importance of becoming aware of the psychological processes of learning, motivation, and perception, particularly as they relate to the behavior of dentist and patient in the delivery of dental care, as well as the behavioral and interaction processes of interpersonal and group relationships, communications, conflict, and influence cannot be overemphasized. By understanding how these psychological and behavioral concepts can be applied to the diagnosis and treatment of dental patients, by experiencing the role of these processes in the dentist-patient relationship through a series of exercises, and by improving individual interpersonal skills through practice and feedback, you will be able to take the first steps toward establishing a smoother and more productive dentist-patient interaction.

Chapter 6

THE PSYCHOLOGICAL CONTRACT

A dentist, seated on the stool, and his assistant are laughing over an amusing incident that must have just happened, when a patient appears at the doorway. Somewhat hesitatingly, the patient makes her way between the dentist and his assistant toward the dental chair, sits down, and waits. At that moment the receptionist sticks her head in the door, says something inaudible to the patient, and the three of them (the dentist, the assistant, and the receptionist) begin laughing together. Almost absentmindedly, the dentist reaches for a mouth mirror, which the assistant has placed on the instrument tray, and still half attending to what is going on between the assistant and the receptionist, asks the patient to open her mouth. The patient, instead, asks, "but aren't you going to wash your hands, Doctor?" The laughter immediately stops. The dentist and assistant exchange embarrassed glances, and the dentist gets up and washes his hands.*

This brief vignette demonstrates several key factors that operate in all interpersonal relationships. The dentist must understand and accommodate these factors if he or she is to be effective in working with patients, other dentists, and co-workers in the dental office. These factors include the following:

1. Definition of group membership—who is in the group and who is not. The camaraderie among the dentist, assistant, and receptionist and the obvious tension that the patient feels in disrupting their activity demonstrate the psychological impact of being "in" the group and of not being in! Obviously, the dentist, assistant, and receptionist share a common membership from which the patient is excluded. There are several levels of groups or relationships within the dental office, some with overlapping membership. The dentist, the hygienist, and other members of the office staff form a professional work group with specific tasks, methods of operation, and patterns of relationships. The dentist and the patient form a two-person group with a different set of tasks, operations, and relational patterns. Typically, these groups function simultaneously with considerable interaction. It requires thought and effort on the part of the dentist to manage effectively the demands of these several levels of group interaction and to avoid the embarrassing tensions that surfaced in the vignette. The dynamics of group behavior will be discussed in greater detail in Chapter 11.

2. Tendency to provide personalized explanations for observed behavior. Individuals typically seek to generate interpretations of behaviors that they observe, and these interpretations tend to have a personalized tone, particularly if the observer is anxious about the situation. Thus the patient who enters the dental office and sees the members of the staff laughing and joking together might easily be led to the interpretation that "They are laughing at me or about my case because there is some-

*From Froelich, R. E., Bishop, F. M., and Dworkin, S. F.: Communication in the dental office, St. Louis, 1976, The C. V. Mosby Co.

thing about my case that is either funny or bizarre." Although the "true" explanation may be quite different from the patient's interpretation, the fact that this interpretation was generated gives it a certain credence in the patient's mind and will undoubtedly color her attitudes toward the dentist. The role of perception and communication in shaping these interpretations of the world is discussed in greater detail in Chapters 9 and 12.

3. Existence of implied contracts in all interpersonal relations—and the tensions that arise when it appears that those contracts have been violated. There is evidence of at least two implied psychological contracts in the vignette. First, the dentist, the assistant, and the receptionist obviously have established a mutually agreed on relationship that involves the informal sharing of humor and a work pattern that permits social interaction to continue while the patient is present. There is also, however, an implied contract between the dental team, particularly the dentist, and the patient. This contract includes both the dentist's and the patient's attitudes about the proper levels of respect and attention to which the patient is entitled and the procedures that will be followed in providing treatment. The laughter and the lack of attention provided the patient (until she interjected herself into the conversation) appear to suggest a violation of the first part of this contract, and the dentist's failure to wash his hands before beginning treatment suggests a violation of the second part. Although neither of the contracts are likely to have a formal, written existence anywhere, the psychological commitment of the participants to them is readily apparent.

In this chapter, we will consider the process by which people come to join groups and form relationships. We will particularly focus on the process of contracting and seek to discriminate those parts of the process that are explicit from those that are implicit. Finally, we will explore some of the problems that occur when too much of the contract is left implicit. We will be using the formation of the contract between the instructor and the members of this class as an ongoing clinical example. We shall see in Part three that therapeutic relationships become the major lever that dentists apply when they want to change a patient's behavior to easier acceptance of dental treatment and toward increased prevention of new dental disease.

OBJECTIVES

The objectives of this chapter are as follows:

1. To examine the role of implicit and explicit psychological contracts in the establishment of interpersonal relationships and to define the ways in which the contract shapes the interpretation and effectiveness of interpersonal behavior
2. To practice negotiating a psychological contract by exploring the formation of a specific contract, reflecting the expectations and attitudes held with regard to this course

IDEAS ABOUT THE PSYCHOLOGICAL CONTRACT

Groups are common in society, and each of us participates in many groups (family, circles of friends, church, study groups, work groups, relationships with other individuals—a two-person group). Task-oriented groups exist for the purpose of *jointly* accomplishing certain specific tasks. Such groups are common in industrial organizations and are becoming increasingly more common in the professions.[5] In this chapter, we will be focusing on *three* task-oriented groups: the dental office staff, the dentist and the patient, and a learning group—this class.

In dentistry, task-oriented groups of several types exist. The traditional group centers around dentist and patient with, perhaps, a hygienist or a receptionist. More recently, formal *teams,* composed of dentists, hygienists, assistants, and technicians working in concert to provide improved patient care, have developed. The emergence of team practice, with its pooling of expertise, enhances the individual dentist's ability to provide a fuller scope of care to more patients.

Although it is not our purpose at this time to discuss the different strengths and weaknesses of individual, group, and team practice, it is useful to distinguish among the several types. **Individual practice** is, of course, readily definable and observable and is quite different from group and team practice. **Group practice** typically involves several dentists, each providing individual treatment to patients but sharing common facilities and supporting staff. The members of the group may also provide backup coverage for others in the practice. The typical group practice would not be an example of a task-oriented group as previously defined. In group practice, different members of a group do not share responsibility for accomplishing the *same* task. In **team practice,** on the other hand, dentists and staff share the responsibility for the accomplishment of specific tasks with each patient. These several levels of interaction should be kept in mind as we discuss the dynamics of group relationship in this and subsequent chapters.

The examination of the formation of relationships begins with an individual's decision to join a group or pursue a particular relationship with another individual. Individuals have their own goals and normal ways of doing things, their experiences, their attitudes and biases, and their expectations. Groups also have norms of behavior, habits, values, and expectations about new members. Whenever a group is formed or an individual enters a group or forms a relationship, a mutual adjustment process is initiated.

Significance of the psychological contract

The adjustment process that "prepares and qualifies individuals to occupy organizational positions," is called **socialization.**[1] Most discussions of socialization emphasize the resources and techniques available to the group in its efforts to shape a new member into a predetermined mold. Practically speaking, of course, the ability of an individual to alter dramatically the norms, traditions, and behavior patterns of a large, long-established organization is limited. However, the relationship of the individual to work groups, even established ones within a large organization, is more open to mutual influence. The process of establishing new groups or relationships has considerable impact on the quality of the mutual adjustment process and particularly on the developing of norms of openness, cooperation, and respect, all of which are needed to guide effective effort.

Forming a relationship involves achieving some level of compatibility and understanding between participants as to the purposes and procedures of each party. It also requires an implicit balance of expectations, goals, and values. The relationship —the group—is held together, and joint effort is made possible by a shared perception that Schein[5] refers to as a **"psychological contract."** In the process of "drawing up" this "contract," each individual forms an understanding of what role he or she will play in terms of responsibility, influence, and interaction with the other members. This understanding includes a conception of what the individual is expected to contribute and what he or she will receive for that contribution. What members provide through their participation is their **contribution;** what the relationship or the group provides for the individual members are its **inducements** to them. People join and remain as participating members of a group or relationship when they perceive that the inducements exceed the contributions required of them.[3]

Considerations in negotiating a psychological contract

The existence of a psychological contract does not mean that members must write a legally binding agreement specifying criteria and procedures for all aspects of the relationship. This would not only be impossible, but it would also interfere with the health and vitality of the relationship. On the other hand, it is reasonable, for example, in the first examination of a new patient for the dentist to devote time to an explicit, well-thought-out discussion of the treatment practices, work schedules, and billing procedures that provide the structure for that particular dentist-patient relationship.

Groups are social entities that grow and develop over time through the interaction of members. The psychological contract reflects this dynamic, adaptive character and is constantly being "renegotiated." In many groups and relationships, a psychological contract is not achieved by open discussion and explicit sharing of understanding but by assumptions made privately by individuals that *such a balance* exists. Much of the potential for conflict comes from this reliance on independently formed individual perceptions. When an individual's expectations as to responsibility or rewards or any other aspect of activity are not realized in practice, disillusionment sets in, and the stability and effectiveness of the relationship are threatened.

Forming a group and bringing a new member into an existing group are particularly critical activities. The point at which the patient entered the operatory in the earlier vignette was a key moment. The manner in which that moment was handled—in this case apparently badly—will shape the form, direction, and effectiveness of the relationship from then on. The success of a relationship and the satisfaction its participants derive from participation depend heavily on feeling that the contract is being honored. Individuals who feel misled or cheated or insulted are not likely to perform effectively; individuals who do not fulfill their responsibilities also violate the contract. It is therefore vital to devote time and effort to agreeing on and monitoring periodically the shared set of expectations about the nature of the relationship—its mores, tasks, procedures, values, and objectives—and the responsibilities, rights, and obligations of members. To the degree that critical expectations are not shared, effectiveness in task accomplishment is threatened.

PRACTICE NEGOTIATING A PSYCHOLOGICAL CONTRACT

In this section, you will have the opportunity to explore the psychological contract as it is being formed for this portion of the class. This exercise has been designed to allow the group and the instructor to explore each other's understanding of the purpose and approach to this section of the course. This exploration is intended to make explicit the role of expectations in forming the psychological contract and to give the group experience in expressing and examining uncertainties.*

Group interviews instructor

In this part of the exercise, the group will have the opportunity to question the instructor as to his or her goals for this section of the course. The group will be able to examine the instructor's approach to learning and expectations as to the role he or she will play in the group meetings. The group will also be able to explore the instructor's attitudes and feelings toward the members of the group. In this part, the group will interview the instructor.

*This exercise is based on a format presented in Kolb, Rubin, and McIntyre, ORGANIZATIONAL PSYCHOLOGY: An Experiential Approach, 2nd edition, © 1974, pp. 23, 25, 27, 28, and pages for the submitted text. Reprinted by permission of Prentice-Hall, Inc., Englewood Cliffs, N.J.

Preparation (approximate time—15 minutes)

1. To facilitate the interviewing process, the group should be broken up into subgroups of four or five persons.
2. These subgroups should meet separately to prepare to interview the instructor. A record should be kept of the questions that the members wish to raise. (NOTE: It is essential that *any* questions that are of real concern to members be raised; this is the only way that sources of potential conflict can be identified and examined. Note should also be taken of any assumptions underlying questions and the reasons for raising questions; in this way, it will be possible to test the instructor's reactions to the assumptions and reasons.)
3. Each subgroup should select a representative who will join with the representatives of the other subgroups to interview the instructor. The representative should clearly understand the questions that the subgroup wants raised as well as the reasons and assumptions behind the questions.

Procedure (approximate time—15 minutes)

1. The representatives, one from each subgroup, should meet with the instructor to conduct an interview in accord with the plans formed by the group.
2. The rest of the group should act as observers to the interview, paying particular attention to the following questions:
   - How do the instructor's theories of learning compare with yours?
   - How do you feel about the instructor's intended role in this section of the course as he or she describes it?
   - How do you feel about the contributions that the instructor expects you and other group members to make to the learning process?
   - How do you think the instructor feels about the course and the group members?
   - What are the instructor's goals, and how do they compare with yours?

Instructor interviews group

In this part of the exercise, the instructor will have the opportunity to explore the group's expectations and objectives. The instructor will be able to examine the feelings group members have about the approach to this section of the course and their expectations as to the contributions of the instructor. The instructor will also be able to learn the group's reactions to his or her responses in the first interview. In this part, the instructor will interview the group.

Preparation (approximate time—15 minutes)

1. The groups should break up into the same initial subgroups.
2. Each subgroup should select a different representative to join with the representatives of other groups to be interviewed by the instructor.
3. The subgroups should discuss the reactions of the members to the first interview; note should be taken of points that were not clearly understood or with which the members disagree. In addition, members should discuss their responses to matters that will be raised by questions the instructor might ask, such as:
   - What are your goals for this course? What do you hope to learn, and how do you expect to use this knowledge?

- What role do you feel the instructor should play in the course? What do you expect the instructor to contribute?
- What are you prepared to contribute?
- How do you feel about the instructor's responses to the first interview?

Again, the representative should clearly understand the responses the members wish to make.

Procedure (approximate time—15 minutes)

1. The representatives, one from each subgroup, meet with the instructor to be interviewed.
2. The other members of the group act as observes, again attending to the relation between the instructor's theories, attitudes, and expectations and those of the group members.

Group discusses interviews (approximate time—15 minutes)

The group should reconvene as a whole, with the instructor, to discuss and compare the interviews. In this discussion, the group should try to develop ways to resolve any conflicts that have emerged. Finally, the group should seek to restate explicitly the psychological contract that has resulted from the interviews.

SUMMARY

We all experience anxiety in joining a new group or forming a new relationship. Will we be able to perform? Will we like and be liked by our new colleagues? Will the job or the relationship be stable and provide security? Will we like the dentist? Will we like the patient? These anxieties often lead us to behave in ways that interfere with obtaining reliable answers to our questions. We worry more about making a good impression and about being accepted than about gaining clear and explicit statements of responsibilities, norms, and objectives. This may lead us to accept values and perspectives without examination, or to give the impression that we do, in order to gain acceptance.

Similarly, any individual or group tries to put the "best foot forward" when meeting new patients or co-workers. Groups like to make a good impression also, and the first several encounters are usually marked with conviviality and the promise of a glowing future.

Thus the psychological contract is often formed under false pretenses. An adopted air of self-assurance and a willingness to assume that both parties share the same understanding of the new relationship may reduce anxiety initially. Patients nod knowingly or repress asking questions to avoid showing ignorance, answering embarrassing questions (How long since your last visit?), or wasting the dentist's time. The masking of feelings and the failure to expose and clear up uncertainties pave the way for future difficulties. Every game has its rules, and the rules should be clearly understood and accepted by all players.

In a democratic society, where relationships and memberships in groups, even work groups, are voluntary, a common sense of the rules of the game is essential for individuals and groups to choose their relationships intelligently. The anxiety experienced in hammering out a mutual perception at the outset is a small price to pay for avoiding subsequent costs in bruised feelings, shattered expectations, and lost confidence and trust.

The responsibility for developing a shared, explicit psychological contract and for monitoring and revising it through experience falls equally on every individual. Some organizations such as the military tightly control the socialization process, and the individual must either agree to submit to being shaped in the desired mold or relinquish membership. In other relationships, each individual will contribute heavily to the culture and atmosphere. At either extreme, however, the potential of the relationship will be realized only if its rules, expectations, and demands are explicitly known to all and if participants openly and freely express their true feelings, motives, and uncertainties.

The failure of individuals to assert themselves actively in the socialization process is, perhaps, the greatest threat to the quality of future relationships. Feelings of dissatisfaction and betrayal arise when expectations are not met; very often, however, expectations are not met because they were not made explicit at the beginning or because faulty assumptions were made about the content or firmness of commitments. Individuals often ask no questions or ask questions unrelated to their most valued goals and expectations. New employees often focus on the *context* of the job—pay, hours, location—to the neglect of its *content*—what will I be doing, and will it be challenging, stimulating, consistent with my values? In his or her professional capacity, the dentist possesses powerful resources, including control of rewards, social acceptance, and knowledge, for shaping other persons' behavior. Moreover, these resources are defenses for the dentist's own anxieties and uncertainties. Thus it is natural to press for conformity, passive compliance, and acceptance of professional omniscience in socializing (orienting) new patients, even though what may be most necessary for an effective treatment experience is inquisitiveness, independence, and enthusiasm on the part of the patient.

Individuals who approach relationships passively and with a too-ready acceptance of ill-defined arrangements in order to mask their own anxiety lead themselves into a self-reinforcing chain of disappointments. Passivity is often interpreted as a sign of weakness and induces pressure to restrain independent behavior; the individual feels excessively controlled and finds initial expectations of challenge and responsibility thwarted, leading to further passivity or withdrawal; the relationship is denied the potential creativity and zeal of the individual, and the individual finds his or her needs for emotional and intellectual growth stymied.

Group and interpersonal relationships are delicate affairs and require frank and explicit discussion if they are to be preserved. Relationships are psychological as well as physical phenomena. Every party to a relationship must feel that the benefits he or she receives for participation compensate for what is given. Since each of us possesses our own criteria for evaluating objects and relationships, it is possible for everyone in a relationship to feel that he or she is profiting. The perception that the balance of inducements to contributions is positive, at least relative to available alternatives, is a first condition for an individual to consider in initiating or maintaining a relationship.[3]

In the preceding exercise, you have had the opportunity to participate in forming the psychological contract for this class. This is an unusual activity to engage in as part of a course, and you may feel bewildered or frustrated that the instructor has not taken a stronger role in organizing the class. The student role, as most of us have experienced it, is typically passive, and the organization (here represented by the instructor) controls the socialization process. You are now being asked to take responsibility not only for defining your goals and expectations for this course but also for establishing the norms and procedures for the class as a whole. Of course in the brief time spent on this exercise, it has not been possible to examine and shape a consensus on all the issues that will arise for the class nor is it reasonable to expect that everyone fully understands and accepts the contract tentatively worked out in your discussion. The group has begun, however, to establish its identity; to develop norms for raising questions, admitting uncertainties, and confronting differences; and to assume responsibility for its future.

At the same time, you have received a brief exposure to the complex and delicate nature of the relationships that you will be forming with patients and colleagues throughout your professional career. Recognizing the importance of setting the contract for those relationships carefully is the first step in effective interpersonal behavior; in the subsequent chapters you will be able to acquire the concepts and develop the skills needed to follow through on this recognition.

REFERENCES

1. Caplow, T.: Principles of organization, New York, 1964, Harcourt Brace Jovanovich, Inc.
2. Froelich, R. E., Bishop, F. M., and Dworkin, S. F.: Communication in the dental office, St. Louis, 1976, The C. V. Mosby Co.
3. March, J. G., and Simon, H. S.: Organization, New York, 1956, John Wiley and Sons, Inc.
4. Schein, E. S.: Organization psychology, Englewood Cliffs, N.J., 1965, Prentice-Hall, Inc.
5. Schein, E. S.: Socialization and the profession of management. In Kolb, D. A., Rubin, I. M., and McIntyre, J. M.: Organizational psychology: an experiential approach, Englewood Cliffs, N.J., 1971, Prentice-Hall, Inc.

Chapter 7

LEARNING STYLE

The dentist and his or her staff are particularly concerned with the how and why of learning, since much effort is directed toward shaping the behavior of patients (to avoid harmful foods or other sources of disease, to adopt proper brushing techniques, etc.). A portion of the effort is exerted through conventional direct teaching methods—the patient is shown how to brush, how to floss, etc. and is given information on the pathology of plaque formation or of peridontal disease. However, much more is accomplished or attempted through less formal, more subjective means such as persuasion, fear, "motivation." The dentist must constantly assess how a patient "learns" (how that patient adapts to his or her environment) in order to produce conditions (to adopt a strategy or approach) that will produce the learning (the behavior change) that the dentist desires. To accomplish this, the dentist needs a general model of how individuals learn and of how they learn differently.

Since learning cannot be treated as distinct from doing and since we cannot fully control the flow of stimuli, we need to translate unsystematic learning into consciously usable knowledge. This becomes an attainable goal when learning is viewed as an ongoing process of renewal and refinement—a process that feeds back on itself and goes through definable, although overlapping, stages. At the level of conscious behavior, the learning process involves the acquisition and processing of information and experience and the application of the output to subsequent situations.

OBJECTIVES

The objectives of this chapter are as follows:

1. To describe some characteristics of the learning process
2. To explore your own approach to learning and to identify your learning style
3. To demonstrate how familiarity with the concept of learning styles is related to more effective interpersonal behavior

LEARNING

Learning occurs when a stimulus and a response are paired

For the psychologist, learning involves the development of associations between *stimulus* and *response*—between, for example, the sound of a piano key being struck (the stimulus) and identification of the note as C sharp (the response) by a student. This relation is *learned*—it does not come naturally, as does blinking one's eye when air is blown into it—and the learning takes place through repeated association of the stimulus and response. The basic premise of learning theory is known as the **law of effect,** which states, in essence, that an act may be altered in strength by its consequences.[3] In the previous example, the response "C sharp" by the student is strengthened or reinforced by the piano teacher saying "correct"; other responses such as "B flat" are weakened by the teacher saying "wrong." The inclusion of any behavior in a person's repertoire thus depends on rehearsal of the behavior under appropriate conditions of reinforcement.

Learning is natural and continuous

In the previous example, the student is conscious that learning is taking place and could probably describe the process. Every individual is constantly experiencing a vast array of stimuli—sound, light, tactile sensation—and responding in various ways. These interactions of stimulus and response are constantly reshaping or adapting behavior patterns. It is in this basic sense that we say that learning is a natural process that goes on continuously without the conscious involvement or intention of the learner. As a psychological process, learning is natural and continuous.

In common social discourse, we tend to use the term "learning" to refer to the planned acquisition of knowledge such as presumably goes on in the schoolroom. We tend to treat learning as a discrete activity that is detached from the real world of events. Learning is presumed to take place in schools, training programs, and the like; once it is completed, the individual can get on to "really doing something."

This distinction between learning and doing is artificial, and individuals often blind themselves to what they have learned by not allowing themselves time to sort out the behavior patterns they have developed. We are continually acquiring information from the environment and adapting our behavior to incorporate that information. We develop attitudes and habits, consciously and unconsciously. Whether we recognize it or not, we are constantly learning.

There is nothing evaluative about this concept of learning. It is neither good nor bad that we learn—it is inevitable. The problem is, first, to appreciate the reality of the learning process, and, second, to gain control over it. There is clearly a difference between learning resulting from the unsystematic flow of externally generated stimuli and learning resulting from the output of a systematic, purposeful analysis of a controlled flow of selected information. The former does not lend itself readily to application in future situations and is typically not recognized as learning. The latter is highly desirable when it can be arranged, as in the classroom, but is often mistakenly thought of as the only form of learning.

How learning occurs: a cycle

The learning process may be thought of as a cycle (Fig. 7-1) that begins with the **acquisition** of information and concrete experience—this is the "doing" stage and provides the data for learning. The acquired data then go through a **processing** stage where they are sifted, manipulated, and compared to other data; in this stage, judgment is withheld while reflection on emotions, observations, and attitudes pertinent to the acquired data is recorded and ordered. The processed data are ready, in the third stage, for **analysis and synthesis,** which are the most abstract aspects of learning and the most physically removed from doing; the object of this stage is to "make sense" of the acquired data by forming or revising concepts, spinning theories, and formulating hypotheses. The final stage, in one loop through the cycle, is **application** of the results of the analysis and synthesis in a concrete situation; it is a stage of experimentation, the testing of hypotheses, and the practicing of skills. This stage also restarts the cycle, since it provides information and experience for a new acquisition stage and so around the loop again.

Individual differences in learning stages

The foregoing is, of course, an idealized view of learning in that it implies that the four stages occur in some optimal

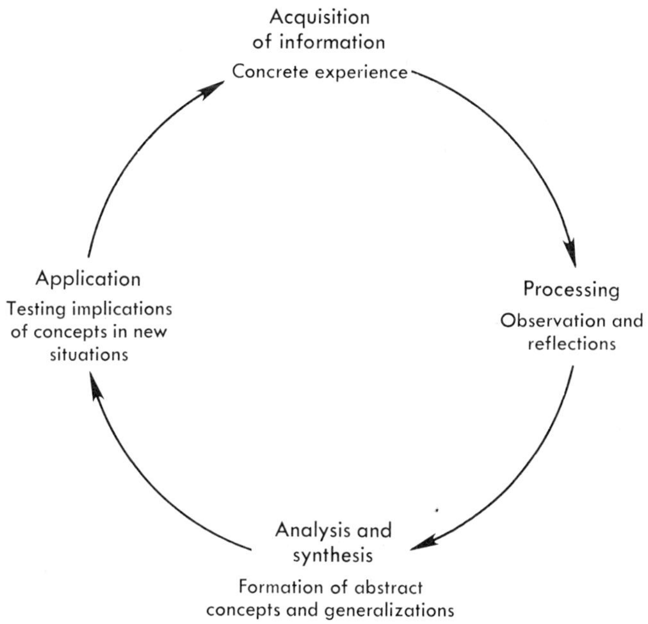

Fig. 7-1. Model of the learning process.

manner. Among different individuals, however, the emphasis placed on a particular stage may vary greatly. One patient may learn only through repeated demonstrations (concrete experience), whereas another may require empirical data—research reports, theories—and the time to analyze. Some of us leap from experience to experiment with little attention to processing or analysis; others never seem to pass beyond observation and reflection to action; and still others are content to trust their theories without subjecting them to empirical testing. The familiar charge that someone "learned nothing from his or her experience" may reflect a breakdown at any of the stages in the process. Further, there is little evidence that allows us to define what an ideal allocation of energy to the several stages might be.

It would seem, however, that many persons fail to learn from experience, that is, to improve in the pursuit of their goals, because they devote insufficient time to ordering and recognizing experience so that its lesson can be identified. In other words, they do not manage their processing activities efficiently. Processing is time consuming, particularly since our society seems to value doing and to look askance at those who take time to reflect.[6] Unless time is allocated for the processing stage and unless the processing effort is oriented toward the solution of problems or the development of skills, the learning cycle will spin along randomly.

Learning need not be random. It can be guided by the learner. Learning is strategic, or problem-solving, behavior: it involves a recurring process of forming hypotheses (abstract conceptualization), testing them in practice (active experimentation), experiencing the results (concrete experience), observing these outcomes (reflective observation), and adapting the hypotheses after interpreting the results (abstract conceptualization).[1] Research has shown that subjects learning to cope with a complex environment do engage in efforts "to identify and interpret critical events in the sequence of decisions and to employ these in selecting subsequent responses."[2] By attending consciously to the goals of learning—by developing learning strategies—learning can be systematic, purposeful, and internally controlled rather than erratic and controlled by the flow of external stimuli.

Before completing the Learning Style Inventory in the following exercise, remember that it was developed to help you define the characteristics of your own approach to learning. Your scores should be treated as data for processing, analysis, and application and not as indicators of competence. It is not possible to identify an ideal profile, and even a balanced profile has no immediately discernible advantages. It is probably closer to truth to assume that some profiles are more appropriate to one set of tasks or situations than to others and that the importance of the stages may also vary with the situation.

Recent research suggests that there is a relationship between learning style and career choice, and perhaps with selected aspects of career success.[4] However, rather than suggesting that there is a best style, the research indicates that some styles are more appropriate than others for specific career situations. Although it is quite early to guess what subsequent research will reveal, there are probably advantages to being consciously aware of your own style, so that you can predict what situations will be relatively easy for you to learn and to perform well in (where you will "fit"). Additionally, we might assume that individuals who are able to alter their learning styles according to the requirements of differing situations are more likely to be effective learners in a variety of situations than are individuals who adhere firmly to the one style with which they are most familiar and comfortable.

You may wish to experiment with your profile to devote more time to processing or to acquisition; the central point is to clarify your objectives in order to provide purpose and focus to your learning. Now you are ready to begin your small group discussion about learning styles.

LEARNING STYLE EXPERIENCE*

This exercise is designed to allow you to explore the structure of the learning process and to become familiar with the notion of individual learning styles. The concept of learning is characteristic of all human behavior; individuals, however, develop their own personal patterns and approaches to learning—their uniquely individual *styles*. Differences in individual styles—of perception, decision making, influence, etc.—occur in other common aspects of human behavior. Such interpersonal differences are natural and result from differences in personality, experience, and many other factors. Individual styles provide richness and variety to social interaction; the effectiveness of interpersonal interactions can be greatly enhanced by the diversity of styles that individuals bring to the relationship. This exercise is designed to assess and examine the learning styles present in the class and to introduce you to a way of looking at your own learning style.

*This exercise is based on Kolb, Rubin, McIntyre, ORGANIZATIONAL PSYCHOLOGY: An Experiential Approach, 2nd edition, © 1974, pp. 23, 25, 27, 28, and pages for the submitted text. Reprinted by permission of Prentice-Hall, Inc., Englewood Cliffs, New Jersey.

Learning style profile (norms for the learning style inventory)

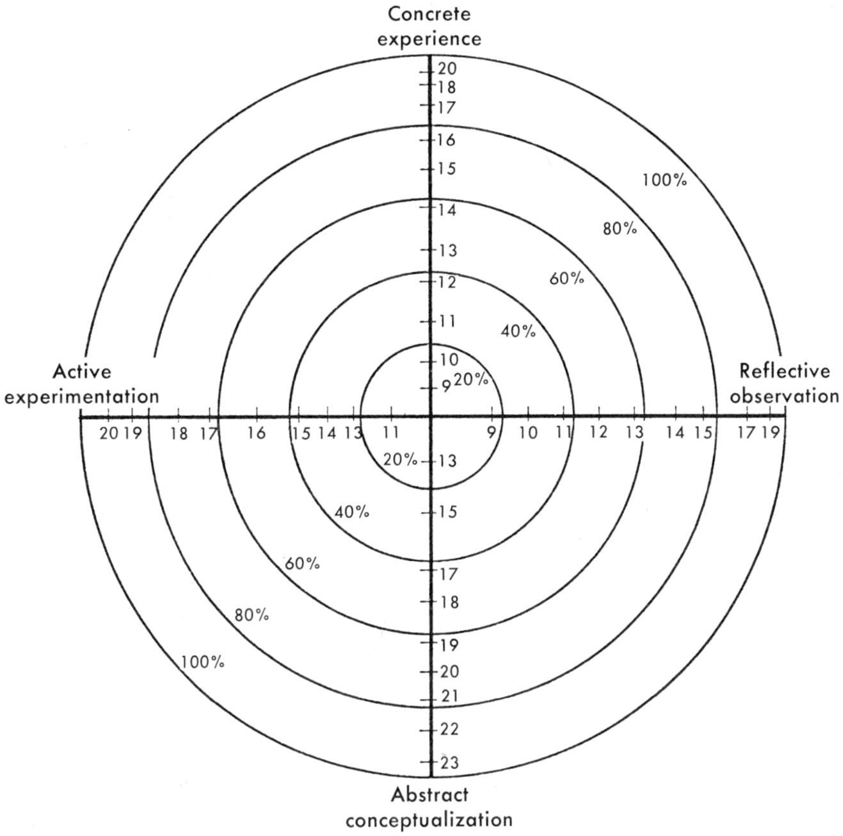

The concentric circles represent percentile scores based on the combined responses of 127 practicing managers and 512 Harvard and MIT graduate students in management. (For example, a raw score of 21 on abstract conceptualization means you scored higher on this dimension than 80% of the managers and students tested, whereas a score of 24 would indicate you scored higher than anyone in the population on which these norms are based.)

Preparation (approximate time—30 minutes)

Each student should complete the Learning Style Inventory on p. 78 and, following the instructions on p. 79, compute his or her scores. These scores should then be recorded on the Learning Style Profile, p. 77.

Procedure (approximate time—50 minutes)

1. When everyone is finished with the inventory and the reading, groups of six to eight members should convene to report on and discuss the individual styles. This can be done conveniently by having each member record his or her scores for each of the four stages of the learning cycle on the blackboard or flip chart. After all the scores have been recorded, it is useful to compute an average score for each stage.
2. After recording the scores, each member in the group should be asked in turn to comment on his or her style; among the topics that might be considered are the following:

- How accurately do you feel your learning style is portrayed by your scores? Why do you think you have adopted your particular style? What, if any, aspects of your style would you like to work on changing?
- How do you feel about the learning opportunity provided by this course? Is it compatible with your style? What would you like to learn about the styles of the other group members?
- What does your learning style imply about your career interests, and how can you explore this relationship further?

Each person should feel free to question each speaker but should take care to ensure that all members of the group have ample time to present their thoughts.

LEARNING STYLE INVENTORY*

This inventory is designed to assess your method of learning. As you take the inventory, give a high rank to those words which best characterize the way you learn and a low rank to the words which are least characteristic of your learning style.

You may find it hard to choose the words that best describe your learning style because there are no right or wrong answers. Different characteristics described in the inventory are equally good. The aim of the inventory is to describe how you learn, not to evaluate your learning ability.

Instructions

There are nine sets of four words listed below. *Rank order* each set of four words assigning a 4 to the word which best characterizes your learning style, a 3 to the word which next best characterizes your learning style, a 2 to the next most characteristic word, and a 1 to the word which is least characteristic of you as a learner. *Be sure to assign a different rank number to each of the four words in each set.* Do not make ties.

1.	____discriminating	____tentative	____involved	____practical
2.	____receptive	____relevant	____analytical	____impartial
3.	____feeling	____watching	____thinking	____doing
4.	____accepting	____risk-taker	____evaluative	____aware
5.	____intuitive	____productive	____logical	____questioning
6.	____abstract	____observing	____concrete	____active
7.	____present-oriented	____reflecting	____future-oriented	____pragmatic
8.	____experience	____observation	____conceptualization	____experimentation
9.	____intense	____reserved	____rational	____responsible

For scoring only

CE____	RO____	AC____	AE____
234578	136789	234589	136789

*From Kolb, Rubin, McIntyre, ORGANIZATIONAL PSYCHOLOGY: An Experiential Approach, 2nd edition, © 1974, pp. 23, 25, 27, 28, and pages for the submitted text. Reprinted by permission of Prentice-Hall, Inc., Englewood Cliffs, New Jersey.

INSTRUCTIONS FOR SCORING THE LEARNING STYLE INVENTORY*

To obtain your score on the four dimensions measured by the inventory—concrete experience (CE), reflective observation (RO), abstract conceptualization (AC), and active experimentation (AE)—sum each column, including only those words whose item number appears under the place for the total score. For example, for CE, total the ranks you have given for words 2, 3, 4, 5, 7, and 8 in the first column. For RO, total the ranks for words 1, 3, 6, 7, 8, and 9 in the second column and so on for AC and AE. Ignore the non-scored words in each column. Transfer the four raw scores to the Learning Style Profile by placing a mark next to the number you scored on each of the four dimensions. Connect these four marks with straight lines.

*From Kolb, Rubin, McIntyre, ORGANIZATIONAL PSYCHOLOGY: An Experiential Approach, 2nd edition, © 1974, pp. 23, 25, 27, 28, and pages for the submitted text. Reprinted by permission of Prentice-Hall, Inc., Englewood Cliffs, New Jersey.

SUMMARY

The learning model that you have examined in this chapter was chosen because it provides a basis for experiencing and applying concepts that will be introduced in later chapters and because it offers important input to your future strategy for establishing good relations with patients and colleagues. This model also provides a useful framework for considering the development of this class. The four stages of the learning cycle can be reviewed in terms of the process of forming a psychological contract. In formulating a contract, you have had the experience of consciously developing the norms, traditions, and behaviors of a new group—the **acquisition** stage. Between the first and second class meetings you had the opportunity to reflect on and sort out this experience—the **processing** stage—and to compare your insights with the writings of various experts in order to formulate theories and hypotheses—the **analysis** stage. Finally, you had an opportunity to practice what you learned and to test your ideas in a class meeting—the **application** stage.

Both this course and your subsequent professional experiences will also provide opportunities to apply these concepts to the management of future relationships. You will be gathering information about yourself and the work environment through exercises, cases, and readings; reflecting on what these data imply about you and how you will fit into and respond in different situations; and developing hypotheses about the "type" of person you are and about the implications of treating a specific patient. You will be testing the quality of these hypotheses through interviewing, in bull sessions with individuals familiar with these situations, and by actually working in a finite (and probably small) number of specific clinical situations.

This chapter, particularly the text material, has been kept brief deliberately. You have become involved with a learning process, and, in the remaining chapters, you will be acquiring the concepts, skills, tools, and experience needed to shape and direct the outcomes of that process for you and for your patients.

REFERENCES

1. Bruner, J. S., Goodnow, J. J., and Austin, G. A.: A study of thinking, New York, 1956, John Wiley & Sons, Inc.
2. Ference, T. P.: Induced strategies in sequential decision-making, Hum. Relations **25**(5):377, 1972.
3. Keller, F. S.: Learning-reinforcement theory, New York, 1954, Random House, Inc.
4. Kolb, D. A.: On management and the learning process. In Kolb, D. A., Rubin, I. M., and McIntyre, J. M.: Organizational psychology: a book of readings, Englewood Cliffs, N.J., 1974, Prentice-Hall, Inc.
5. Learning and problem solving. In Kolb, D. A., Rubin, I. M., and McIntyre, J. M.: Organizational psychology: an experiential approach, ed. 2, Englewood Cliffs, N.J., 1974, Prentice-Hall, Inc.
6. Odiorne, G.: The activity trap. (Mimeographed.)

Chapter 8

MOTIVATION

This brief but familiar conversation demonstrates the critical role that an understanding of human motivation plays in dental practice. Dr. Williams is speaking to Fred Bradley as Fred is leaving the office as follows:

> Well, Fred, that takes care of everything for now. Before you go, I'd like to say a few things. I have been your dentist for over 8 years now, and I feel I can speak frankly. I am concerned that you have not followed my instructions on taking proper care of your teeth and your mouth. We had a lot more work to do this time than we should have. For someone in your line of work, appearance is very important, and yet you seem to neglect even something as simple as regular brushing. Also, you really should come in more often. You know that you canceled three appointments over the last 6 months, and that's why that problem in the upper left molar got so bad. I must insist that you do better. I want to schedule an appointment tonight for you to come in 3 months from now for a checkup. I'd like to keep a closer watch on you; there are some problems developing that I would like to head off.

Fred replied as he put on his coat as follows:

> I know that you are concerned, Doc, and don't think that I don't appreciate it, but I have to devote all my attention to running my business. I have set goals for myself and I have got to push hard to make them. Those broken appointments were cases of staying at work and pushing myself a bit or coming here after dinner. When I have that kind of choice, work comes first. Besides, you know that I don't like all that regular routine of brushing, visits, and so on. That's why I left big business—to avoid routines and be in control of my own time. I trust you to worry about my teeth. As for that appointment, I can't say what my schedule will be like 3 months from now. Let me call you.

Dr. Williams is concerned with changing Fred Bradley's behavior and is apparently frustrated by the results to date. Dr. Williams' remarks reflect considerable difficulty in understanding the causes of Fred's behavior. In a few short sentences, Dr. Williams has attempted to change Fred's behavior by expressing displeasure, by associating good dental practice with career success, and by suggesting that serious problems may occur. These several lines of attack reflect a variety of assumptions about the sources of Fred's behavior—that he is motivated by a need for approval, by a need for achievement, or by a need to avoid pain or future expense.

The success of the effort to change Fred depends, of course, on the validity of these assumptions about the sources of his behavior. There is more to the conversation, however; in their remarks, both Fred and Dr. Williams provide some significant clues to the sources of their own behavior. Fred's concern for the success of his business and Dr. Williams' desire to change Fred's behavior help us to understand why they behave as they do.

Our present concern is not whether you

agree with Dr. Williams' approach to Fred nor even whether the effort is likely to be successful. One might seriously question whether Dr. Williams' effort to place Fred on a tight schedule is consistent with Fred's expressed desire for freedom. The key point here is to understand why Fred and Dr. Williams behave as they do, to understand their motivations. In this chapter, we will be examining a variety of explanations of the motives that underlie human behavior.

Perhaps the question that the science of behavior has answered least adequately is "Why do we behave in the first place"? More specifically, we would like to know the conditions necessary for arousing the wide variety of thoughts, feelings, and actions of which humans are capable.

It seems clear that much of our behavior is learned. Experience reinforces our knowledge that a particular behavior is appropriate or rewarding under the right conditions. For example, by now we have all learned that soup is better eaten with a spoon than with a fork. We have, of course, also learned far more complex behaviors. In the dental education setting, we have learned complicated sets of technical procedures for improving the oral health of patients. In our day-to-day experience, we have learned even more complicated behaviors—how to make someone happy and, unfortunately, how to make someone angry or frustrated.

Learning can be thought of as a process by which new behaviors are added to our repertoire of methods for dealing with the world. But not all our behaviors are learned, in the usual sense of the word. Some of our complex behaviors seem to be inherited as part of our endowment as human beings. We do not learn to experience hunger or thirst or relief from hunger or thirst. It seems more accurate to view some of our basic responses as inherited ones on which we later build through the learning process. Each of us can be looked on as a repository of an almost infinite number of behaviors, whether inherited or learned, that include thoughts and feelings as well as overt actions. Yet at any particular time we are exhibiting only a tiny fraction of the behaviors available to us.

In asking "Why do we behave at all?" we are seeking to determine the conditions necessary for the performance of certain behaviors. Put another way, we can talk about a person's repertoire of behaviors and ask why at a given point in time is one behavior performed and another not? Psychologists use the concept **motivation** to explain *the forces that compel a particular behavior to be exhibited whereas others are not.*

OBJECTIVES

The objectives of this chapter are as follows:

1. To examine different theories of motivation
2. To explore how motivation influences behavior, focusing specifically on the individual and the situation
3. To investigate the relationship between shifting hierarchies of need and consistent motive patterns
4. To discuss how motivation relates to perception, thoughts, and actions
5. To examine achievement motivation and its relation to the dentist as entrepreneur
6. To practice assessing the motivational needs of others by exploring our individual motivational patterns

DIFFERENT THEORIES OF MOTIVATION

In every important psychological theory, from Freudian psychoanalysis to Skinnerian behaviorism, a motivational concept has been required, although the label "motivation" does not usually occur in Skinnerian theory. The relevance of different psychological theories in relation to dentist-patient interactions is examined in Part three. In Chapter 8 we will discuss how different theories of behavior handle specifically the problem of motivation.

Behavioral versus psychoanalytical theories of motivation

Behavioral theorists use terms such as **"drive"** or **"need"** to provide a theoretical accounting for behavior. The problem with the term "motivation" for many behavioral psychologists is that it implies that non-observable unconscious forces are ruling our choice of behaviors and that these non-observable forces can be inferred from visible behavior.

The conflict between behavioral versus psychoanalytical theories of motivation resides in how behavior is defined. If the focus of study is overt performance, the description of someone's performance is equivalent to the description of their behavior. This is essentially the viewpoint of behavioral theorists. In Chapter 8 we develop a definition of behavior that emphasizes intentionality, or purposiveness. If the focus of study is the intent or purpose of behavior, the description of visible performance is not a sufficient description of a person's behavior. This is essentially the view first suggested by Freud. He theorized that motivation has a fundamental role in determining behavior. Freud focused almost exclusively on unconscious motivation. He claimed that individuals do things without really knowing why.

How would these different psychologists describe the behavior of a dentist working at his or her chair? The behaviorist might say the dentist is drilling a specially shaped hole into a first molar and restoring the tooth with a silver amalgam filling material. Contrast this description of behavior with an interpretation of the same event that might be rendered by a psychoanalyst. A so-called Freudian might describe the dentist as achieving gratification of oral aggressive needs by sublimating his or her unconscious hostility in a socially useful and acceptable fashion.

An objection to the latter description of one's behavior is that its validity rests on a whole set of theoretical assumptions that may not be justified or even testable. An opponent of psychoanalytical theory would ask how oral aggression, which is an interpretation of someone's behavior, could, in fact, be demonstrated to exist at all.

Hierarchy of needs theory

A level of analysis of behavior that seems more useful for our purposes than either of the extreme positions just illustrated has been provided by Abraham Maslow (Chapter 1).[5] He has formulated a positive theory of human motivation proposing that individual differences in personality and behavior arise from the arrangement of needs in a hierarchy of priorities. The chief dynamic principle of his theory of motivation says that less important needs emerge after gratification of more potent ones. In other words, a person's current motivational state will be a reflection of the needs that are strongest at that time. Behaviors that follow will be those that will meet a person's current needs.

Basic needs are the starting point for motivating behavior. According to Maslow, **physical needs** (hunger) and **safety needs** (freedom from pain or threat of bodily harm) are the basic needs. As physical and safety needs are met, the need for **belonging** and **love** emerge as high-order needs. The need hierarchy continues with **ego** or **self-esteem** needs (self-respect and respect of others) and ends with **self-actualizing** needs at the top.

Many studies that have inquired into the motivational, perceptual, and cognitive functioning of health care providers have come to similar generalizations about the particular needs that seem most important to such persons. The following needs have been identified:

1. *Need for achievement (n ach):* A desire to accomplish difficult things; to overcome obstacles; to reach a high standard; to compete in order to surpass
2. *Need for affiliation (n aff):* A desire to be with and enjoy people; to cooperate with others; to please and win affection; to love and trust others
3. *Need for power (n pow):* A desire to

control or influence others; to obtain and hold the means of influence; to be superior to subordinates

4. *Need for autonomy (n aut):* A desire to resist restriction or coercion; to avoid activities or situations in which others dominate; to be independent and free to act, even according to impulse or against convention

It is obvious that these four needs are not unique to health care providers. We do wish to stress, however, that these four needs, whatever their general status for most persons, have been reported as important determinants of the behavior of personnel in the health professions.

Variation in the potency of each of these needs can be expected, both among different individuals and within the same individual, as different roles in the health field are assumed. For example, a dentist's need for autonomy and power may gain importance and increased visibility in his or her private office. The needs for achievement and affiliation may become more important determinants of behavior in a hospital or dental clinic setting.

Clearly, the roles we are currently assuming and our need to satisfy role expectations will serve to modify our individual need hierarchies. However, the utility of this approach to understanding motivation lies in its ability to allow observable behavior together with associated thoughts and feelings to be examined in the total context of one's purpose or intention when behaving.

Maslow, viewing the same dentist cited earlier, might reject equally the behaviorist's observational analysis and the psychoanalyst's in-depth interpretations. He might say, instead, that the dentist was meeting self-actualizing needs because he was doing what had to be done.

MOTIVATIONAL INFLUENCES IN BEHAVIOR: INTERACTION OF PERSON AND SITUATION

Different needs and motive patterns can be elicited by different situations. Although each of us may have dominant motive patterns, a variety of motives is potentially operative in our behavior. A person functioning primarily at the self-actualizing level in Maslow's hierarchy may still be motivated in different situations by needs for security or ego gratification. Similarly, a person with a generally high level of need for achievement may experience needs for power, affiliation, security, etc. Motivational influences in behavior represent a dynamic balance of the characteristic motive patterns of the individual and the unique aspects of the situation.

This interaction of individual and situation is assumed in the hierarchical process; the emergence of higher needs depends on the life history of the individual.[5] Self-esteem and self-actualization needs become operative only when lower-order needs are relatively satisfied. When lower-order needs are rearoused, as in times of danger and crisis, higher-order needs lose their potency. For example, most of us have little day-to-day concern for basic survival; our physical, shelter, and other security needs are routinely attended to without much conscious effort. It is not surprising, therefore, that ego, social, and self-actualization concerns influence most of our behavior. This situation is drastically reversed when our secure environment is shattered by natural disaster, accidents, and similar events that threaten survival. As discussed previously, many patients view going to the dentist as a potentially threatening experience. To the extent that this is so for a given individual, lower-order needs (safety, physical) may take precedence while that patient is in the dentist's chair.

An individual's life experiences may result in a characteristic behavior pattern in which achievement and self-esteem needs, for example, dominate. Needs for power, affiliation, ego, self-actualization, etc. would also occur. One of these needs may become dominant under the influence of a particular situation. In dealing successfully with other persons, therefore, we must be aware not only of their general motive patterns but also of the forces operating in a given situation.

The implications of this circular, seemingly obvious conclusion are considerable. For example, a long-standing debate in industrial society concerns the relative potency of economic incentives (higher pay, bonuses, etc.) and psychological incentives (participation in decision making, more challenging tasks, responsibility, etc.) as motivators of work. One can easily find studies that appear to support each of these positions; one can also find studies that show that more money, participation, or job enrichment does *not* lead to higher productivity.[3,9,11] In one sense, these conflicting data should not be surprising; most persons do want more money, pleasant social relations, more control over decisions that affect them significantly, more opportunity to engage in challenging and meaningful activities, etc.

There are several points that might be made about these generalizations. These "wants," or motives, will vary in their strength at different points in time for a given person. One reason for these variations is the operation of the hierarchy of needs; an individual concerned with maintaining a subsistence level of existence would probably be motivated more by a higher piece rate than by a role in decision making. Conversely, an individual whose physical and security needs are well taken care of may be very unhappy in a position that does not allow for some sense of personal achievement.

However, the notion of a uniform hierarchy for all persons is also misleading. The artist may well place creativity, a self-actualizing need, ahead of social and ego needs, that is, lower in the hierarchy.[2] Similarly, a scientist may neglect social and even physical needs until achievement needs have been relatively satisfied.

Finally, what "satisfies" a need for one person may be inadequate for another. What is enough money, challenge, or social interaction for one person may not be enough for another. The assumption that all persons will be motivated to greater effort by higher economic rewards or more opportunities for achievement overlooks differences in characteristic motive patterns. Not everyone has strong, persistent needs for achievement, power, or affiliation, and it makes little sense to base motivational programs on idealized notions about how individuals are or ought to be.

This point is underscored by recent studies showing that many workers resist having their jobs enlarged or enriched; they resist attempts to increase the potential for self-actualization on the job. This may be because the lower-order needs of these individuals are not being satisfied or because their needs for social interaction (affiliation) dominate their achievement needs. It may also be that higher-order needs are operative for these individuals but are being pursued in nonwork situations. This suggests that work may not be the only means to satisfying needs but may be instrumental in allowing individuals to pursue other means of satisfaction.[11] It is unreasonable to assume that individuals seem to satisfy all their needs through their work, and yet many motivational theorists make this assumption!

Thus debate over whether persons in general are more motivated by needs for survival, power, affiliation, or achievement are irresolvable and possible irrelevant. These several motives are present to some degree in most persons. It is equally clear that some situations are more powerful than others in eliciting certain needs in most persons.

CONSISTENT MOTIVE PATTERN VERSUS SHIFTING HIERARCHIES

There is some difficulty in arguing that a hierarchy of needs is operative in human behavior and simultaneously arguing that individuals exhibit consistent motive patterns. If higher-order needs come into play only when more basic needs are met, does it make sense to claim that an individual is generally motivated by a need for achievement or power? Hampton et al.[2] attempted to reconcile this apparent conflict by placing affiliation, power, achievement, and autonomy within the hierarchy of needs; affiliation is seen as a social need, and power, achievement, and autonomy as expressions of a self-actualizing need. Thus the arousal of needs for achievement, power, autonomy, and affiliation is presumably controlled by the same factors controlling the emergence of other needs in the hierarchy. How is it, then, that some individuals have higher needs for affiliation, achievement, or power than others? Two possible explanations follow:

1. The first explanation suggests that the strength of a need reflects the stage in the hierarchy at which the individual is functioning at any one point in time. This would imply that a need for achievement could be raised by satisfying lower-order needs, thereby allowing achievement needs to emerge. This explanation, which suggests that everyone would exhibit a high need for achievement given appropriate conditions, is consistent with the position of Herzberg and other motivational theorists.[3,9]
2. The second explanation suggests that dominant needs reflect enduring motive patterns that are characteristic of the individual's behavior across situations and through time. In this sense, a strong need for power or for achievement is a *trait* of the individual; he or she may function at different levels of the hierarchy as circumstances vary, but his or her behavior would typically reflect the persistent need for power or achievement. Achievement, affiliation, power, and autonomy are, in this view, treated as acquired needs; they represent the outcome of prior learning and experience. Individuals have different life histories, and some histories induce the

THE HIERARCHY OF NEEDS*

Higher ↑

Self-actualization: The desire for self-fulfillment, the need to know who and what we are and to achieve our full potentials

Ego: The need for prestige, for self-respect and the respect and admiration of others; the desire for esteem

Social: The need for the company and the acceptance of others; the desire for affection and a feeling of belonging and of not being alone

Safety: The need for security and order, for stability and protection from uncertainty and danger

Physical: The need to satisfy the physiological conditions of survival, including control of hunger, thirst, etc.

↓ Lower

*Based on Maslow, A.: A theory of human motivation, Psychol. Rev. **50:**370, 1943.

DOMINANT MOTIVE PATTERNS*

Need for achievement

A person with a high achievement need wants to take personal responsibility for success and failure; develops and aspires to personal standards of excellence; functions well in situations with moderate levels of risk; wants and responds well to immediate, concrete feedback on performance.

Need for affiliation

A person with a high affiliation need desires warm, friendly relations; is uncomfortable with interpersonal conflict; enjoys the company of others and wants to be liked and accepted; is sensitive to and concerned about the feelings of others.

Need for power

A person with a high power need is concerned about getting and maintaining the means of influencing others; is comfortable in situations where status relations are clear; desires to dominate and hold positions of control; wants to convince others in arguments.

Need for autonomy

A person with a high autonomy need is concerned about freedom from restriction or coercion; is comfortable acting on impulse or with disregard for convention; greatly values independence.

*Based on McClelland, D. S.: The achieving society, New York, 1961, D. Van Nostrand Co.

need for achievement more than others on the basis of past experience, parental behavior, etc.[6,8] Therefore it is not natural that everyone exhibit a high need for achievement. This would explain why some individuals resist job enrichment and other programs seeking to tap achievement motivation.

The second explanation seems the more likely. Characteristic motive patterns result from complex social learning processes. Some individuals will acquire a strong need for achievement; others, a need for power; and still others, strong power and achievement needs. These learned motives are alternative expressions of higher-order needs. We should not be surprised if one or the other (or even both) is absent in a given person.

Although this view of the acquisition of *specific* motives belies the simplistic hierarchical model in that needs for power and achievement will not emerge merely with the satisfaction of lower-order needs, there remains a certain inevitability in the notion. Circumstances can produce the dominance of lower-order needs. The individual with a high achievement need would probably seek to satisfy security or ego needs through different behaviors and activities than would an individual who had dominant power needs.

HOW MOTIVATION RELATES TO LEARNING, PERCEPTION, AND ACTIONS

Motivational theory provides a framework for a dynamic concept of personality. It provides an understanding of which needs are at the top of a person's hierarchy, thereby explaining the types of behaviors that might occur initially.

It is, of course, not a simple thing to determine if the behavior we observe in ourselves and others is prompted by physical and safety needs or by higher-order needs for belonging or esteem. It seems safe to conclude that, for most of us, basic needs are not uppermost in our individual hierarchies.

The individual need hierarchies of most persons arise instead from differences in the way we attempt to meet needs for belonging, love, and esteem. Indeed, each

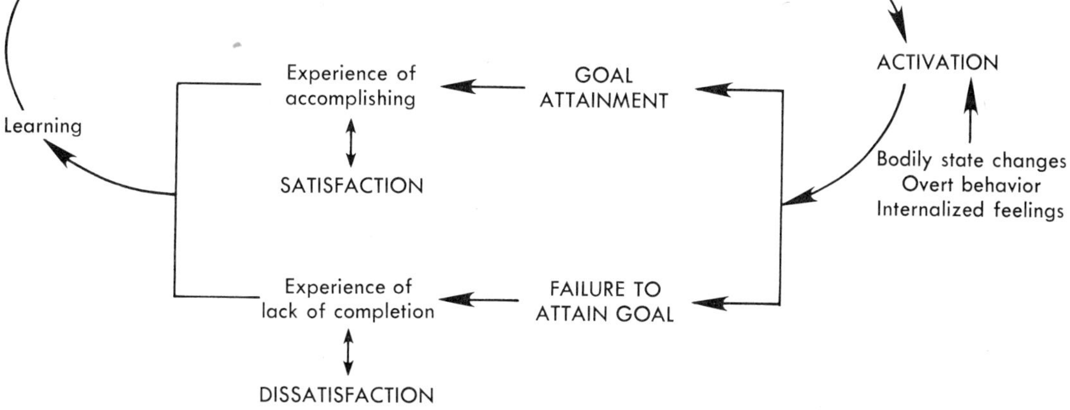

Fig. 8-1. The determinants of goal-directed behavior.

person's need hierarchy seems to have certain characteristics that endure over time, even though within that hierarchy changes do take place.

Our personalities are perhaps best understood as the relationship among motivational states that influences our patterns of perception and that, in turn, determines how we think and act. A simple model is schematically outlined indicating the sequence of events leading to behavior (Fig. 8-1). This model suggests that how we organize our perceptions depends on our motivational state. Viewing perception as motivated by need states helps us understand the individual differences that may arise when the same situation is viewed by different individuals. In effect, we see what we need to see, screening and filtering our perceptions to meet our uppermost needs.

Not only is our perceptual apparatus adaptable to our needs, but, apparently, we also develop *cognitive styles* to convert our perceptions into thoughts and actions. Our cognitive style—the interaction of our needs and our perceptual style—"sets us up" to deal with the world. The intellectual deep-thinker who contemplates every alternative and makes lists of what to do first, second, and third, exhibits one kind of cognitive style. The impulsive person who flits from one task to another and who always appears disorganized and harried represents quite a different cognitive style. In both cases, the most pressing needs determine how the world will be perceived and how the resources of the person—memory, thinking, etc.—will be marshaled so that decisions can be made about which behavior should come next. This process is examined in detail in Chapter 9.

MOTIVATION AND THE DENTIST-ENTREPRENEUR

The need for achievement is a particularly fascinating aspect of human behavior. Individuals with high achievement needs tend to outperform others in pursuing long-term academic and occupational goals. Achievers are more than normally interested in tangible feedback in concrete performance terms. They like to assume personal responsibility for solving problems and are interested in excellence for its own sake: "It is the challenge of the job itself that rewards the achiever people."[7] They pay more attention to the *realistic* probabilities of success and treat both success and failure as learning opportunities. They prefer situations in which they have control over outcomes to situations ruled by chance. They are relatively unconcerned with other individuals, pick experts rather than friends as co-workers, and function better when they can concentrate on tasks rather than on developing and coordinating others.[4] They are described by David McClelland as follows:

> They're entrepreneurs, kind of driven—always trying to improve themselves and find a shorter route to the office or a faster way of reading the mail . . . (need achievement) includes taking personal responsibility to solve problems and achieve moderate goals at calculated risks—in situations that provide real feedback. You can see why most innovative businessmen score high on n ach.*

There is evidence that the level of achievement motivation can be increased through training.[6,8] This is consistent with our view that motives such as power and affiliation are acquired and that conscious learning strategies can be applied to changing human behavior. The social implications of achievement training are considerable; McClelland and his colleagues have accumulated considerable evidence of a strong correlation between levels of achievement need in a population and subsequent levels of economic growth and entrepreneurial activity. Their methods hold forth intriguing possibilities for stimulating economic activity in underdeveloped areas. This is not to say that a high achievement need score is necessarily indicative of individual or national superiority; a research

*From McClelland, D. S., and Harris, T. G.: Psychol. Today **4**(Jan.):35, 1971.

scientist or an artist whose work may consume years before feedback is available would probably be hampered by a high achievement need. Like other motive patterns, the need for achievement is related to success in particular kinds of endeavor and is aroused by particular environmental conditions.

The entrepreneur is an unusual person in the corporate world or elsewhere. The professions contain many entrepreneurs—individuals who prefer to rely on their own resources, who strive for excellence, and who thrive on work. The dentist in an independent practice is, in many ways, a classic entrepreneur. He or she is motivated by the work itself and receives immediate feedback from comparing the treatment provided patients with professional standards of quality.

For the dentist (as for many other professionals and managers) the work environment provides an opportunity to function at several levels of the needs hierarchy simultaneously. Hampton et al. suggest the following:

> The labor which a man performs to gain the physiological necessities of life may also be the work he does to express his higher level drives. The idealistic MD cures the sick, obtains the necessary victuals, pays for his Cadillac, and expresses his creativity—all with the same activity. This perhaps accounts for the long hours that professionals and executives work, and their oft-quoted statements that they have recreation and fun in their work, that their work is their life, etc.*

This utopian view is not always realized in practice. Research has shown the potential for alienation and disillusionment is as high in entrepreneurial fields as in blue-collar work, if not higher![10] Perhaps this is so because the promise of self-actualizing work is more explicit, and, consequently, the frustrations of repetitive, nonchallenging, meaningless tasks are correspondingly greater.

The problem, therefore, is to design work environments that provide opportunities to satisfy personal motive patterns for the dentist, the patient, and the staff. For the dentist, as for other professionals, this may mean freeing oneself to do professional work. Paraprofessional teams represent one approach to this design problem; the team approach allows the dentist to delegate aspects of the total treatment to other team members while concentrating personally on tasks that require his or her specific competence. Working effectively in such teams may be uncomfortable for dentists accustomed to independent (entrepreneurial) practice, particularly if the need for achievement or autonomy is a dominant part of their motive patterns. Task-oriented groups can, however, facilitate the satisfaction of achievement and other higher-order needs by treating the group interaction as an ongoing learning experience for improving task performance.

A dental environment providing opportunities for the patient and the dental staff to satisfy their own personal motive patterns will probably increase the level of the dentist's work satisfaction as well as his or her ability to provide effective treatment. However, being aware of one's own motivations is hard enough, let alone being aware of and responding to those of others. The following exercises are designed to assist students in clarifying for themselves what their individual need hierarchies might be. In later chapters, the motivation principles discussed in this chapter will be utilized when methods of changing other persons' (patients' and staff's) behavior are considered.

Text continued on p. 97.

*From Hampton, D. R., Summer, C. E., and Webber, R. A.: Organizational behavior and the practice of management. Glenview, Ill., 1968, Scott, Foresman, & Co.

PRACTICE IN ASSESSING MOTIVATIONAL NEEDS

Individual exercises

IMPORTANT: Each person should read the following instructions and do the exercise *before taking the next step.*

1. In this exercise you are asked to think up a story about each of the pictures that follow. You should use your imagination freely. There are no right or wrong or good or bad stories. You should try only to capture what comes to mind as you look at each picture. To help you, we have provided some guidelines that are useful in creating a story. You may use these guidelines or not, remembering that the objective is to obtain a short but continuous story.
   - What do you think is happening?
   - Who are the people involved?
   - What led up to the situation? How did it begin?
   - What is going to happen next?
   - How will it end?

   Write three brief stories. Do not take more than 10 minutes per story. Do not go on until you have completed three stories.*

*Based on Atkinson, J., ed.: Motives in fantasy action and society, New York, 1958, D. Van Nostrand, Co.

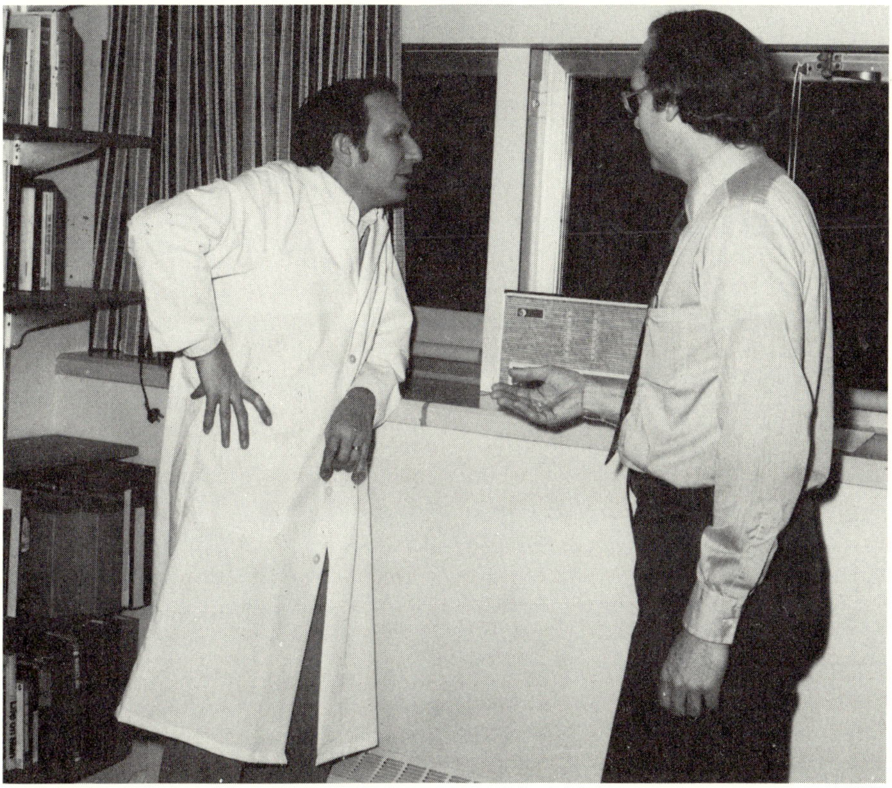

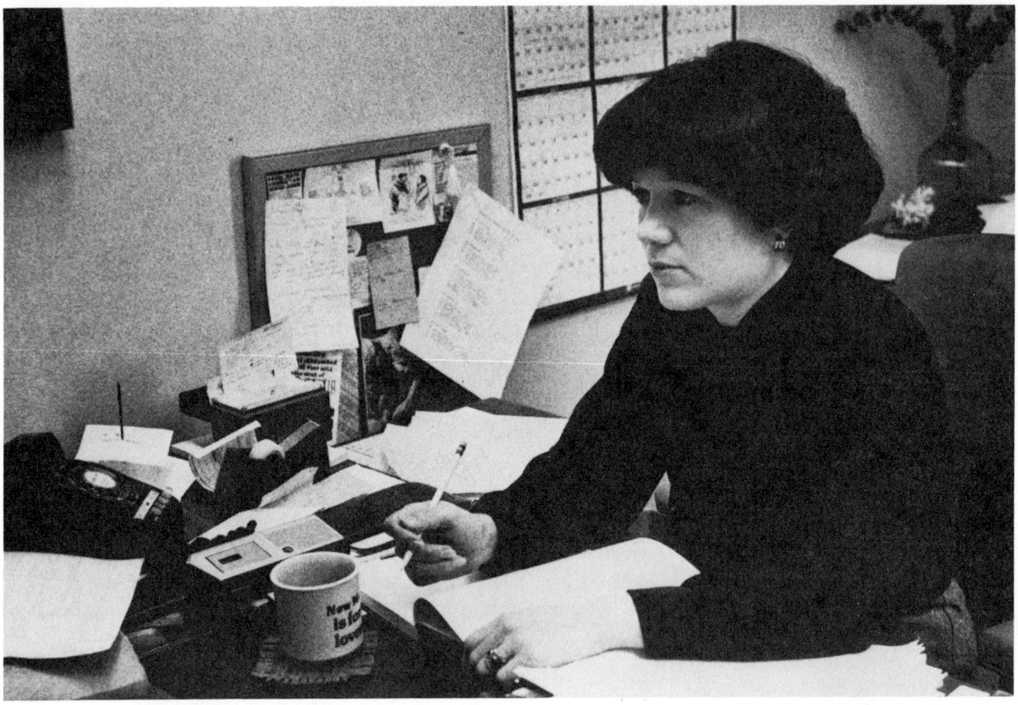

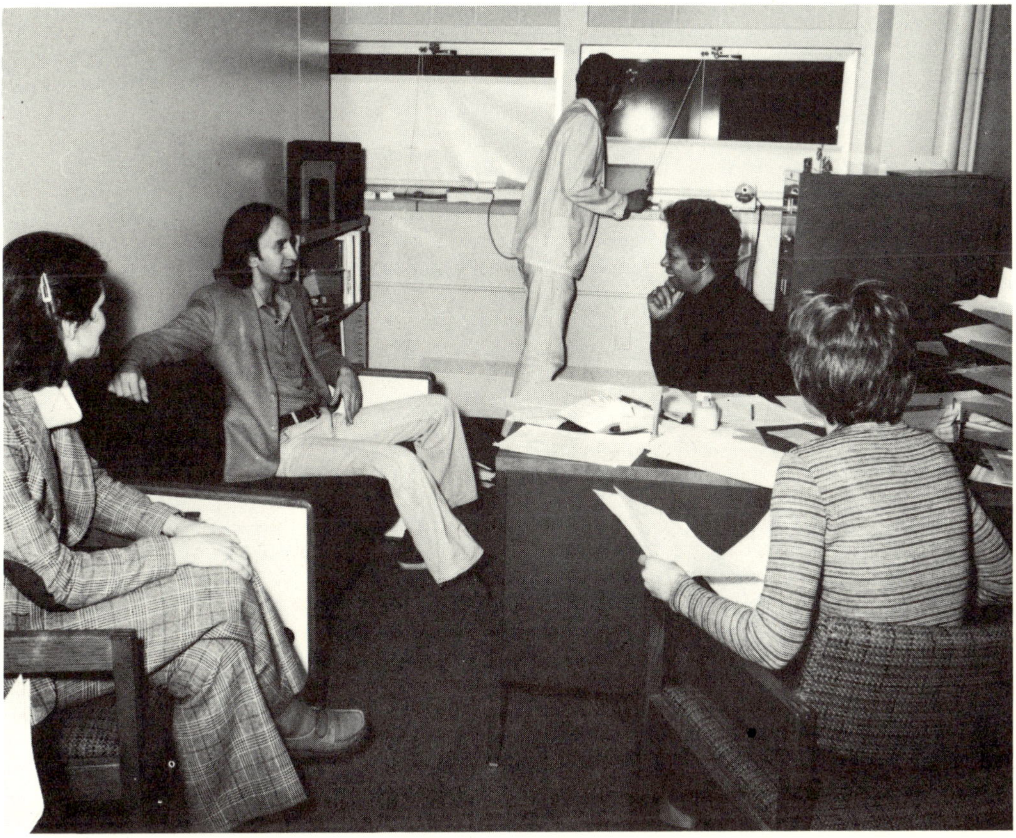

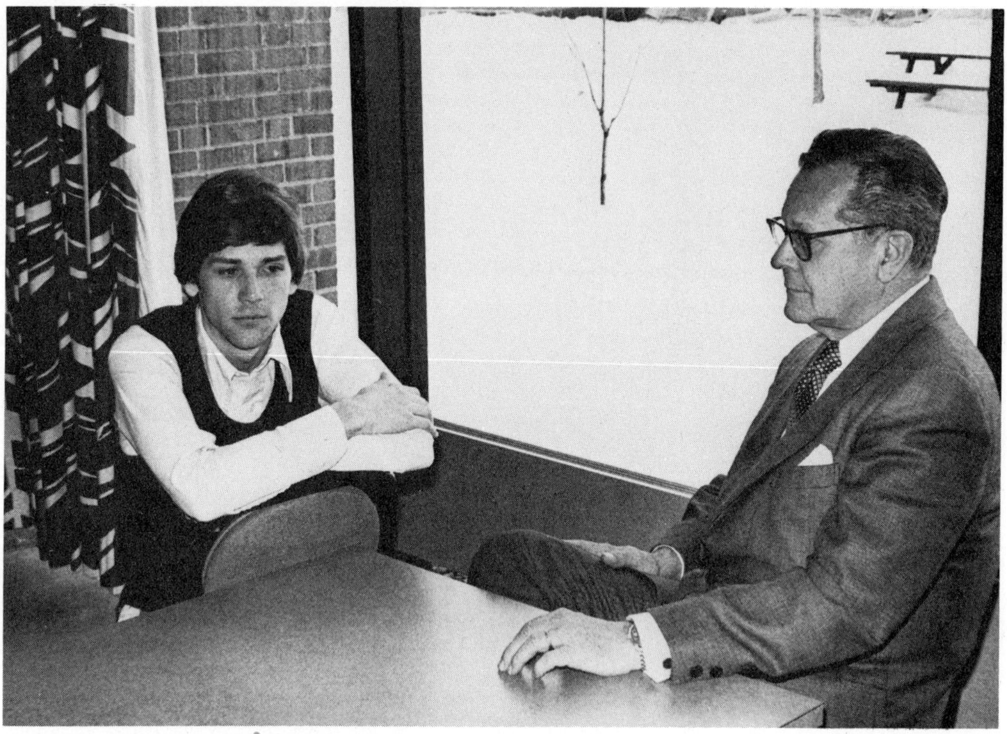

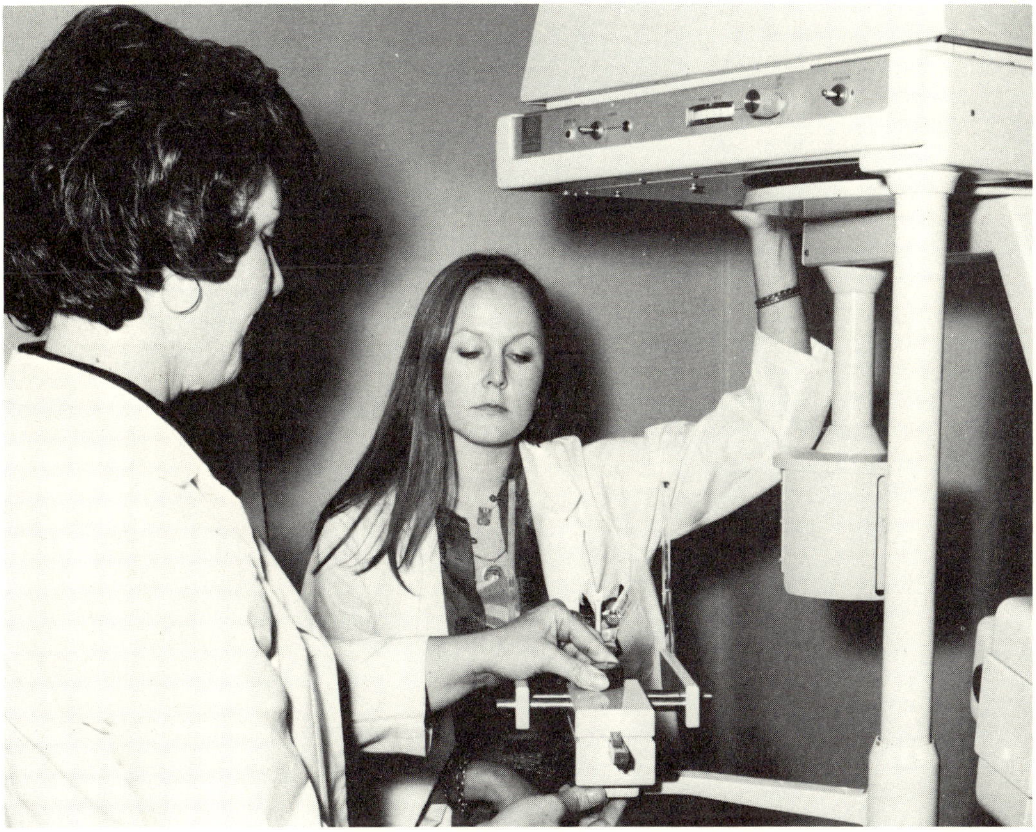

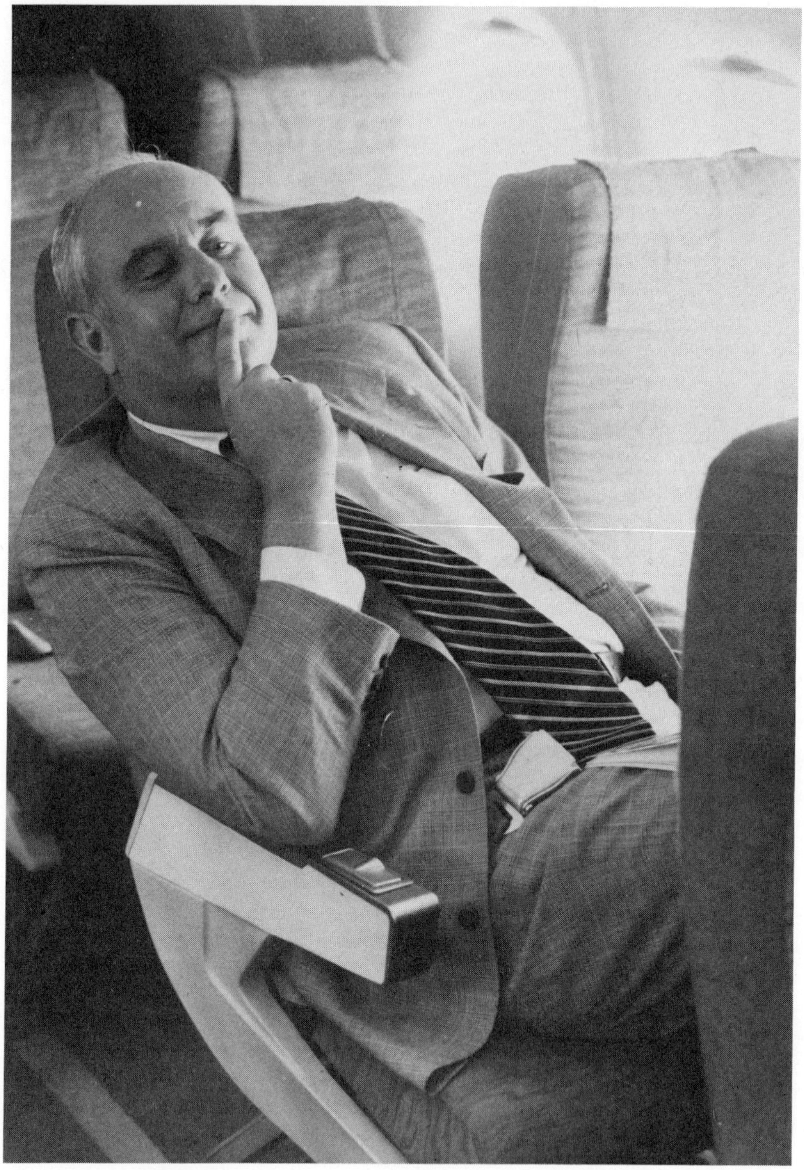

2. Definitions of four important personal and social needs are given below. Arrange them in a hierarchy from most to least important for you. Your hierarchy should provide a ranking, from 1 to 4, of your most descriptive through least descriptive needs. Let the most descriptive need in your hierarchy be ranked first and the least descriptive need, fourth. Please work quickly. Do not spend more than 15 minutes arranging your need hierarchy.

Group exercise

After completing the stories and your own need hierarchies, you should form groups of three persons each. Each person in turn should read his or her stories to the others, who will score them for the presence of (1) need for achievement, (2) need for affiliation, (3) need for autonomy, and (4) need for power. Refer to the definitions of each of these needs as provided on p. 86 to help you identify those parts in the story that might reflect these needs.

Use the scoring sheet provided on p. 98 to record how other individuals score each of your stories for each of the preceding needs. Total the number of stories, including each of the needs. Determine you own need hierarchy for individual exercise 1, as indicated by your stories.

Enter your own need hierarchy on the scoring sheet, as you determined it from the rankings you gave each need in individual exercise 2. Make note of any differences you discovered between your need hierarchies in the different exercises. What might be learned from these exercises?

PERSONAL AND SOCIAL NEEDS

achievement: I accomplish difficult things. I try to overcome obstacles and to achieve a high standard. I compete with others and try to surpass them. I am ambitious and aspiring.

affiliation: I like to be with and enjoy cooperating with other people. I like to please and win the affection of others whom I like. I like to be with friends and am loyal to them. I love and trust others.

power: I control my environment. I influence others. I am forceful, masterful, assertive, and authoritative. I am confident in my relations with others.

autonomy: I resist coercion and restrictions. I avoid or leave activities in which others try to dominate me. I am independent and free to act according to impulse. I defy convention.

SUMMARY

The assessment of human needs is a complex process and requires considerable skill. Despite the difficulty of the process, however, we all engage in it continuously in our everyday lives. The actions that we take are stimulated by our present needs, and our explanations of those actions are guided by our understanding of those needs. Further, we base our explanations of the actions of others on our assessments of their needs. A motivational analysis helps us to decide how to behave toward others.

INDIVIDUAL EXERCISES SCORING FORM

Story	Motives	Needs present	Comments on other motives present
1	Achievement Affiliation Power Autonomy		
2	Achievement Affiliation Power Autonomy		
3	Achievement Affiliation Power Autonomy		

Summary

Exercise 1 Ranking of *your need hierarchy*

1. ____________________
2. ____________________
3. ____________________
4. ____________________

Number of stories with

Achievement ______

Affiliation ______

Power ______

Autonomy ______

Exercise 2 Ranking of *your need hierarchy*

1. ____________________
2. ____________________
3. ____________________
4. ____________________

Note any differences between your need hierarchies in exercises 1 and 2.

The dentist who is concerned with changing a patient's behavior must be particularly attuned to the patient's motive patterns. The patient's present behavior is a consequence of complex motivational forces, some of which reflect lifelong learning processes, whereas others reflect primarily the present situation. To the extent that the dentist can assess these motivational forces, he or she will be more likely to be successful in steering the patient's behavior in a desired direction. After we have added some elements to our analysis of human behavior, the role of assessments of the patient's motives in selecting change strategies will be developed in greater detail in Chapter 13.

The assessment of the motives of others is only part of the story, however; we also need to understand and accept our own motive patterns. The exercise that you have just completed has afforded you an unusual opportunity to deepen your understanding of your own motivations and, at the same time, to develop skills in assessing and evaluating the motives of others. The discussion of motives and needs is a very personal and challenging process. You and the other members of your group were probably uncomfortable initially in discussing each other's needs. Most of us do not have much practice in talking about ourselves or others in such intimate terms. Thus the process that you have just completed was, hopefully, very exciting and gratifying, as you were able to obtain the help of interested others in acquiring a better understanding of yourself.

This brief exercise is, however, only a first step in developing your understanding and acceptance of motivational processes. In the remaining chapters of Part two, you will have the opportunity to explore the other elements of the model shown in Fig. 8-1. Hopefully, these chapters will assist you in better understanding the linkages between motivation and behavior and in applying an understanding of motivation to the effecting of behavioral change.

REFERENCES

1. Atkinson, J., ed.: Motives in fantasy action and society, New York, 1958, D. Van Nostrand Co.
2. Hampton, D. R., Summer, C. E., and Webber, R. A.: Organizational behavior and the practice of management, Glenview, Ill., 1968, Scott, Foresman & Co.
3. Herzberg, F., Mausner, B., and Snyderman, B.: The motivation to work, New York, 1960, John Wiley & Sons, Inc.
4. Kolb, D. A., Rubin, I. M., and McIntyre, J. M.: Organizational psychology: an experiential approach, ed. 2, Englewood Cliffs, N.J., 1974, Prentice-Hall, Inc.
5. Maslow, A.: A theory of human motivation, Psychol. Rev. **50:**370, 1943.
6. McClelland, D. S.: The achieving society, New York, 1961, D. Van Nostrand Co.
7. McClelland, D. S., and Harris T. G.: To know why men do what they do, Psychol. Today **4** (Jan.):35, 1971.
8. McClelland, D. S., and Winter, D.: Motivating economic achievement, New York, 1969, The Free Press.
9. Myers, M. S.: Who are your motivated workers? Harvard Bus. Rev. (Jan./Feb.):73, 1964.
10. Ritti, R. R., Ference, T. P., and Goldner, F. H.: Professions and their plausibility, Sociol. Work Organizations I, pp. 24-51, 1974.
11. Vroom, V. H.: Work and motivation, New York, 1964, John Wiley & Sons, Inc.

Chapter 9

PERCEPTION

Dr. Jones, a practicing dentist, has just completed a first visit with a new patient. The entire visit took place in Dr. Jones' private office and not in the operatory; the patient sat in an ordinary chair throughout the visit. Dr. Jones provided the patient with a fairly full explanation of the manner in which the office is run, the approach that Dr. Jones and the staff attempt to take with patients, and what the patient can expect by way of diagnostic information gathering and full disclosure of treatment plans. Dr. Jones also collected a detailed dental and medical history from the patient during the interview. Before the meeting ended, a brief examination of the patient's mouth was conducted, using a mouth mirror, an explorer, and a small bib to protect the patient's clothing.

When asked why the initial visit with the patient was conducted in this manner, Dr. Jones responded as follows:

> When I arranged the first visit with the patient over the telephone, the patient seemed to express a great deal of apprehension and anxiety about undergoing dental treatment. I felt that my private office would be a more comfortable setting for the patient—less likely to trigger anxiety and to recall past dental experiences that the patient might have if seated immediately in a dental chair. By going over procedures in a comfortable setting, I think that a lot can be done to reduce the patient's anxieties.
>
> I prefer having the first visit in my office if I sense any tension because I have found it to be a very effective method. Patients like full explanations of what you have in mind and how you go about your work; they are more likely to understand what you are trying to say if you do it in a comfortable setting and demonstrate some sensitivity and concern for them.
>
> I really want the patient to feel I am a different kind of dentist who is willing to take the time to explain, who is concerned for the patient, and who is thoughtful enough to provide information to help the patient know what is going to happen. Patients tend to think of dentists as mechanics who are too busy to do anything but jump right into the work. The first visit is probably the single most important encounter that I will have with the patient, and I want things to get started properly.
>
> That is also why I feel it is necessary to do something before the visit is over. I could probably conduct the initial examination of the mouth more effectively in the chair—and I will repeat it—but the patient expects you to do something on every visit. The patient is paying for me to do something, not just for me to talk, and, if I examine the mouth, the patient feels that I have provided treatment.

Whether you agree with these particular methods or not, this behavioral description, particularly as Dr. Jones interprets and explains it, provides a clear example of the issues and perceptions that are the key concerns of this chapter. Dr. Jones' behavior has been influenced strongly by at least four major sets of perceptions, as follows:

1. Dr. Jones perceives patients in general (as a class) in certain ways: Pa-

tients like information and appreciate having dental procedures and treatment plans explained; patients come to dentists for specific reasons with specific problems and expect the dentist to do something directed toward those problems.

2. Dr. Jones perceives this particular patient as having an unusual amount of anxiety and apprehension with regard to dental treatment.
3. Dr. Jones perceives that patients perceive dentists in certain ways: Dentists are mechanics who are primarily concerned with their work and devote little time to providing information to patients; dentists treat patients physically in each visit.
4. Dr. Jones wants to be seen in a certain way by patients, as a "different kind of dentist."

Again, our concern here is not whether you agree with Dr. Jones' perceptions or not, but that you understand that these perceptions describe reality to Dr. Jones and, therefore, strongly influence behavior. It is precisely because of this set of perceptual patterns that Dr. Jones has chosen to approach this particular patient in the manner described.

In the remainder of this chapter, we will be exploring the forces that influence and shape our perceptions of the world and the ways in which those perceptions shape our behavior. Specifically, we will be concerned with the following:

1. *How we perceive others:* Our perception of others as individuals and as parts of groups or classes and how our behavior follows from those perceptions.
2. *How we perceive others' perceptions of ourselves:* Our perceptions of others' perception of us as individuals and as members of classes or groups.
3. *How we attempt to present ourselves:* How we can influence the perception that others have of us.

In Chapter 4, we discussed how perceived need of dental care, different from objective need (that is, observable pathological condition), is often the prime factor that determines whether or not a patient will or will not seek dental care.

OBJECTIVES

The objectives of this chapter are as follows:

1. To examine the cognitive factors influencing our perceptions of ourselves and others
2. To discuss the functions of perception
3. To examine some factors influencing perception
4. To explore the relation of perception to behavior
5. To gain experience with the process of perception by identifying and practicing the skills needed to improve the accuracy of perception

PERCEPTION AS A COGNITIVE PROCESS

To the physiologist or the experimental psychologist, perception may be very much of a science. Variations and patterns of neural response to different levels of sound or light can be measured precisely, and the data used to build increasingly sophisticated models of neurological processes. Analyses of differential reactions of the tympanum in the right and left ears to sounds emanating from different locations or of differential firings of rods and cones in response to visual stimuli of differing hue or intensity are of only modest value to the student of human behavior. To the cognitive or behavioral psychologist—and to the dentist who must work daily with different individuals—the perceptual process provides ample evidence that the "facts" do not speak for themselves.

It is obvious that accurate perception involves more than good eyesight or hearing—or an accurate mapping of the objective stimuli on the appropriate cells of the brain. Consider the simple line drawing shown in Fig. 9-1. Look at it closely for a minute or two, and note what you see. Without revealing your own perceptions,

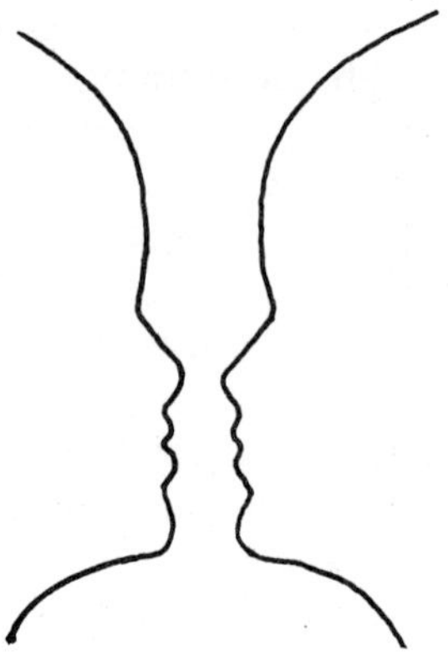

Fig. 9-1. Ambiguous perceptual stimulus.

ask a few friends to describe what they see. Now compare your perceptions. If you and your friends are like most groups of people, you have probably suggested several different interpretations of the picture. Some of you may see it as a vase, others may see it as a table leg, and still others might be convinced that the figure represents two facing profiles about to kiss. Finally, some of you may perceive the figure as alternating between a vase and two profiles and may be experiencing some difficulty in getting the figure to "hold still."

This old psychology textbook figure is deliberately ambiguous and drawn to illustrate problems in perception. The "fact" as perceived by one viewer differs greatly from the "fact" as perceived by another. Further, these different images or interpretations that the same objective drawing raises in the mind of different individuals stem from a complex series of factors. Past learning, present needs, our most recent experiences—perhaps a song heard on the radio or a table lamp sitting on a desk—all shape this picture perception that we have of a given situation at a particular point in time.

There may be some level of generalization or abstraction at which all observers could agree on a description of Fig. 9-1. A mathematician, for example, might describe the figure as a succession of curves drawn symmetrically around an imaginary center line. Although most of us could agree with this perception, we would probably not find it very useful or satisfying. Stated in neutral mathematical terms, the perception would lack substance, interpretation, and a variety of other attributes that make most of our perceptions psychologically interesting. We are accustomed to think that pictures, words, and actions have meaning, and, where meaning is absent on the surface, we seek to provide or infer it. Thus it is psychologically more comfortable for us to perceive Fig. 9-1 as a vase or as two profiles, since these images have meaning; we can associate them with past experience and can extrapolate them to further instances, behavioral predictions, etc.

Unfortunately, when we study perception at this level, we have moved away from the simple world of the mathematician and the physiological psychologist, where a common, objective description of perceptions is possible. Once we acknowledge the role of interpretation and extrapolation in perception, the facts no longer speak for themselves, and it is not at all surprising that different individuals will have sharply differing perceptions of the same "stimuli."

Consider one further implication of Fig. 9-1. What we perceive becomes for us a definition of external reality and the basis on which further thoughts, perceptions, and behaviors are based. Examine Fig. 9-1 again. If you have become convinced that the figure represents a table leg, it will probably require considerable effort on your part to see the two faces. On the other hand, if your initial perception was of two faces, you have come to impute intention and personality to those faces, perhaps identifying one as male and the other as female; thus it will probably require a major act of will not to see the faces.

Incidentally, if you are having trouble changing your perceptions of Fig. 9-1, you are acquiring firsthand experience of a "need" as described in Chapter 8. The tension or discomfort that follows from missing something that others can see or from realizing a gap in knowledge is what is meant by a need, and you will probably find it difficult to concentrate further until you satisfy that need by "finding" the second image in Fig. 9-1.[7]

Initial perceptions exert a powerful influence on subsequent cognitive and behavioral processes. An understanding of the perceptual process is, therefore, fundamental to understanding the dynamics of human behavior. As we will see, perceptual processes provide a link between the internal processes of learning and motivation discussed in previous chapters and the external or interpersonal behaviors of communication, influence, and group behavior discussed in subsequent chapters. Our perceptions are greatly influenced by our needs and our past learning and, in turn, influence our subsequent behavior.

FUNCTIONS OF PERCEPTION

The basic point of this chapter is that "the world as it is perceived is the world that is behaviorally important."* The basic physiological process of perception (the transference of external stimuli into internal neurological patterns) provides the raw material on which a variety of psychological forces operate. Cognitively, the **process of perception** is a complex interplay of objective stimuli that are external to the receiver and internal, idiosyncratic procedures for processing these stimuli. In cognitive terms, the perceptual process has at least three distinctive elements, as follows:

1. **Identification:** The reception and processing of external stimuli provide a physical basis for identifying and sorting stimulus objects into classes or categories; thus our perceptions enable us to identify an object as a rock or a chair or a person as a child or an adult. This identification may or may not be accurate—what we perceive as signs of anxiety in a patient may represent fatigue or psychological disorder—but it does trigger and shape the remaining steps of the process.
2. **Interpretation:** The identification of an individual or an object leads immediately to a further set of judgments about the remaining characteristics or attributes of that individual or object; the perception that a person is a child, a lawyer, or any other class identity calls forth an entire network of expectations and evaluations of other characteristics. Thus the perception is itself a stimulus that elicits a file of interpretive information.
3. **Extrapolation:** Having identified the person or object as a member of a particular class and having examined the interpretive file associated with that class, we move readily to predictions about as yet unobserved characteristics or behaviors. Thus our perception of the identity and characteristics of an individual leads us to make predictions as to how the individual will act in a certain situation or will respond to actions of ours.

These three elements of perception provide the basis for translating perception into behavior. Once we have used our perception of a particular characteristic to identify an individual or an object, used that identification to form expectations and evaluations of other characteristics that we have observed to be associated with that characteristic, and then used that interpretation to extrapolate to other unobserved characteristics or predictions of subsequent behavior, we have formed a basis for determining how we will behave with regard to that individual or object.

For example, we may, on the basis of certain stimuli such as size and general physical appearance, identify an individual as a child. Our previous experience with children leads us to interpret this perception in terms of characteristics that we have observed in other children—they are

*From Leavitt, H. J.: Managerial Psychology (ed. 3), Chicago, 1972, The University of Chicago Press. © 1972 by The University of Chicago Press.

restless in a dental chair, they do not understand complex explanations—and then to extrapolate from these general perceptions to specific predictions about the behavior of this particular child—he or she will fidget and will not listen attentively to descriptions of good brushing techniques. Given this complex cognitive process, we then determine how we will behave with regard to the child: we will position the child's head firmly and securely in the chair; we will repeat descriptions of the brushing techniques several times over. Note that this entire process, from the initial perception to the determination of a treatment approach, has taken place without any direct interaction or communication between dentist and patient. A great deal of information has been employed by the dentist, including present observation, past experience, and a fair amount of judgment and guesswork. Moreover, this complex process and effort has taken place in a very short time, as the dentist brings the patient from the doorway into the chair. Yet it will set the tone for the entire future relationship between the dentist and the patient.

FACTORS INFLUENCING PERCEPTION

It is because of the central role perception plays in the determination of behavior that we need to be aware of factors that influence what we perceive. We are concerned with the factors that act as filters between the objective stimulus we observe and the set of perceptions that are cognitively real for us.

Perceptual filtering

At any given instance, the individual sensory system is confronted with a wide array of stimuli—visual, auditory, tactile, and olfactory. The processing capacities of the individual are limited, however, and the individual necessarily organizes these stimuli into coherent perceptions. Although psychologically necessary, the organizing process is not totally conscious. We automatically organize a set of stimuli into the perception of a person rather than into a series of colors, intensities, and shapes. The end result of the organizing process may not include all the stimuli potentially available in the situation and certainly does not give equal emphasis and weight to all the stimuli present. Thus the very complexity of stimulus situations necessitates perceptual filtering. Two consequences of perceptual filtering are as follows:

1. We are not aware of all the factors influencing our perceptions.
2. We perceive selectively in that we do not make use of the entire array of stimuli available.

Aspects of perceptual filtering outside individual awareness. Johnson,[4] in a review of research on object perception (where psychological sources of distortion may be less operative than in person perception), identified the following aspects of perceptual filtering that may be operating outside the explicit awareness of the perceiver:

1. The perceiver may be responding to cues that are below the threshold of awareness; thus judgments of size may be influenced by color, even though the perceiver may not be aware of and conscious of color.
2. The perceiver may be responding to related cues in making perceptual judgments; thus a firm handshake is often used as a cue for judging another's sincerity.
3. The perceiver may be influenced by emotions in making ostensibly intellectual judgments; thus what is liked or desired often seems correct.
4. The perceiver will give more weight to cues provided by respected or admired sources than to those provided by others; thus the opinions of friends are often given more weight than those of the dentist, even on matters for which the dentist clearly has a higher level of objective knowledge.
5. The perceiver may not be able to

identify all the factors influencing personal judgment or to assess the weight given those judgments; thus a patient who feels he or she has gotten over early childhood fears of the dentist may still be subconsciously influenced by those fears in reaching a judgment that the next visit to the dentist can be delayed.[2,4,10]

Note that not all these factors are subjective. Although emotions or attitudes based on past experience may subjectively influence present perceptions, the influence of irrelevant or subthreshold cues is a consequence of the complexity of the present objective stimulus situation.

Factors influencing selective perception. The complexity of the stimulus situation also produces the second major consequence of perceptual filtering: selective perception. Stimulus complexity and processing limitations make stimulus sampling necessary. This sampling is not, however, a random process but represents a cognitive effort to make sense of the world. We organize our perceptions of persons and things in order to deal with the world as sensibly as possible. If our perceptions are organized accurately, we can make sensible discriminations concerning what is going on about us, and we have a better chance of responding in a way that will best meet our needs and the needs of others. If our sampling process is ineffective (in that it overlooks significant cues) or inaccurate (in that it interprets cues incorrectly), we are likely to experience difficulty in satisfying our needs and possible conflict with others who see the world differently.

Perceptual readiness. The most common consequence of stimulus sampling is that different persons come to different organized perceptions of the same objective stimulus situation. Consider again Fig. 9-1. One person sees a table leg, another sees a vase, and a third sees two profiles; yet all three are observing the same objective situation. In general, our selective sampling of a total array of available stimuli is mainly influenced by the following forces:

1. *We perceive what we expect to perceive:* Our sampling of the stimulus array is guided by our expectations of what is available to be perceived. Our past experience, however limited and nonsystematic, has led us to anticipate that particular objects will appear or that particular words will be spoken in particular situations. The accumulation of learning leads us to make predictions about present and future situations and to attend specifically to cues that support these predictions.
2. *We perceive what we want to perceive:* Active needs such as hunger, thirst, and the desire for recognition or achievement focus attention on identifying possible ways to satisfy those needs. When we are motivated by a need for recognition, we are more likely to perceive consciously cues indicating that another approves of our action. This does not imply that our perceptions are biased or that we are responding to cues that are not there. Although cues indicating recognition may frequently be part of the available stimulus array, it is the focusing effect of the need for recognition (the motivational state) that brings the cue past the threshold of awareness.

Selective perception is, therefore, a necessary response to the complexity of the stimulus environment. The particular pattern of selection that an individual exhibits is strongly influenced by expectations (the consequence of past learning) and desires (the focusing effect of motivation). The joint effect of motivation and learning is to place the individual in a state of **perceptual readiness.**[1] Thus if we are hungry, we look for cues signaling the availability of food, and our past experience guides us as to where to look for those cues, for example, restaurant signs or rooms that look like kitchens.

Individual needs. There is considerable evidence that individuals' perceptions are determined largely by their needs. Thus changes in internal states of hunger and thirst modify our desires for food. Hungry people often find that foods that ordinarily are distasteful have become appealing or highly desirable. Our perception of what is good to eat depends, at least in part, on the strength of our hunger needs. The focusing effect of needs can add efficiency to behavior by drawing our attention to ways to satisfy those needs; it can also distort perceptions by leading us to overestimate the potential of a situation to satisfy our needs.

Freud claimed that all errors in perception such as mistaking the face in a crowd for someone familiar or slips of the tongue (the so-called Freudian slips) were, in fact, complex perceptual errors dictated by inner needs. Forgetting a face was a significant failure of perception and was dictated by a sexual or aggressive motive. Freud saw perception as an active organizing process, intervening between unconscious needs and conscious thoughts, feelings, and observable behavior—a position consistent with the cognitive interpretation of perception that we have taken in this chapter.

Although more recent research suggests that the Freudian view is focused too narrowly on sexual and aggressive motivation, the general consensus is that perceptions are largely determined by inner physiological needs. Although Freud dealt almost exclusively with pathological consequences of perceptual processes, the ability to focus perceptions in the pursuit of needs can also provide an effective way of dealing with stimulus environments.

Perceptual styles. Another major influence on individual patterns of selective perception is the personal "perceptual style" that each of us has developed in our lifetime. The interweaving of needs with perceptions in guiding behavior and the experiences of success and failure that result from that behavior shape preferred patterns of perceiving. Individuals tend to develop styles that permit a more or less efficient and consistent reconciliation of inner needs with the outer world. Some perceptual styles—the cockeyed optimist and the hard-nosed realist—are mainly identifiable by their extremeness and unidimensionality. Although such extremes of style may not be typical, learned predispositions and dominant motive patterns are evident in the perceptual behavior of most individuals. If we perceive people as warm and friendly, we tend to pick up cues that support that perception and, in response, to be warm and friendly ourselves. Similarly, individuals with strong power needs may interpret most situations in competitive terms, while individuals with strong affiliation needs may, in the same situations, focus on views that indicate the possibility of cooperation.

Perceptual defenses. The use of perceptual defenses is the final major influence on individual patterns of selective perception. We have described perception as a cognitive process that enables us to organize and manage the complex array of stimuli provided by our environment. The psychological and behavioral value of perception lies in this ability to organize complexity and to reduce uncertainty by identifying reliable patterns of relationships among stimuli, needs, and behavior. Thus conceptual structures play a major role in behavior, and individuals are naturally motivated to conserve those structures and the investment of learning that has gone into their development. In particular, individuals are motivated to reject information that does not fit into existing perceptual systems.

Individuals with a strong fear of dental treatment and a perception of dentistry as painful and expensive may ignore or deny cues such as discoloration of the teeth, swelling of the gums, or even severe tooth pain in order to avoid seeking dental treatment. Not all perceptual defenses are negative, however; the ability to ignore background noise such as music or conversation or to deny the perception of such noise can facilitate concentrating on the work at hand. Similarly, the ability to ignore the threat of the hydrogen bomb and to go on eating and sleeping as though this danger were not there is a very useful defensive reaction to perceptions over which we have no control and yet that could seriously disrupt behavior.[7] The following paragraph illustrates this point:

> We have at our disposal a host of perceptual defenses. These defenses act like a screen or filter, blocking out that which we do not want to see and letting through that which we do want to see. The closer we get to conceptual systems and our concern with our self-perceptions (self-image) and our relationships with others, the more likely we are to call upon these defensive screens.*

Thus perceptual defenses may have a positive or a negative impact. On the one hand, they enable us to ignore distractions that might block us from achieving our goals, and on the other hand, they may lead us to overlook information that could have serious consequences.

• • •

The combination of perceptual readiness, individual needs, perceptual styles, and perceptual defenses provides the following general set of guidelines for understanding the process of perception:

1. Individuals perceive what they feel will help satisfy needs.
2. Individuals ignore what is disturbing and distracting in the pursuit of needs.
3. Individuals perceiving disturbances that persist and strengthen first attempt to force the disturbance to fit into the pattern of existing perceptions and second, to change behavior to accommodate new perceptions.[7]

PERCEPTION AND BEHAVIOR

Perception of others

With this understanding of selective perception, we can examine patterns of perception typically observed in human behavior. Turning first to patterns in the perception of others, much attention has been given to the identification stage, the forming of first impressions. The tendency is to look for cues that allow us to classify new persons, things, and objects into existing categories in order to preserve our presently developed perceptual structure. This tendency to focus on cues that seem to indicate a relationship with existing categories may lead us to ignore cues that, if perceived accurately, would have necessitated an entirely different classification or even the creation of a new category.

First impressions also provide a basis for identifying and extrapolating to additional characteristics and likely future behaviors of the stimulus object. Thus in a famous study subjects were shown pictures of individuals and asked to describe the character traits of these individuals and also how they might act in specific situations. Different groups of subjects were shown the same picture—the only difference being that, for one group, the individual in the picture was identified as a senior executive and, for the second group, the same individual was described as a union leader. On the basis of this identifying variable, subjects attributed to the individual in the picture sharply different sets of values and responses to specific behavioral situations.[3] The lesson in this example to the dentist is clear: take care that normal perceptual habits do not induce premature judgments of patients—judgments as to characteristics and likely behavior based on a limited sample of available cues and not on observed behavior. In this way, significant data that might lead to the development of more effective treatment plans may be overlooked.

Two particular aspects of the perception of others have received considerable attention and are worthy of note: stereotyping and the halo effect.

Stereotyping. Stereotypes represent rigid, judgmental perceptions of individuals based primarily on group membership. Thus bankers are conservative, professors are absentminded, etc. These stereotypes

*From Kolb, Rubin, McIntyre, ORGANIZATIONAL PSYCHOLOGY: An Experiential Approach, 2nd edition, © 1974, pp. 23, 25, 27, 28, and pages for the submitted text. Reprinted by permission of Prentice-Hall, Inc., Englewood Cliffs, New Jersey.

are typically based on limited, carefully selected perceptions of reality. The dentist who perceives that women are concerned primarily with appearance or that children are unable to understand the reasons for recommended dental practices is unlikely to take the time to discover that a particular female patient is motivated primarily by concern for dental health or that a particular child is very interested in technical explanations. If the dentist acts primarily on the basis of stereotypes, he or she is likely to miss opportunities for a truly effective treatment of patients.

The dentist who is concerned with improving the level of dental care in society must also overcome a variety of stereotypes about dentists and dentistry. The common images of dentistry and dentists are that dentistry is an expensive and painful procedure and that dentists are concerned primarily with making money. There is considerable evidence demonstrating that, after financial obstacles, negative perception is the major reason why many people do not avail themselves of regular dental care.[5] The dentist who wishes to be effective with patients must recognize that his or her approach must acknowledge and respond to these negative perceptual barriers. This means that technically competent work will not be sufficient to change a patient's behavior or perceptions of dentistry. Possible approaches for shaping existing perceptions that others have of us will be discussed on p. 119 and will be examined in the exercise for this chapter.

Halo effect. The concept of a "halo effect" refers to the tendency to attribute a variety of traits and characteristics to an individual on the basis of the possession of other (desirable) traits. Thus we may attribute such characteristics as honesty, intelligence, and integrity to an individual whom we perceive as sincere. This tendency to generalize on the basis of limited information can produce many of the same distortions and generalizations that were previously noted for stereotyping. The principal difference is that stereotyping attributes characteristics to individuals on the basis of group membership, whereas the halo effect attributes qualities to an individual based on other (positive) qualities possessed by that specific individual. Thus a dentist whose skills and professional status are respected by patients may acquire a "halo," leading the same patients to seek advice and guidance on nondental matters such as local politics or education.

Presentation of self

This analysis of stereotypes and the halo effect immediately raises questions as to how we can induce others to perceive us as we would like to be perceived. Our effectiveness in dealing with others is affected by the perceptions they have of us. This perception comes in part from objective characteristics over which we have little control (for example, a young dentist may have difficulties with older patients because of the perceptions they have with regard to the dentist's age; frustrating as this may be, there is very little the dentist can do about it); in part by the other individual's patterns of perceiving other persons, again over which we have very little control (for example, the patient who sees the world primarily in conflict terms will approach the dentist as an antagonist, independent of any perceptions he or she has of that particular dentist); and in part by the way in which we present ourselves (for example, the dentist who wishes to be seen as serving an adult clientele would do well to remove rock music from his or her office). The effective presentation of self requires first, learning who we really are, and second, learning how to present ourselves so that others will see us as we want to be seen.

The process of self-learning involves identifying the ways in which the world defines our attributes and the expectations that the world has of us as well as the ways in which the world responds to specific actions on our part. In the following exercise, you will have the opportunity to learn something about how others see you and to compare this viewpoint with your perceptions of yourself. Where discrepancies between your self-image and the image others have of you exist, you will have the opportunity to explore actions that might reduce such discrepancies and to test your plans against the reactions of classmates.

Presenting yourself so that others will see you as you wish to be seen is a delicate process. There is ample evidence that not only do others not perceive us as we wish to be perceived or even as we "really are," but also that we do not perceive ourselves as we really are. Webber provides the following example of how sixty pairs of managers and their subordinates perceive the amount of time per week they communicated with each other:

1. Superior perceives: 4.1 hours a week communicating with his subordinate
2. Subordinate perceives: 3.0 hours a week communicating with superior
3. Actual (estimated from sample observations): 2.8 hours a week that superior and subordinate communicated with each other*

The key point here is not that superior and subordinate had different perceptions of the amount of time they spent together, but that each was incorrect and overestimated the contact time.

Leavitt provides the following description of the difficulty of effective presentation of the self:

> You are trying to tell me that you are strong, worldly, and decisive (and you may be—or you may not), but I am just as busily trying to communicate to you that I am the sagacious, understanding, and intellectually stimulating character that I would like to be (and may actually be—or may not). We have both been practicing our acts for a long time so we have both developed clever ways of being convincing, ways that the poor inept adolescent has not even dreamed of. But we have also developed further ways of spotting the other guy's act. . . . While you stand there trying to radiate strength and decisiveness, I see you as brash and immature. And you, wanting action and recognition, see my efforts at quiet, pipe-smoking wisdom as dullness and lack of imagination. . . . The first big problem then is . . . estimating the discrepancy between the actor and the "real" person. The second problem is to estimate how well our act is working.*

In the exercise that follows, you will have the opportunity first, to explore the patterns of perceptions that you and your classmates have of groups within society, and second, having completed this exercise, to explore the perceptions that you have of each other. A useful framework for organizing this experience is shown in Fig. 9-2. The diagram describes what is known

*From Webber, R. A.: Hum. Relations **23:**235, 1970.

*From Leavitt, H. J.: Managerial psychology, ed. 3, Chicago, 1972, The University of Chicago Press. © 1972 by The University of Chicago Press.

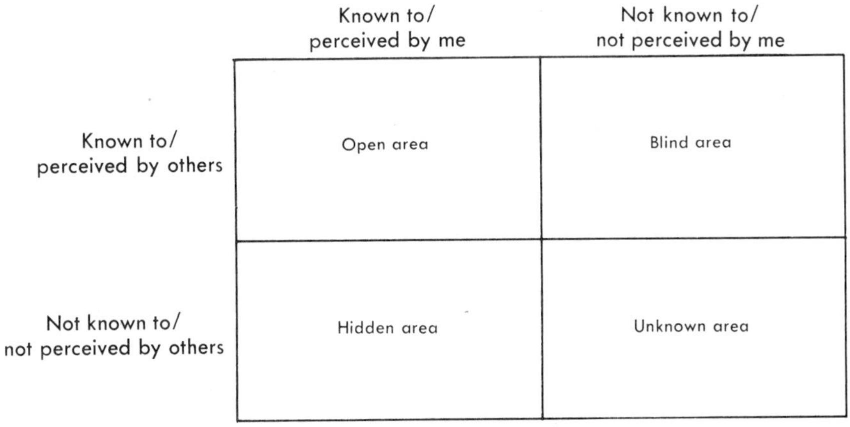

Fig. 9-2. The Johari window.

as a Johari window and has two main dimensions: those attributes of ourselves that are known or not known to ourselves and those attributes that are known or not known to others. In combination, these attributes define the following four areas of joint perception:

1. *Open area:* In this area, your self-perception and the perception that others have of you are consistent—people see you the way you see yourself with respect to these characteristics.
2. *Unknown area:* This area includes those attributes or characteristics that neither you nor others see in yourself.
3. *Hidden area:* This area includes attributes or characteristics that you see in yourself but that are hidden from others—"I am basically a shy person, but I hide this in public by being gregarious, and nobody has recognized my basic shyness." There may be, of course, considerable strain involved in maintaining this role in order to prevent others from seeing the "real you."
4. *Blind area:* This area includes those attributes and characteristics that others see in you but that you do not see in yourself—"Others see me as aggressive and power seeking, but I either do not recognize or deny such motives, because I have been led to believe that they are socially unacceptable."[6]

In the following exercise, you will have the opportunity to fill in these areas for yourself and to assist your classmates in identifying the attributes that fit each of the four areas in their windows.

EXPERIENCE WITH PERCEPTION

This exercise provides an opportunity first, to explore the differing perceptions that individuals have about familiar ideas and roles, and second, to experience the challenge of understanding and reconciling differences in individual perceptions. The exercise will also help you in identifying your personal perceptual style. Finally, by providing you with information about how others perceive you, you will be able to judge the effectiveness of your presentation of self—to estimate "how well your act is working." In the exercise, you will be asked to do the following:

1. Rank a series of social roles (physician, secretary, hygienist, etc.) in terms of your perception of their status in society and then meet with a group of your classmates and come to a common agreement on the ranking.
2. Record your perceptions of yourself and a group of your classmates and then share these perceptions with the group in order to identify your perceptual style and to explore the reasons why others see you as they do.
3. Construct a Johari window for yourself (p. 111).

Group meeting preparation

1. Before class, rank the fifteen social roles shown in the chart on your perceptions of different roles, p. 113, in terms of their status in society as you perceive them. Record your judgments in the first column, using 1 for the highest rank role and 15 for the lowest. At the bottom of the column, note the criteria that you used in reaching your judgment and any significant perceptions that influenced your judgment.

MY JOHARI WINDOW

	Known to/perceived by me	Not known to/not perceived by me
Known to/ perceived by others	Open area	Blind area
Not known to/ not perceived by others	Hidden area	Unknown area

2. The class should be divided at the meeting into groups of four to six members. Record the names of the other members of your group at the top of the columns in the chart on your perceptions of others, p. 114. Before class, complete the matrix of this chart, recording your perceptions of yourself and the other members of your small group. In completing the matrix, work quickly, recording the first perception or impressions that come to mind when you think of either yourself or the other individuals in your group. In the first column of the chart, record the image you have of yourself in terms of the following categories:
   - The first five or six key words that come to mind when you think of yourself
   - The type of dentist you think you will become
   - The type of dental patient you think you are

Repeat this process for each of the other members of your small group.

Group meeting procedure

Discussion of perceived status ranking

1. Small group meeting (approximate time—30 minutes). The small group should meet to reach a group consensus on the perceived status ranking of the fifteen social roles. Individual members should explain their personal ranking, the criteria they used, and whatever significant perceptions may have influenced their judgments. The group should then discuss differences that exist among the individual perceptions in order to agree on a common ranking. The group ranking should be recorded in the second column of the chart on p. 113. During the discussion, a record should be kept of the following possible sources of differing perceptions:
   - *Objective differences:* Is the group able to agree on what an individual in a given social role actually does? Are there differences in perceived objective reality?
   - *Criterion differences:* Are there differences within the group on the criteria that should be used to assign status to social roles? For example, do some members feel that status should be assigned in terms of service to society, whereas others feel influence or power should be the criterion? Do some members wish to rank the roles in terms of the criteria they perceive society is actually using, whereas others prefer to use the criteria they believe society should use?
   - *Evaluation differences:* Do members differ in their assignments of how individuals in a given social role measure up against an agreed on criterion? For example, do some members feel that lawyers rank high in terms of service to society, whereas others feel that lawyers do not measure well on this criterion?

   Note that the first of these sources of differences includes both objective and cognitive aspects of perception. Although it may be possible to resolve objective differences by gathering information on the activities of a particular social role, factual information alone will not resolve differences over the choice of criteria or the assessment of performance against criteria.

YOUR PERCEPTIONS OF DIFFERENT ROLES

Social roles	Your initial rank	Final group rank	Rankings by other groups		
			Group 1	Group 2	Group 3
Physician					
Lawyer					
Legal stenographer					
Registered nurse					
Dentist					
Hygienist					
Carpenter					
Physical therapist					
Office receptionist					
Engineer					
Accountant					
Secretary					
Housewife					
Steelworker					
Working mother					

Criteria used to form ranking

Significant perceptions

YOUR PERCEPTIONS OF OTHERS

	Individual					
Area	**Self**	**Person A:**	**Person B:**	**Person C:**	**Person D:**	**Person E:**
Five or six key words						
Type of dentist or paraprofessional						
Type of dental patient						

PERCEPTION OF SELF BY OTHERS

	How I am seen by				
Area	**Person A:**	**Person B:**	**Person C:**	**Person D:**	**Person E:**
Five or six key words					
Type of dentist or paraprofessional					
Type of dental patient					

2. Class meeting (approximate time—30 minutes). After the small groups have reached consensus on their rankings of social roles, the class should reconvene to discuss differences in the group ranking. Each group should present its rankings, which can be recorded on chalkboard and also in the columns provided in the chart on p. 113. In discussing differences in the group ranking, each group should report on the particular set of objective descriptions of the social roles, criteria, and performance against the criteria it used in forming its ranking. This discussion should further illuminate the impact of perceptions on differences in fact, criteria, and performance and should identify clearly the several levels of difficulty that have to be overcome in reconciling perceptual differences.

Interpersonal perception. With the experience of reconciling perceptions gained in discussing perceived status rankings, the small groups should now reconvene to discuss the interpersonal perceptions.

1. Each member of the group should read his or her perceptions of self and of the other group members as recorded on the chart of your perceptions of others, p. 114. The other members should record that individual's perceptions of them in the appropriate column of that chart. The total pattern of the individual's perception of self and other group members should be recorded on a chalkboard for group examination.
2. After each individual has presented his or her perceptual matrix from the chart on p. 114, the groups should discuss the patterns of perception as they emerge in order to formulate a description of each individual's personal perceptual style. In examining the pattern of perceptions, the following questions should be considered:
   - Are the perceptions largely objective? Do the descriptions of self and others focus on objective characteristics such as height, weight, sex, etc. that would be available to other observers? Are descriptions provided in terms of behaviors that might be available to other observers?
   - Are the perceptions stated largely in judgmental or evaluative terms? Do the descriptions reflect interpretations of characteristics and behavior influenced by the values, feelings, and opinions of the perceivers? Do the descriptions refer to general attributes of the person (effective, honest, likeable, etc.) rather than to observable, specific behaviors?
   - Are the perceptions stated largely in terms of values and motive patterns of the perceivers? Do the descriptions of different group members reflect a consistent pattern, for example, a tendency to describe persons in terms of their power, their achievements, or their integrity? Do the concepts and concerns appear in the list of the different individuals?
3. After the group has discussed the perceptual style of each member (the way in which that individual tends to organize the world, as demonstrated in the chart on your perceptions of others, p. 114, the group should devote the remainder of its time to a discussion of the perceptions that the group has of each of its members (as recorded on the chart on perception of self by others, p. 115). In this part of the exercise, each individual should receive from the other group members an explanation of why they perceive

him or her as they do. This is a difficult task. You will have to explain your perceptions of another to them in a way that will be useful to them without arousing their defenses. This requires considerable tact and sensitivity, and you should plan your remarks carefully in terms of the perceptions that you have of that individual. The group should provide feedback on the perceptions that each has of a given individual before going on to the next member. Thus members B, C, D, and E would discuss their perceptions of A with A, then members A, C, D, and E would discuss their perceptions of B with B, etc. until everyone has received feedback from the rest of the group. In presenting your perceptions of them to other group members, try to include the following:

- Point to specific behaviors that lead to your perception.
- Explain your perception of the behavior of others in terms of your own feelings and reactions.

In the discussion, each individual might want to explore the following questions with the group:

- If different members of the group perceived me differently—why? What are the sources of their different perceptions—my behavior, the nature of my relation with them, their values?
- If others see me differently than I see myself—why? Do the differences lie in what I know about myself but do not reveal to others or in different interpretations of behaviors and characteristics that we both observe?

4. At the end of the group discussion, each individual privately (or perhaps with the assistance of other group members) should complete a Johari window for himself or herself. Use the information recorded on the charts on pp. 114 and 115 and any other insights that may have come to you during the group discussion.
5. Looking at your completed window, consider the following questions:
   - Do you see elements that surprise you, particularly in the blind area? Would you like to change these perceptions that others have of you? If so, how would you go about doing so?
   - Do you see things in yourself that you wish others would see, particularly in the hidden area? How might you bring these out and to the attention of others? In what ways is your presentation of yourself at this time effective and ineffective? Would you like to change how others perceive you? If so, how might you accomplish this?

SUMMARY

Perceptions, whether of physical, social, or interpersonal events, form the basic data that we use to organize the world. What we perceive is filtered through a complex system of needs, past experience, and personal perceptual styles. We perceive what we want to perceive or expect to perceive, and we often ignore, deny, or reject cues that might force us to alter our present perceptual structure. Perceptual selectivity is a necessary accommodation to the complexity of stimuli provided by the environment, and our present needs and personal style make us perceptually ready to attend to some stimuli and to ignore others. Perceptual defenses are necessary, but potentially distorting, elements of this efficient cognitive organization. The process of perception is, therefore, complex and tenuous; the facts do not always speak for themselves. The significance of perception in dentist-patient interactions is probably self-evident. We will be referring to this phenomenon directly and indirectly when we discuss selecting strategies for behavior change in the dental treatment setting in Chapters 13 and 15.

Perceptual categories based on group characteristics

Sensitivity to differences in perception that exist, even when people are apparently discussing the same objective event, should lead us to a continuing examination of our perceptual patterns—how we perceive others and how others perceive us. In the exercise you have just completed, you have had the opportunity to examine the complexities of perception at several levels. By looking at the status attributed to social roles, you have seen how objective information forms the basis for the perceptions that we have of specific classes or groups of individuals. Knowing that an individual belongs to a certain class or group stimulates a complex network of associated perceptions: lawyers are well educated, are physically weak, wear three-piece suits, speak effectively; steelworkers are not well educated, are physically strong, wear working clothes, and speak gruffly. The social roles or category labels that individuals carry around with them greatly influence perceptions of their characteristics, lead us to make predictions about their behavior, and enable us to assign social value or status to them. The social roles that we have described represent one set of category labels that we use to organize our perceptions. The organization of stimuli into perceptual categories is a necessary response to the complexity of the stimulus environment.

How perceptual style relates to perceptual categories. The particular set of perceptual categories that we employ is typically not objectively valid but based on our own unique cognitive experiences and patterns, our perceptual style. The practical consequences of our perceptual styles were demonstrated in the exercise by the differences in perceptions of several social roles held by different group members. More importantly, the accuracy of your perception was probably improved through the process of reconciling your perceptions with those of the other group members.

The list of social roles provides one set of perceptual categories; you had the opportunity to examine a second set of categories when you dealt with the group's perception of specific individuals. In this part of the exercise, you experienced two different patterns of perceptual organization.

The first pattern of perceptual organization that you observed was the unique perceptual style each group member possessed. If the members of your group were like most of us, each individual probably organized his or her perceptions of the rest of the group in terms of a specific set of categories. These perceptual styles might differ from person to person, perhaps with one individual organizing his or her perceptions around emotional concepts and another around intellectual concepts. Although different individuals might favor different concepts, they undoubtedly tend to use the same concepts in their perceptions of the other group members.

The second pattern of perceptual organization that you observed was the perceptions the group members had of each individual. Although there undoubtedly were differences in the perceptions that the several members of the group had of a specific individual, there were probably also perceptions on which there was general agreement. Further, the general set of perceptions that the group had of member A probably differed noticeably from those they had of member B, member C, etc.

There is a certain irony in this last point when you consider the members of your group as individuals; the individuals were probably sharply differentiated, and yet you are all members of the same social role or category—dental students. If the group had been asked to give its perception of dental students, you would have likely come to a description on which there was general agreement and that attributed common characteristics to all members of the group. This demonstrates the subjective nature of perceptual concepts and perceptual organization. At one level, dental students do share a set of common traits, and a category that treats students as a homogeneous group can be perceptually useful. At another level, however, dental students in the group are not homogeneous, as you have seen in the exercise, and a perceptual category that treats them as such would fail to identify meaningful individual differences.

Uses of perceptual categories. In considering the uses of perceptual categories, the lessons are twofold. First, different patterns of perceptual organization are appropriate and useful for different purposes; it is not a question of whether one form of perceptual organization is better than another but rather of selecting which form will be most useful to the needs of the present situation. Second, perceptual categories based on group characteristics (stereotypes) are of minimal value when dealing with specific individuals, since such categories obscure individual differences in identifying common denominators. This critical and seemingly obvious point is frequently overlooked in normal behavior. The pressures of a busy schedule or mere laziness frequently lead us to treat patients as members of a class rather than as separate and distinct individuals with separate and distinct needs, feelings, and other personal characteristics. The frequently heard comment that "Dr. Jones does good work but is so impersonal" reflects this tendency to perceive individuals as members of a homogeneous class.

Just as all dental students are not alike, all patients, or even all child patients, are not alike. You have had the opportunity in this exercise to observe your own tendencies to perceive in terms of categories or stereotypes rather than in terms of unique characteristics of specific individuals; careful monitoring and restraint of this tendency is essential to effective interpersonal relations with patients and co-workers.

Perception of self-image

In the second part of the exercise, you received a considerable amount of information on how others perceive you. Hopefully, this was a stimulating and exciting experience, but it could also have been very frustrating and, perhaps, upsetting. Each of us has a detailed and complicated image of ourselves—our abilities, characteristics, needs and values, and appearance. We have both an ideal self (what we would like to be) and a real self (what we perceive ourselves to be at present). Much of our behavior is typically directed toward bridging whatever gap exists between our real and ideal selves. In recording your perception of yourself, you have taken a preliminary step in explicitly defining your self-image.

Our self-image derives from many sources. We can observe our own characteristics, our physical and psychological attributes, and our behavior and, on the basis of these observations, describe the kind of person we are. We also know that part of our self-image comes from our conception of our ideal self or from our imagination or anticipation of how we would behave in situations. For example, our belief about how we would act should our house catch fire is, for those of us who have not actually experienced a house fire, based in part on the sense of how we would like to think we would behave and on how we should behave (our ideal self). Many of the elements of our self-image that provide us with the greatest satisfaction and ego gratification are based on similar anticipations of how we would respond nobly to tragedies. A final part of our self-image is based not on our own observation or imagining but on descriptions of ourselves provided by others. From childhood on, parents, teachers, and friends provide us with descriptions and evaluations of ourselves. We are told that we are handsome, intelligent, artistic, funny, etc., and these descriptions become part of our self-image.

In the exercise, you have received a rather heavy dose of this last sort of information about yourself. Probably the descriptions provided by your group members do not coincide entirely with the self-image that you brought to the exercise. This is understandable, since each of the members of your group have had only limited contact with you relative to the knowledge you have about yourself. Further, their descriptions of you are inevitably influenced by their own values and perceptions of themselves as well as by objective observations of your character and behavior. Before completing this chapter, consider taking the time to decide to what extent you are concerned about the discrepancies between your self-image and the image that others have of you and whether you want to do anything about these discrepancies in terms of the following questions:

- □ To what extent are the perceptions others have of you a function of their own needs and concerns and, therefore, not really reliable information about you?
- □ Do others see in you traits that you do not see in yourself? Now that you have become aware of them, do you want to change them because they are undesirable? Do others perceive traits you would like to add to your self-image because they are desirable?

Influences on our perception of others

A number of general observations about the major influences on how we perceive others can be made based on extensive research.[10] They are as follows:

1. *The characteristics of the perceiver influence the characteristics that he or she is likely to see in others.* We tend to use the significant elements of our own self-image as a guide to the characteristics that we look for in others and as a point of reference for the assessment of those characteristics in others. Similarly, the importance that certain characteristics have in our own self-image influences the weight that we give to those characteristics in our perception and evaluation of others. Thus if we see ourselves as sociable, we tend to use assessments of the sociability of others as a critical element in our perception of them, and, in addition, we stress their sociability in proportion to the importance of sociability in our own self-image. Dentists are likely to pay more attention to individuals' attitudes toward dental hygiene and toward dentistry in forming impressions of these individuals than they may pay to other characteristics.

2. *Individuals who accept themselves—who are comfortable with their self-image and with others' perceptions of them—are more likely to perceive favorable characteristics in other persons.* If we are relatively secure with ourselves, we are more likely to be open to a more objective and thorough analysis of others; if we do not feel the need to establish our own status, we are less likely to look for ways to criticize others. This characteristic is relevant to assessing the opinions provided by others; we often depend on other persons for information and assessment of new acquaintances and new patients. It is sensible to take into account the security of the provider of the information in making judgments about the validity of the information.

3. *The status and position of individuals influence our perceptions of their abilities and judgments of their behaviors.* There is a tendency to perceive favorable qualities in high-status individuals and unfavorable qualities in low-status individuals. Further, there is a tendency to supply more favorable interpretations of the behavior of persons in authority than of those in positions of little influence. This characteristic very often works on the dentist's behalf. For many patients, the dentist is a high-status individual of considerable expertise, and the dentist's opinions and suggestions are likely to be given enhanced credence for this reason. Differences in status can present a problem for the dentist, however, in dealing with patients who are seen by either the dentist or the patient as having higher status than the dentist. Attempts to influence these individuals through appeals to status or expertise are less likely to be effective than approaches that acknowledge their (real or perceived) higher status.

4. *Our perceptions of individuals and events are influenced by the social roles we perform.* We tend to perceive things in terms of the particular responsibilities, perspectives, philosophies, and methods of our particular social role or activity. Thus educators may perceive all examples of ineffective performance as evidence of inadequate training; marketing managers see all organizational issues in marketing terms, etc. The dentist is equally susceptible to perceiving all oral difficulties as indicative of dental pathology. This tendency is exaggerated for those who specialize in particular activities, and the dentist is well advised to consider carefully whether diagnosis of treatment needs is based on the condition of the patient's teeth or on the desire to apply favorite solutions such as extraction or orthodontics.

Importance of perceptual accuracy

The influence of the preceding characteristics on our perceptions raises the question of whether we should be concerned with the accuracy of perception. If our perceptual activity were limited to passive observation, the many potential sources of perceptual inaccuracy would be of only limited interest. Our perceptions are, however, related to our subsequent behavior. What we perceive largely determines how we will act. Our perceptions, first of all, allow us to identify situations, and this identification guides us in selecting appropriate potential behaviors from our repertoire. Further, our initial perception guides whatever additional gathering of information or sampling of cues that we might undertake in order to make behavioral decisions. For example, if we enter a large room in which a social event such as a cocktail party is taking place, our initial perception of the room and its ambience will largely shape our behavior at the party and our subsequent evaluation of our participation. We pick up a series of cues such as size of the group, style of dress, composition (in terms of age group, sex, etc. represented), and type of music being played to form an initial judgment about the party (naturally, this judgment is also influenced by our general attitude toward cocktail parties). Having made these judgments (that it is a good party or a bad party) we proceed to look for information that confirms our judgment. If we have decided that it is a good party, it will require a considerable amount of negative information or experience to overturn that judgment. Similarly, if we decide that it is going to be a bad party, it will take a considerable amount of pleasant experience, conversation, etc. to revise our initial impression.

The relation between perceptual accuracy and behavior is important also in that what is perceived in us by others tends to shape the manner in which they behave toward us and the opportunities to behave that they have to offer us. Students who are perceived by teachers as having high potential are typically given more challenging work, more opportunities to perform, and more personal attention than are students with lower perceived potential.[8] Perceptions of potential are also positively related to subsequent evaluations of performance, with the result that more rewards are directed toward persons of perceived high potential, thus reinforcing their behavioral patterns.

The development of leaders is a good example of this process. Typically, children and teachers choose leaders from among classmates on the basis of perceived characteristics such as height, appearance, or enthusiasm rather than demonstrated performance. The children so chosen are given the opportunity to perform leadership functions and are often praised for their efforts. As this process is repeated throughout the developmental years, with children who have served as leaders before being chosen to lead again, now on the basis of their experience, the behaviors that they engage in in their leadership roles are reinforced. More importantly, the image of themselves as leaders becomes increasingly reinforced in their self-image and in the perceptions that others have of them, and they develop greater confidence in seeking leadership positions in new situations. Thus by the end of the school experience, the division of the student body into leaders and non-leaders can represent a psychological reality that is a good indication of the subsequent behaviors of individuals, even though the division does not represent inherent differences in the possession of some intangible known as "leadership."

Improving perceptual accuracy

Given the importance of accurate perception in the development of effective behavior, it is sensible for individuals to attempt to assess the accuracy of their perception and to sharpen their perceptual skills. The best, and perhaps the only available, mechanism for improving the accuracy of our perceptions is that of *feedback*. In the exercise you have just completed, feedback was the primary means employed to provide you with information about the accuracy of your perceptions and to sharpen your perceptions through practice. It is only by sharing our perceptions with others, by comparing our perceptions with their perceptions, and by thoroughly discussing the reasons for the similarities and differences that we can hope to improve the accuracy of our perceptions of specific persons, objects, or ideas and, more importantly, to sharpen our ability to form accurate perceptions. The process of feedback and discussion helps to increase perceptual accuracy in the following three ways:

1. The exchange of perceptions with others provides direct information, first, that others may see the world differently than we do, and second, that others may possess facts of which we were unaware.
2. The discussion of differences forces us to examine the sources of our perceptions: are they factual and associated with objective and observable data or are they interpretations? If they are interpretations, have they been developed through a process of logic or do they represent the action of subjective preferences?
3. The process of sharing perceptions helps us to identify patterns, habits, and biases in our typical perceptual behavior, thus identifying the need to attend to how we perceive (how we sample cues and organize stimuli).

Despite the great value of feedback and discussion in improving perceptual accuracy, we often fail to utilize the process. As you saw in the exercise, feedback and discussion are time-consuming activities and can be threatening and frustrating. Further, we often do not recognize the need to improve the accuracy of our perceptions because we believe that our present perceptual structure is accurate and adequate. Because these barriers to seeking feedback exist, we will be devoting a considerable amount of time in subsequent chapters to working on improving perceptual and concept-forming abilities as well as to practicing communications, influence, and group leadership skills. In Chapters 10 and 11 we will be focusing on the dynamics of relationships within groups in the performance of problem-solving and conflict resolution tasks, and in Chapters 12 and 13 we will be working on patterns of influence and interpersonal communications.

REFERENCES

1. Bruner, J.: Social psychology and perception. In Maccoby, E., Newcomb, T., and Hartley, E., eds.: Readings in social psychology, New York, 1958, Holt, Rinehart & Winston, Inc.
2. Ference, T. P.: Organizational communications systems and the decision process, Management Sci. **17:**83, 1970.
3. Haire, M., and Grunes, W. F.: Perceptual defenses: processes protesting an original perception of another personality, Hum. Relations **3:**403, 1950.
4. Johnson, D. M.: A systematic treatment of judgment, Psychol. Bull. **42:**193, 1945.
5. Kegeles, S. S.: Why people seek dental care: a test of a conceptual formulation, J. Health Soc. Behav. **4:**166, 1963.
6. Kolb, D. A., Rubin, I. M., and McIntyre, J. M.: Organizational psychology: an experiential approach, Englewood Cliffs, N.J., 1971, Prentice-Hall, Inc.
7. Leavitt, H. J.: Managerial psychology, ed. 3, Chicago, 1972, The University of Chicago Press.
8. Rosenthal, R.: Experimenter effects in behavioral research, New York, 1966, Appleton-Century-Crofts.
9. Webber, R. A.: Perceptions of interactions between superiors and subordinates, Hum. Relations **23:**235, 1970.
10. Zalkind, S. S., and Costello, T. W.: Perception: implications for administration, Admin. Sci. Q. **7:**218, 1962.

Chapter 10

GROUP AND INDIVIDUAL APPROACHES TO PROBLEM SOLVING

Despite the inherent difficulties of solving problems in groups, joint problem solving is frequently called for by the nature of the problem. Although the dentist can repair a damaged tooth with minimal cooperation from the patient, he or she cannot prevent such damage from occurring again without the full cooperation of the patient. The symptom can be treated independently, but the problem that has generated the symptom cannot be "solved" without a joint effort. The dentist may lead in developing the solution, but the patient retains responsibility for implementation. This example demonstrates both the necessity for and the demands of effective joint problem solving. Different individuals bring different resources and responsibilities to the group effort, and effective communication and shared commitment to the solution and its goals are necessary for success.

Many other situations in a dentist's normal work life require similar group effort. Consultation with colleagues on difficult cases is an invaluable tool for polling information, checking observations, and exploring a range of possibilities. The interaction among dentists, hygienists, and assistants in the delivery of services to the patient is also inherently of a group nature.

OBJECTIVES

The objectives of this chapter are as follows:

1. To explore the problem-solving and decision-making behavior of individuals and groups and to understand the ways in which past experience, values, and personal needs affect the interpretation of problems and the nature of participation in groups
2. To practice group and individual problem solving
3. To develop guidelines for using individuals and groups effectively to elicit creativity and innovation in solving complex problems

PROBLEM-SOLVING BEHAVIOR

In one of his famous tales of Tevye the Milkman, Sholem Aleichem describes a scene in which Tevye comes upon two friends arguing in the street. The first friend appeals to Tevye for support, and Tevye responds, "You're right." The second friend, on hearing this, attacks Tevye's judgment and restates his position, to which Tevye again responds, "You're right." A third friend, who has overheard this exchange, exclaims to Tevye, "But they hold opposite opinions. They cannot both be right." Tevye once again nods in agreement and says, "You're right."

Tevye is confronted with a problem common in many group discussions. As we learned in Chapters 7, 8, and 9, there are often as many different beliefs, opinions, or recommended actions as there are members of a group. Further, these several positions are normally either incompatible or only partially overlapping. There may even be disagreement as to the definition of the problem or issue that these positions seek to resolve. This is particularly evident when dentists face the problem of implementing preventive dental programs. These programs, as analyzed in Chapter 18, seriously test the dentist's skills at problem solving. Unfortunately, there is often no ready means for discriminating that one solution is "correct" or even for ranking the positions in some order of "correctness." It is more likely that each of the several positions contains elements of wisdom, insight, and usefulness.

Typical approaches used in group problem solving

There are usually three approaches to resolving the dilemma of group problem solving: political, democratic, and rational.

Political. The first approach is political —to follow Tevye and agree with everybody. Although utilizing this approach may be a problem when all the participants are present, it is, in fact, a frequently used method for dealing with individuals one at a time. We often expect politicians and others in the public eye to behave this way, altering their positions on various issues in order to win approval from different audiences. This tactic is not limited to politicians, however; we all frequently deal with uncomfortable interpersonal situations in the same manner. Thus the dentist caught in the middle of an altercation between patient and receptionist or between technician and hygienist may take each party aside individually, listen sympathetically to their position, and indicate agreement that they have been aggrieved. Obviously, this can be an effective way to buy time and allow tempers to cool; when actual decisions of which the parties are aware must follow, however, the political approach is likely to be ineffective.

Democratic. A second approach to resolving differences of opinion within a group might be called the democratic approach. Agreement among the participants is sought either through extensive discussion, which persists until there is a meeting of the minds, or through the adoption of a method of choice such as voting or drawing of lots that is seen as treating each of the positions equitably. In the purest forms such as town meetings, these democratic processes are firmly rooted in tradition and appeal to many deeply held values. In practice, extended discussion among several individuals of goodwill seeking a "good" resolution can sharpen issues and emphasize common goals and interests. This can often produce agreement on one position or lead to a compromise that satisfies everyone. The democratic approach is, however, time consuming, and the distinction between objective discussion and partisan persuasion is easily blurred. There is, moreover, no guarantee that the democratic choice, either by compromise or vote or lot, is necessarily "the best" response to the problem at hand.

Rational. A third approach might be called the rational approach. Resolution is achieved not through temporizing or subjective deliberations of group members but, instead, through submission of the various positions to a formal, analytical method or model where selection is based on abstract criteria of correctness or optimality. In mathematics and economic theory, formal models that test all possible alternatives against formal optimality criteria are common. Unfortunately, many problems, particularly those the dentist deals with in diagnosing pathological conditions or in influencing patient behavior, are not so neatly and cleanly defined. The full range of alternative courses of action is generally not known. Full information is generally not available, and, most importantly, neither are formal models for performing the analysis. Clinical situations seldom attain the purity and rigor of mathematical formulas or laboratory experiments. Thus there are limitations in the application of formally rational approaches to many human problem situations.

There is, however, another aspect to rationality—the emphasis on reaching decisions through logical, objective analysis. In this sense, much group behavior can be "intendedly rational,"[64] in that alternatives are considered on their own merit and not in terms of the political influence of proponents or the number of proponents. It is frequently difficult, however, for a group to be consistently rational when dealing with human problems. In fact, the dentist who discusses treatment needs with the patient in purely objective, clinical terms is often criticized for being insensitive to the emotional and attitudinal considerations. In group problem solving, it is equally difficult to keep the discussion at a detached, clinical level on issues that involve judgment and deeply held philosophies and values. Moreover, many traditional mechanisms such as voting or persuasion, which focus on reaching *a* decision rather than *the best* decision, are more conducive to arguing for and sticking to positions than to analyzing, seeking new alternatives, and compromising. Staking positions produces debate over the relative merits of specific alternatives rather than consideration of the substance of the issue itself. Thus rational decision making, although highly desirable in principle, is difficult to obtain in practice, both because problems frequently do not fully satisfy the demands of rational problem-solving methods and because it is difficult for human problem solvers to adhere rigorously to the demands of rationality.

• • •

Each of these approaches to group problem solving—political, democratic, and rational—has inherent deficiencies. The political approach seeks to keep everyone happy at the expense of resolving the problem. The democratic approach makes decisions but runs the risk of sacrificing quality in the interests of resolution and equity. The rational approach makes a quality decision but only for those problems that satisfy strict conditions of information and theoretical understanding. Group processes that satisfy members' needs for participation and equitable treatment of their views and also produce quality decisions are difficult to sustain. These difficulties lead many persons to avoid groups altogether.

Approach used in individual problem solving

Advantages and disadvantages. Much traditional thought focuses on the individual professional—dentist, physician, manager—as a solitary figure, assuming full, personal responsibility for problem solving and for decision making. This "individual" approach to problem solving is appealing on several grounds: it clearly assigns the burden of responsibility; it is less time consuming and emotionally draining than the negotiating and bickering of group meetings; and, seemingly, it avoids the emotions and interpersonal tension that often accompanies the "win-lose" atmosphere of group discussion. There are, however, two major sets of considerations that limit the use of this approach. First, most human problem-solving situations are inherently of a group or joint nature in the sense that more than one person is involved in the problem, in the analysis, and in the implementation of solutions. Second, the problem-solving capabilities of the individual are limited by a complex of objective and psychological factors.

Limitations. Certain tendencies that are commonly observed in individual problem-solving behavior also suggest the desirability of joint effort. The limitations of individual efforts are most evident when the complexity of problems extends beyond the experience and information possessed by a single person. Less obvious are characteristic elements of cognitive behavior that may block the individual from using his or her resources to the fullest extent. The following three patterns are commonly observed.

1. *The tendency to equate old and new experiences.* Much of our cognitive life is devoted to synthesizing past experience in order to develop concepts and frameworks for analyzing new situations. The ability to recognize similarities between old and new situations and to apply past experiences is the essence of the learning process. Much of education is designed to equip us to handle new situations in the context of accumulated knowledge and experience. Thus we learn that the symptoms of incipient periodontal disease are such and such or that a patient who grips the arms of the chair will have to be dealt with differently from one who relaxes. Learning of this sort enables us to act in a given situation after a limited sampling of the total set of cues or stimuli available in the situation; we can behave efficiently because we do not have to treat each situation as totally new. We can behave effectively, however, only to the extent that the cues sampled provide an adequate picture of the similarities and differences between the present situation and past experiences with which we associate it. Identical symptoms in patients with different histories may stem from different underlying sources. Past experience, whether individual or the accumulation of an entire profession, is necessarily imperfect. An individual's experience is strongly influenced by the particular idiosyncratic set of cases that he or she has encountered. It is deceptively easy to see this set of cases as representing all possible cases and to force new situations to fit into this set of already learned categories. Joint problem solving is an effective mechanism for enlarging these sets of cues or symptoms and for bringing a broader range of experience and knowledge to bear on the problem.

2. *The tendency to begin with value judgments or preferred outcomes.* We all have strong values, well-developed skills that we enjoy using, and favorite interpretations of how the world really works. Thus the free market economist will find evidence in support of his or her viewpoint in the same situation that the proponent of a planned economy interprets as supporting his or her position. Similarly, educators will tend to seek out situations that require teaching skills and, more importantly, will tend to diagnose a need for educational solutions to cure most problems. The cue-sampling process previously described is influenced by preference as well as by learning. There is a tendency to look for evidence that supports our beliefs or suits our expectations—for problems that fit our favorite solution, that are consistent with our beliefs and theories, and that allow us to exercise skills for which we have been rewarded. Thus a dentist with skill in extracting teeth might overlook cues suggesting other forms of treatment; another dentist might habitually recommend orthodontic work. Much effort is extended in constructing analytical processes that justify solutions based on preferences or value judgments. Group efforts provide some insulation against the tendency to short-circuit the diagnostic process.

3. *The tendency to become locked into a particular solution or solution path.* We often find it difficult to "shift gears," to think of more than one way to approach solving a particular problem. We acknowledge the tendency to become locked into a particular approach in a number of ways; we speak of individuals who try the same solution over and over again unsuccessfully as "beating their heads against a wall" and make helpful suggestions that they "go at a problem in a different way." Anyone who has ever attempted to correct a 5-cent error in a checkbook balance by checking and rechecking calculations will recognize the frustration of repeating the same mistake over and over. It is difficult, however, to discard an initial insight or approach to a problem or to break out of a pattern established by early efforts. The more common response to an unsuccessful solution such as punishing a disobedient child is to apply "more of the same" solution, thus increasing the severity or duration of the punishment. In Chapter 19 when we dis-

cuss the younger dental patient, it should become clear that the problem-solving approach to pursue is to introduce deliberately an approach to child/patient management that the younger dental patient has probably not experienced previously. It is deceptively easy to follow *old* patterns in many situations. Thus if we initially diagnose the source of the patient's problems as psychological, it becomes increasingly difficult for us to recognize symptoms or to adopt approaches that indicate a physiological or genetic base. Bringing the perspective of more than one person to bear on the problem can help insulate against becoming locked into a single, unproductive approach.[3]

Conclusion—a comparison

To summarize, there are several informational, psychological, and environmental conditions that argue for the use of joint problem-solving techniques. They are as follows:

1. Groups can bring a greater sum of knowledge and information to a problem than any single individual and can circumvent deficiencies in individual information processes.
2. Group discussion can produce and identify a greater number of approaches to a given problem, and multiple perspectives provide some defense against inadequate sampling of significant cues and premature funneling and commitment to a single solution path.
3. Participation in the problem-solving effort increases the willingness of participants to accept the eventual solution, even when the participants may play different roles (dentist-expert, patient-implementer) in the process.
4. Group processes generally require a fuller, more extensive discussion of analysis and solution and can, therefore, produce a better understanding of conclusions.[2]

The fundamental question is not whether groups or individuals are more effective as problem solvers, but rather under what conditions or for what sort of problems are groups or individuals likely to be more effective. In the following exercise, you will have the opportunity to experience both group and individual problem-solving approaches to the same set of problems. This experience will provide a basis for deciding when groups are necessary, when groups are likely to be more effective than individuals, and what conditions must be met for groups to function effectively.

EXPERIENCE WITH GROUP AND INDIVIDUAL PROBLEM SOLVING*

This exercise provides opportunities to experience group problem solving both as a member of a problem-solving group and as an observer and to compare decisions made by individuals acting independently with decisions made by those same individuals acting as a group. Before the class begins, each member should read through carefully and reach a personal decision about each of the 12 problems in the exercise. Note that *for every problem* the lower choices in the scale (0 chances in 10, 1 chance in 10) indicate a greater willingness to accept risk—to accept the higher reward but also the potentially more dangerous or difficult alternative—than do the higher choices in the scale (9 chances in 10, 10 chances in 10). In the group meeting, the class will be broken into a series of small groups. Each small group will be asked to reach a group consensus on six of the problems in the exercise and to observe one of the other small groups

*From an exercise and problem set developed by Prof. James A. F. Stoner; used with permission.

performing a similar task. The entire class will then reconvene to discuss and evaluate observations.

Premeeting preparation

Read the 12 problems in the exercise carefully, and form an individual decision on each problem. Record your decision on a sheet of paper in the same format as the answer sheet provided with the exercise (below). Be prepared to discuss these problems again with a group of classmates for the group meeting.

INSTRUCTIONS

On the following pages you will find a series of situations that could occur in everyday life. The central person in each situation is faced with a choice between two courses of action. We want your opinion as to how desirable it is for the person to follow one of the two courses of action. Read each situation carefully before giving your opinion. Do not write in the book. Record your answers on a sheet of paper in the same format as the answer sheet on this page; the answer sheet will be collected at the beginning of the session.

Please do not discuss the material in this questionnaire with any of your colleagues.

ANSWER SHEET

Name ______________________________

Please follow the above instructions for the problems. However, instead of writing your answers in the space provided for each problem, record them on a sheet of paper in the following format.

This sheet will be collected at the beginning of the session.

Answers

1. Dr. A ____________	7. Mr. G ____________
2. Mr. B ____________	8. Mr. and Mrs. H ____________
3. Dr. C ____________	9. Mr. I ____________
4. Mr. D ____________	10. Leslie and Lee J ____________
5. Mr. E ____________	11. Mr. K ____________
6. Mr. F ____________	12. Mr. L ____________

Do not forget to write your name in the space provided.

1. Dr. A, a 45-year-old dentist with two children in high school, has recently been informed by his physician that he has a partially plugged artery (sclerosis) in his right arm. The condition causes continuous severe pain, but he is able to carry out his work with no reduction in skill. The physician informs Dr. A that there is a new surgical operation that, if successful, would completely relieve the condition. If the operation failed, his hand would be left useless, and it would be impossible for him to go on with his work as a dentist.

Imagine that you are advising Dr. A. Several probabilities or odds that the operation will prove successful follow. **Please check the lowest probability that you would consider acceptable for the operation to be performed.**

_____ The chances are 0 in 10 that the operation will be a success, that is, the operation is certain to be a failure.
_____ The chances are 1 in 10 that the operation will be a success.
_____ The chances are 2 in 10 that the operation will be a success.
_____ The chances are 3 in 10 that the operation will be a success.
_____ The chances are 4 in 10 that the operation will be a success.
_____ The chances are 5 in 10 that the operation will be a success.
_____ The chances are 6 in 10 that the operation will be a success.
_____ The chances are 7 in 10 that the operation will be a success.
_____ The chances are 8 in 10 that the operation will be a success.
_____ The chances are 9 in 10 that the operation will be a success.
_____ The chances are 10 in 10 that the operation will be a success, that is, the operation is certain to be a success.

2. Mr. B is about to board a plane at the airport to begin his overseas vacation. Although he has been looking forward to this trip for some time, he is troubled because he awoke in the morning with a severe abdominal pain. Because he has never flown before, he thinks that the pain may simply be an upset stomach brought on by anticipation of the flight. Although he is not far from a hospital where he knows he would obtain quick attention, he realizes that a visit to the hospital would cause him to miss his flight, which, in turn, would seriously disrupt his vacation plans. The pain has gotten more severe in the last few minutes.

Imagine that you are advising Mr. B. Several probabilities or odds that Mr. B's adbominal pains will *not* become more severe during his trip follow. **Please check the lowest probability that you would consider acceptable for him to board the plane.**

_____ The chances are 0 in 10 that Mr. B's abdominal pains will *not* become more severe during the trip, that is, the pains are certain to become more severe.
_____ The chances are 1 in 10 that Mr. B's abdominal pains will *not* become more severe during the trip.
_____ The chances are 2 in 10 that Mr. B's abdominal pains will *not* become more severe during the trip.
_____ The chances are 3 in 10 that Mr. B's abdominal pains will *not* become more severe during the trip.

_____ The chances are 4 in 10 that Mr. B's abdominal pains will *not* become more severe during the trip.
_____ The chances are 5 in 10 that Mr. B's abdominal pains will *not* become more severe during the trip.
_____ The chances are 6 in 10 that Mr. B's abdominal pains will *not* become more severe during the trip.
_____ The chances are 7 in 10 that Mr. B's abdominal pains will *not* become more severe during the trip.
_____ The chances are 8 in 10 that Mr. B's abdominal pains will *not* become more severe during the trip.
_____ The chances are 9 in 10 that Mr. B's abdominal pains will *not* become more severe during the trip.
_____ The chances are 10 in 10 that Mr. B's abdominal pains will *not* become more severe during the trip, that is, the pains are certain not to become more severe.

3. Dr. C has recently received his doctor of medicine degree. He plans to pursue a career in medical research. Because of the high quality of his academic work, he realizes that he will be able to obtain a substantial grant for virtually any promising research project he wishes to undertake. Two very different projects have occurred to him during the course of his studies. Both projects will take from 5 to 10 years to complete. The first project has many separable components, and Dr. C can be assured that with his capabilities he will be successful in developing enough of the components to establish for himself a substantial reputation in his field as well as related financial benefits. There will be some net benefit to the practice of medicine from this project, but the related discoveries are not likely to be of major importance. The second project is likely to be either a complete success or a complete failure. If successful, the project will lead to a cure for a crippling disease that leaves children blind and mentally retarded.

Imagine that you are advising Dr. C. Several probabilities or odds that the second project (the one involving the crippling disease) will be a success follow. **Please check the lowest probability of success that you would consider acceptable to make it worthwhile for Mr. C to undertake the second project.**

_____ The chances are 0 in 10 that the second project, the one involving the crippling disease, will be a success, that is, the project is certain to be a failure.
_____ The chances are 1 in 10 that the second project will be a success.
_____ The chances are 2 in 10 that the second project will be a success.
_____ The chances are 3 in 10 that the second project will be a success.
_____ The chances are 4 in 10 that the second project will be a success.
_____ The chances are 5 in 10 that the second project will be a success.
_____ The chances are 6 in 10 that the second project will be a success.
_____ The chances are 7 in 10 that the second project will be a success.
_____ The chances are 8 in 10 that the second project will be a success.

_____ The chances are 9 in 10 that the second project will be a success.
_____ The chances are 10 in 10 that the second project, the one involving the crippling disease, will be a success, that is, the project is certain to be a success.

4. Mr. D, an electrical engineer who is married and has one child, has been working for a large electronics corporation since graduating from college 5 years ago. He is assured of a lifetime job with a modest, although adequate, salary and liberal pension benefits on retirement. On the other hand, it is very unlikely that his salary will increase much before he retires. While attending a convention, Mr. D is offered a job with a small, newly founded company with a highly uncertain future. The new job would pay more to start and would offer the possibility of a share in the ownership if the company survived the competition of the larger firms.

Imagine that you are advising Mr. D. Several probabilities or odds of the new company's proving financially sound follow. **Please check the lowest probability that you would consider acceptable to make it worthwhile for Mr. D to take the new job.**

_____ The chances are 0 in 10 that the company will prove financially sound, that is, the company is certain to fail.
_____ The chances are 1 in 10 that the company will prove financially sound.
_____ The chances are 2 in 10 that the company will prove financially sound.
_____ The chances are 3 in 10 that the company will prove financially sound.
_____ The chances are 4 in 10 that the company will prove financially sound.
_____ The chances are 5 in 10 that the company will prove financially sound.
_____ The chances are 6 in 10 that the company will prove financially sound.
_____ The chances are 7 in 10 that the company will prove financially sound.
_____ The chances are 8 in 10 that the company will prove financially sound.
_____ The chances are 9 in 10 that the company will prove financially sound.
_____ The chances are 10 in 10 that the company will prove financially sound, that is, the company is certain not to fail.

5. Mr. E, a competent chess player, is participating in a national chess tournament. In an early match he draws the top-favored player in the tournament as his opponent. Mr. E has been given a relatively low ranking in view of his performance in previous tournaments. During the course of his play with the top-favored man, Mr. E notes the possibility of a deceptive, although risky, maneuver that might bring him quick victory. At the same time, if the attempted maneuver should fail, Mr. E would be left in an exposed position, and defeat would almost certainly follow.

Imagine that you are advising Mr. E. Several probabilities or odds that Mr. E's deceptive play would succeed follow. **Please check the lowest probability that you would consider acceptable for the risky play in question to be attempted.**

_____ The chances are 0 in 10 that the play would succeed, that is, the play is certain to fail.
_____ The chances are 1 in 10 that the play would succeed.

_____ The chances are 2 in 10 that the play would succeed.
_____ The chances are 3 in 10 that the play would succeed.
_____ The chances are 4 in 10 that the play would succeed.
_____ The chances are 5 in 10 that the play would succeed.
_____ The chances are 6 in 10 that the play would succeed.
_____ The chances are 7 in 10 that the play would succeed.
_____ The chances are 8 in 10 that the play would succeed.
_____ The chances are 9 in 10 that the play would succeed.
_____ The chances are 10 in 10 that the play would succeed, that is, the play is certain to succeed.

6. Mr. F is considering taking his family to Europe for a summer vacation. He has a well-paying job and has recently received a promotion. He realizes that the promotion indicates that he is likely but not certain to experience similar advancement in the years ahead. He has two sons who will be of college age in a few years. A number of years ago Mr. F started a savings account to finance his sons' education. He now recognizes that if his promotion possibilities are realized, he will have no trouble at all in financing his sons' college costs out of his earnings at that time. He and his wife have always wanted to make a family visit to Europe but have never had the spare cash to enable them to make the trip. Mr. F realizes that with the increased responsibilities associated with his promotion, it will be many years before he will have another opportunity to make the trip.

Imagine that you are advising Mr. F. Several probabilities or odds that Mr. F's promotion possibilities will be realized follow. **Please check the lowest probability that you would consider acceptable for Mr. F to take the European trip.**

_____ The chances are 0 in 10 that Mr. F's promotion possibilities will be realized, that is, it is certain that they will not be realized.
_____ The chances are 1 in 10 that Mr. F's promotion possibilities will be realized.
_____ The chances are 2 in 10 that Mr. F's promotion possibilities will be realized.
_____ The chances are 3 in 10 that Mr. F's promotion possibilities will be realized.
_____ The chances are 4 in 10 that Mr. F's promotion possibilities will be realized.
_____ The chances are 5 in 10 that Mr. F's promotion possibilities will be realized.
_____ The chances are 6 in 10 that Mr. F's promotion possibilities will be realized.
_____ The chances are 7 in 10 that Mr. F's promotion possibilities will be realized.
_____ The chances are 8 in 10 that Mr. F's promotion possibilities will be realized.
_____ The chances are 9 in 10 that Mr. F's promotion possibilities will be realized.
_____ The chances are 10 in 10 that Mr. F's promotion possibilities will be realized, that is, it is certain that they will be realized.

7. Mr. G is currently a college senior who is very eager to pursue graduate study in chemistry leading to the doctor of philosophy degree. He has been accepted by both University X and University Y. University X has a worldwide reputation for excellence in chemistry. Although a degree from University X would signify outstanding training in this field, the standards are so very rigorous that only a fraction of the degree candidates actually receive the degree. University Y, on the other hand, has much less of a reputation in

chemistry, but almost everyone admitted is awarded the doctoral degree, although the degree has much less prestige than the corresponding degree from University X.

Imagine that you are advising Mr. G. Several probabilities or odds that Mr. G. would be awarded a degree at University X, the one with the greater prestige, follow. **Please check the lowest probability that you would consider acceptable to make it worthwhile for Mr. G to enroll in University X rather than University Y.**

_____ The chances are 0 in 10 that Mr. G would receive a degree from University X, that is, it is certain that Mr. G would *not* receive a degree from University X.

_____ The chances are 1 in 10 that Mr. G would receive a degree from University X.

_____ The chances are 2 in 10 that Mr. G would receive a degree from University X.

_____ The chances are 3 in 10 that Mr. G would receive a degree from University X.

_____ The chances are 4 in 10 that Mr. G would receive a degree from University X.

_____ The chances are 5 in 10 that Mr. G would receive a degree from University X.

_____ The chances are 6 in 10 that Mr. G would receive a degree from University X.

_____ The chances are 7 in 10 that Mr. G would receive a degree from University X.

_____ The chances are 8 in 10 that Mr. G would receive a degree from University X.

_____ The chances are 9 in 10 that Mr. G would receive a degree from University X.

_____ The chances are 10 in 10 that Mr. G would receive a degree from University X, that is, it is certain that Mr. G would receive a degree from University X.

8. Mr. and Mrs. H have been attempting to have a child for a number of years. Mrs. H is now pregnant, but a complication has arisen. The physician has advised Mr. and Mrs. H that if the pregnancy is allowed to progress, Mrs. H's life will be in danger. If further complications do develop, the physician will not be able to save the child and may not be able to save Mrs. H. If the pregnancy is terminated at this time, it will be impossible for Mrs. H to become pregnant again.

Imagine that you are advising Mr. and Mrs. H. Several probabilities or odds that no further complications will occur during Mrs. H's pregnancy follow. **Please check the lowest probability of the occurrence of no additional complications that you would consider acceptable for Mr. and Mrs. H to allow the pregnancy to progress.**

_____The chances are 0 in 10 that further complications will *not* arise, that is, it is certain that further complications *will* arise.
_____The chances are 1 in 10 that further complications will *not* arise.
_____The chances are 2 in 10 that further complications will *not* arise.
_____The chances are 3 in 10 that further complications will *not* arise.
_____The chances are 4 in 10 that further complications will *not* arise.
_____The chances are 5 in 10 that further complications will *not* arise.
_____The chances are 6 in 10 that further complications will *not* arise.
_____The chances are 7 in 10 that further complications will *not* arise.
_____The chances are 8 in 10 that further complications will *not* arise.
_____The chances are 9 in 10 that further complications will *not* arise.
_____The chances are 10 in 10 that further complications will *not* arise, that is, it is certain that further complications will *not* arise.

9. Mr. I is the captain of College X's football team. College X is playing its traditional rival, College Y, in the final game of the season. The game is in its final seconds, and Mr. I's team, College X, is behind in the score. College X has time to run one more play. Mr. I, the captain, must decide whether it is best to settle for a tie score with a play that would be almost certain to work or, on the other hand, should he try a more complicated and risky play that would bring victory if it succeeded, but defeat if not.

Imagine that you are advising Mr. I. Several probabilities or odds that the risky play will work follow. **Please check the lowest probability that you would consider acceptable for the play to be attempted.**

_____The chances are 0 in 10 that the risky play will work, that is, the risky play is certain to fail.
_____The chances are 1 in 10 that the risky play will work.
_____The chances are 2 in 10 that the risky play will work.
_____The chances are 3 in 10 that the risky play will work.
_____The chances are 4 in 10 that the risky play will work.
_____The chances are 5 in 10 that the risky play will work.
_____The chances are 6 in 10 that the risky play will work.
_____The chances are 7 in 10 that the risky play will work.
_____The chances are 8 in 10 that the risky play will work.
_____The chances are 9 in 10 that the risky play will work.
_____The chances are 10 in 10 that the risky play will work, that is, the risky play is certain to succeed.

10. Leslie and Lee J, who both have doctor of medicine degrees, are taking an airplane flight to South America with their only child. During the flight, engine trouble develops, and the plane is forced down at sea. As the plane crashes, the family is thrown into the water, but only Leslie retains consciousness. The child and Lee are unconscious in the water and will drown if they are not rescued immediately. Leslie must decide whether to attempt to rescue Lee or the child first. If Leslie attempts to rescue the child first, there will be no possibility of failure; but by the time the child has been rescued, it will be too late to attempt to save Lee. On the other hand, if Leslie attempts to save

Lee first and the child afterwards there are two possible outcomes: either both Lee and the child will be saved or both will be lost. No matter which decision is made (whether to attempt to save only the child, with no chance of failure, or to attempt to save both Lee and the child, with the chance that both will be lost), there will be no danger to Leslie.

Imagine that you are advising Leslie. Several probabilities or odds that Leslie will be successful in rescuing both Lee and the child follow. **Please check the lowest probability that you would consider acceptable for Leslie to attempt the double rescue (instead of simply rescuing the child).**

_____The chances are 0 in 10 that Leslie will succeed in rescuing both Lee and the child, that is, Leslie is certain to fail and both Lee and the child will drown if an attempt is made to rescue Lee first.
_____The chances are 1 in 10 that Leslie will succeed in rescuing both Lee and the child.
_____The chances are 2 in 10 that Leslie will succeed in rescuing both Lee and the child.
_____The chances are 3 in 10 that Leslie will succeed in rescuing both Lee and the child.
_____The chances are 4 in 10 that Leslie will succeed in rescuing both Lee and the child.
_____The chances are 5 in 10 that Leslie will succeed in rescuing both Lee and the child.
_____The chances are 6 in 10 that Leslie will succeed in rescuing both Lee and the child.
_____The chances are 7 in 10 that Leslie will succeed in rescuing both Lee and the child.
_____The chances are 8 in 10 that Leslie will succeed in rescuing both Lee and the child.
_____The chances are 9 in 10 that Leslie will succeed in rescuing both Lee and the child.
_____The chances are 10 in 10 that Leslie will succeed in rescuing both Lee and the child, that is, Leslie is certain to rescue both Lee and the child.

11. Mr. K has a well-paying job with a large company. He has been married for 6 months, and his wife has just become pregnant. For a number of years, he has spent many of his summer weekends racing sports cars. He enjoys the sport very much. He is a good driver, and although he races purely for the excitement and fun of the sport, he does win enough to cover all his racing expenses. Mr. K has never been in a racing accident but realizes that such accidents, although rarely fatal for the type of races he enters, can still be quite serious. He is deciding whether or not to give up racing.

Imagine that you are advising Mr. K. Several probabilities or odds that Mr. K will *not* be involved in any racing accidents if he continues to pursue the sport follow. **Please check the lowest probability that you would consider acceptable for Mr. K to continue to race.**

_____The chances are 0 in 10 that Mr. K will *not* be involved in any racing accidents, that is, it is certain that he will be involved in racing accidents.
_____The chances are 1 in 10 that Mr. K will *not* be involved in any racing accidents.
_____The chances are 2 in 10 that Mr. K will *not* be involved in any racing accidents.
_____The chances are 3 in 10 that Mr. K will *not* be involved in any racing accidents.
_____The chances are 4 in 10 that Mr. K will *not* be involved in any racing accidents.
_____The chances are 5 in 10 that Mr. K will *not* be involved in any racing accidents.
_____The chances are 6 in 10 that Mr. K will *not* be involved in any racing accidents.
_____The chances are 7 in 10 that Mr. K will *not* be involved in any racing accidents.
_____The chances are 8 in 10 that Mr. K will *not* be involved in any racing accidents.
_____The chances are 9 in 10 that Mr. K will *not* be involved in any racing accidents.
_____The chances are 10 in 10 that Mr. K will *not* be involved in any racing accidents, that is, it is certain that he will *not* be involved in racing accidents.

12. Mr. L, a married man with two children of school age, has a secure job that pays him about $12,000 per year. He can easily afford the necessities of life but few of the luxuries. Except for a life insurance policy, he has no savings. Mr. L has heard from reliable sources that the stock of relatively unknown Company X might triple its present value if a new product currently in production is favorably received by the buying public. On the other hand, if the product is unfavorably received, the stock might decline considerably in value. Mr. L is considering investing in this company. He can raise $10,000 on his life insurance policy.

Imagine that you are advising Mr. L. Several probabilities or odds that the stock of Company X will triple in value follow. **Please check the lowest probability that you would consider acceptable for Mr. L to invest in Company X stock.**

_____The chances are 0 in 10 that the stock will triple in value, that is, there is *no* chance that the stock will triple in value.
_____The chances are 1 in 10 that the stock will triple in value.
_____The chances are 2 in 10 that the stock will triple in value.
_____The chances are 3 in 10 that the stock will triple in value.
_____The chances are 4 in 10 that the stock will triple in value.
_____The chances are 5 in 10 that the stock will triple in value.
_____The chances are 6 in 10 that the stock will triple in value.
_____The chances are 7 in 10 that the stock will triple in value.
_____The chances are 8 in 10 that the stock will triple in value.

GROUP DECISION-MAKING INSTRUCTIONS

Consensus

Consensus is difficult to reach. Complete unanimity is not the goal—it is rarely achieved. However, each individual should be able to *accept* the group rankings on the basis of logic and feasibility. When all group members feel this way, you have reached consensus as defined here, and the judgment may be entered as a group decision.

Guidelines

1. Avoid arguing for your own ranking. Present your position clearly, *and* listen to the other members' reactions.
2. Do not assume that someone must win and someone must lose. Look for the next most acceptable alternative for all parties.
3. Do not change your mind simply to avoid conflict and to reach agreement and harmony.
4. Avoid conflict-reducing techniques such as majority vote.
5. Differences of opinion are natural and expected.

_____ The chances are 9 in 10 that the stock will triple in value.
_____ The chances are 10 in 10 that the stock will triple in value, that is, the stock is certain to triple in value.

Procedure for the small group meeting

Phase 1 (approximate time—30 to 40 minutes)

1. The class should be divided into small groups. There should be an even number of small groups with, whenever possible, five to seven members in each group.
2. Each group should be assigned a number. The members of each group should place their group number at the top of their answer sheet and hand the answer sheet in to the instructor. While the small group discussions are going on, the instructor should compute the average response of the members of *each* small group to the 12 problems. These averages will be used later in the group discussion to compare group decisions with the average of the initial positions of the members.
3. In phase 1 of the exercise, the *odd*-numbered groups should seat themselves in a small circle. The task of each of the odd-numbered groups will be to reach a consensual group decision on problems one through six (inclusive). In their discussion, the group should follow the above guidelines for group decision making. A record should be kept of the group's final decision on each problem, which should be given to the instructor at the end of the discussion.
4. While the odd-numbered groups are discussing problems one through six, each of the *even*-numbered groups should sit in a larger circle around the discussion group and observe the problem-solving process. Thus group two would observe group one, group four would observe group three, etc. The observers should use the points outlined in the guide for observers, p. 139, and should make note as to important aspects of the problem-solving group's be-

GUIDE FOR OBSERVERS

1. How were decisions actually made?
2. Did the group adopt a procedure? What and how?
3. Was there a leader? Formally selected or emergent? What was the leader's task, behavior, influence?
4. How were "irreconcilable" disagreements, if any, handled?
5. Were there deviants? How were they treated?
6. What did you learn about your group decision-making style? About recognizing and dealing with the styles of others?
7. How do you feel about the decisions your group made? Would you now make a better individual decision?

havior. Observers may not take part in the discussion and should remain silent throughout.

Phase 2 (approximate time—30 to 40 minutes)

1. At the end of phase 1 of the exercise, each pair of groups should switch roles. Thus the even-numbered groups would move to the inner circle and the odd-numbered groups would move to the outer circle. The task for the even-numbered groups will be to reach a consensus on problems seven through twelve (inclusive); the odd-numbered groups should now act as observers. Thus group one would observe group two, group three would observe group four, etc.

Procedure for the large group discussion

When both problem-solving rounds have been completed, the entire class should reconvene to discuss the exercise. Each group should be given an opportunity to comment on the problem-solving behaviors of the group it observed. The points listed in the guide for observers (above) provide a useful basis for beginning this discussion. It may be helpful to list critical points of the processes adopted by each small group on a blackboard or easel chart for comparison.

After a thorough discussion of the problem-solving processes employed, the group should then turn to a consideration of the decisions made by the small groups. The instructor should place the initial average decisions of the groups on a blackboard alongside the final group decisions. The following questions could be used to guide this discussion:

- Do groups tend to make more or less risky decisions than individuals acting independently?
- Are there sharp differences between group and individual decisions? On what sorts of problems? Are any patterns evident?
- What can be learned from the pattern of decisions about the conditions under which problems should be assigned to individuals or to a group?

SUMMARY

Working with other people in seeking solutions to complex human problems can be a rewarding process, particularly if these individuals bring to the discussion new information, insights, and experience from which we can learn and increase our own competence. Participating in groups—whether the group involves the dentist and the patient, co-workers, or other dentists—can also be frustrating, however, as we are often delayed or prevented from implementing our own solutions by the need to gain the acceptance of others. The skills needed to participate effectively in groups do not come naturally to most of us, and it is difficult to mold a group of individuals into an effective problem-solving unit. Kolb et al. point this out as follows:

> . . . it is foolhardy to assume that simply because a group of people assemble to perform a task, they will somehow automatically know how to work together effectively. A comparison between the behavior of a football team and the behavior of a management team highlights the essence of this paradox. The football team spends untold hours practicing team work in preparation for the sixty minutes each week that their performance as a team really counts. In contrast most management teams do not spend sixty minutes per year practicing teamwork in spite of the fact that for forty or more hours every week their behavior as a team really counts.*

This analogy holds equally well for the dentist engaged in joint problem solving with patients, hygienists, and assistants or other dentists with whom he or she consults. Although technical skills are subjected to continual practice and refinement, very little conscious attention and effort are directed toward developing the skills necessary for effective group interaction.

*From Kolb, Rubin, McIntyre, ORGANIZATIONAL PSYCHOLOGY: An Experiential Approach, 2nd edition, © 1974, pp. 23, 25, 27, 28, and pages for the submitted text. Reprinted by permission of Prentice-Hall, Inc., Englewood Cliffs, New Jersey.

Functions necessary for effective group performance

The following three principal functions must be satisfied if the group is going to perform effectively:

task competence Skills and information necessary for the adequate performance of the group task must be present within the group.

process The group should be self-consciously aware of and agree to the procedures to be used in organizing itself and working on its task.

maintenance The group must be aware of and willing to respond to the emotions and needs of the members of the group in order to preserve commitments to the group and its actions.

In the group experience that you have just completed, you have had the opportunity to observe the performance of task, process, and maintenance functions. Most likely, your group devoted most of its attention to task concerns, that is, to moving quickly and aggressively to decisions on each of the problems that the group considered. The procedures that your group used to solicit opinions, generate information, discuss differences, and reach an eventual decision were probably not explicitly adopted by the group before it began working on its task. In most new groups, process issues are not raised, and procedures develop randomly; in many groups, members are either unable to describe the procedures they are using or the description of different members is inconsistent. Finally, if your group was similar to most new groups, very little attention was paid to the feelings of its members, particularly those members whose position on some problems may have differed sharply from the majority of the group.

Your group worked on a frustrating and challenging set of problems for which there are no ready answers; problems that made strong demands on your knowledge, your beliefs, and your values. These are particularly difficult issues to discuss with others whose attitudes or values may differ sharply from your own. Reaching a common decision can often be a stress-producing process. In the exercise, your ability to express your own basic values and ideas clearly; to persuade others of the rightness of your viewpoint; and, most importantly, to respond and work with their needs have been tested. If your views prevailed in much of the discussion, you may be feeling pleased with the group experience; if, on the other hand, your views were not reflected in the group decision, you may be feeling considerable irritation and tension. You may want to sort out your feelings about how your opinions were handled in the discussion with the members of your group. You may also want to take the time now to learn and explore their feelings.

Task competence functions. The particular task that you were asked to perform has an interesting history. The usefulness of groups for problem solving has long been a controversial and emotionally charged topic. Proponents of group methods have stressed the innovativeness, creativity, and flexibility of group discussions; in this view, groups are able to avoid becoming "locked in" to individual thought patterns. The interaction of a group of capable people in a joint problem-solving situation is presumed to produce output that exceeds the capabilities of any of those individuals acting independently. The use of "brainstorming" groups in advertising and research organizations as catalysts to creativity is a direct application of this perspective.

At the same time that brainstorming groups were attracting attention as sources of innovation, critics were pointing to the growing use of committees as a prime source of mediocrity and stagnation in many organizations. These critics of "committeeitis" asserted that the group process produced conformity rather than creativity by forcing members to subject their individuality to the need to find solutions that would satisfy everyone, that is, to "least common denominators." This fear that groups are a threat to individuality and quality performance was expressed succintly by the head of a major consulting firm: "Groups are more cautious than individuals and cannot be used for decision making for that reason."

These two positions, argued with equal vigor by their proponents, are naturally perplexing to the individual looking for an effective problem-solving method. Creativity and the willingness to accept risk are important aspects of problem solving. The set of problems that you have just worked through were designed to research differences between groups and individuals on these dimensions.

The accumulation of data from hundreds of groups like yours reveals a complex pattern of relationships in the willingness to take risk in individual and group problem solvers. If you consider the difference between the average response of individual group members before the meeting and the eventual group decision, you will notice for several of the problems that the group decision was riskier, that is, the group was willing to accept a lower probability of success than the average of the individuals. For example, groups' decisions are usually riskier in the problems dealing with choice of research project (3), chess (5), and the choice of a doctoral degree program (7). This pattern of responses has been repeated across a wide variety of groups and an equally wide range of research settings. The explanations that have been offered for this phenomenon include the notion that the group environment provides for sharing of responsibility, allowing each person to absolve himself or herself for personal accountability for the decision. Other explanations suggest that the group discussion brought more information to bear on the question, that information generally supported a riskier position, or that the group situation aroused social values that supported a riskier approach.

However, this so-called risky shift did not occur for all problems. A closer examination of the data revealed that certain problems produced cautious shifts, that is, groups insisting on higher odds than the average of individuals. This second set of problems had the distinctive characteristic of dealing with essentially life-and-death choices. Examples from this set included the possibility of abortion (8), the amateur automobile racer (11), and the investment of life savings in a new business venture (12).

After considering the critical differences between risky and cautious problems, researchers have been able to write questions that would predictably produce either cautious or risky shifts. This has led to a different position on the potential for groups producing creative or risky solutions. Rather than being inherently risky or conservative, it seems that group performance is controlled by values present in the particular situation at hand. Although there does seem to be evidence suggesting that there is a general value in our society placed on taking chances (being risky), this general disposition seems to be tempered in situations having serious and permanent physical consequences for individuals. Thus groups do tend to be cautious in life-and-death situations.

In general, however, groups will tend to be either more risky or more cautious than the average individual, that is, groups are less prone to tread the middle ground. The explanation for this seems to lie in the dynamics of group discussions. Those members of a group who would generally tend to hold extreme positions on either side of an issue tend to be more committed, more ego involved, more focused on value issues, and more certain of their opinion than their fellows who started from a more balanced perspective. Thus these individuals tend to be more vigorous participants in the discussion and to pull the eventual decision toward one extreme or another.[1] The willingness to take a risk is, of course, only one dimension of the problem-solving process.

Process functions. This examination of the task your group has just performed is also important for highlighting the influence of process on group output. The way in which a group organizes itself to perform its task will have a major effect on the content and quality of the group output and on the willingness of group members to commit themselves to the implementation of that output. For a group that must function over time, for example, a committee that must meet regularly, a dental practice team, or even a dentist and a patient, the development of an agreed on set of procedures for doing the group's work is critical to success. Process issues may be grouped in the following four main categories:

1. *Explicit development of a procedure to get the work done.* Individuals brought together to form a group typically move directly to the task at hand without devoting conscious time and effort to the identification of an explicit procedure for dealing with that task. Groups can often function for a long time without consciously considering process issues. Questions of procedure normally do not infringe on the group's working time until an individual member complains that "I don't like the way we're doing things. I don't think that my opinions are being given a fair chance." When such an outburst occurs, groups are forced to attend to process issues. The attention is often defensive, designed to calm the protesting member with the assurance that "Everyone else is happy with the way we're doing things; let's get back to work." It takes persistence to force a functioning group to attend explicitly to the way it has organized itself to do its work.

To avoid outbursts from frustrated members, accusations that decisions were reached without the full consideration of all important factors, or "wheelspinning" that does not lead to conclusions, groups are well advised at the beginning of their work together to devote time to developing an identifiable process. Further, it is sensible for groups to devote time in future meetings to evaluating the effectiveness of the process in the light of past experience. Although the argument that "We are too busy with the task at hand to devote time to such abstract matters as process" is often made by busy, pressured groups, the adoption of explicit processes will generally improve the quality and efficiency of task performance and increase individual members' sense of fair and equitable participation.

2. *Leadership*. Leadership as applied to groups can be a confusing and complex subject. Generally in a group discussion there are many leadership roles to be performed. Among the most common are those of organizer, influencer, and mediator.

The **organizer** is typically that individual or individuals in the group who is either assigned or assumes responsibility for keeping the group focused on the task it is seeking to perform and for ensuring that the group follows the process or procedures it has established. Thus the organizer role is primarily a structure and process role. The organizer may or may not have a stake in the particular decision or outcome, that is, he or she may or may not be a partisan of a particular viewpoint. The organizer does, however, play the essential role of keeping the group focused on its task and on its commitment to itself as a group.

The **influencer** plays a more familiar leadership role. The influencer has a stake in the outcome of the process, that is, he or she is a partisan on a particular issue and exercises leadership efforts in seeking to persuade others to accept a particular viewpoint.

The **mediator** is more concerned with the personal feelings and relations among members of the group. The mediator is often more concerned with the continuance of the group over time and with the commitment of members to each other and to the group than he or she is with the particular issue at hand. Although the mediator and the organizer may seem to play similar roles and, in many groups, may well be the same person, the concerns are clearly different. The mediator would be quite willing to waive process or to take time away from task performance in order to soothe the injured feelings of a group member.

These three leadership roles are present in any effective group. Different members may play each of the roles at different periods of time. In most groups, only the organizer is specifically identified, although he or she may not be the person with the greatest formal authority in the group. In fact, it is often difficult for an organizer to play the role of influencer, as this can be seen as an abuse of position. All three roles are essential to effective performance—the organizer to keep the group on track, the influencer to bring about a decision, and the mediator to keep the group together to deal with the next task.

3. *Decision-making method*. Numerous groups move directly to their problem-solving task without considering exclusively how they will make a final decision. As alternatives emerge, the group is often uncertain whether to make a choice through voting, through continuing discussion, through a consensus, or through some other method. Decision-making procedures should be identified as part of the self-conscious development process and should be consistent with the nature of the problem with which the group is dealing and the particular demands for implementing solutions. Thus although voting is an almost reflexive response in our society in most situations involving choice, it is not at all clear that the "one person—one vote" system is the best way to deal with problems in which there are different degrees of knowledge in the group or where all members of a group must participate enthusiastically in the implementation of the decision. Voting, particularly as a means for terminating discussion, produces winners and losers, and it is often difficult for losers to put aside their feelings when the time comes to implement the decisions. Further, voting focuses attention on reaching a decision rather than on reaching the best decision and often prematurely terminates discussion that might lead to a fuller understanding of problem situations. Voting can be a desirable method, however, when there is need for immediate action, particularly when members of the group will not

be directly responsible for implementation. The important thing is that the group determine its decision-making procedures before turning to task performance.

4. *Group-building strategy.* All too often, groups not only move directly to task performance, but also take up the series of tasks as presented without any consideration for the development of the competence of the group. This point can be best demonstrated by considering the six problems that your small group has just completed solving. If you behaved like most groups, you worked on the problems one at a time, beginning with the first one presented and going sequentially to the last. This may be a logical approach to problems, but it does not reflect any concern for building the competence of your group. A more reasonable approach, from the team-building point of view, would be to consider the entire set of problems that your group had to deal with, identify positions and potential areas of conflict within each of these problems, and then begin by working on those problems on which there seems to be the greatest amount of agreement within the group. By dealing with "easier" problems first, the group can build a pattern of success, that is, a feeling that "We are a pretty good group and we get things done," that can facilitate dealing with more difficult, divisive problems later. This "success experience" provides a sense of commitment to the group as a whole and to the working out of points of conflict. By allowing process considerations to control the allocation of group efforts rather than simply reacting to externally presented events, the group can greatly enhance its sense of confidence and competence.

In summary, group problem solving is enhanced when the group does as follows:

- Spends time identifying a specific procedure by which the work will get done
- Recognizes that it is helpful to have members who function as organizers, influencers, and/or mediators
- Specifies how a final decision will be made *before* moving to task performance
- Builds competence in the group by starting with "easier" problems before tackling more difficult issues

The previous points are samples of the process issues that a group might consider before turning to task performance; these same issues might be reviewed periodically in order to identify the ways to use experience to improve future performance.

Maintenance functions. In addition to direct task performance and the development of the problem-solving process procedures, groups must also attend to their general working atmosphere and continued effectiveness over time, that is, to group maintenance. Maintenance issues involve the general climate of the group. Is it a happy group? Do members respect and listen to each others' opinions? Are members aware of the effect of their actions and comments on the feelings of others? Is participation in the group a rewarding experience, and are members in the group motivated to put forth their best effort? Sensitivity to the opinions and feelings of others is particularly difficult to achieve in the heat of group discussions. As the discussion progresses, we become increasingly focused on the task at hand and, more particularly, on the defense of our own position. If our position prevails, we experience feelings of elation and accomplishment and are likely to look forward to the next group meeting. If our position does not prevail, we may feel frustrated, disappointed, or angered; these feelings will clearly color our subsequent participation in the group.

Although it is relatively easy to recognize these emotional reactions to the group experience in ourselves, it is much more difficult to be aware of and respond to the experience of others; we only discover well after the fact that another member has been angered or hurt by the outcome and tenor of the discussion. The most graphic example of the failure to attend to group maintenance functions is the manner in which groups deal with members who hold a deviant position on an issue. If a group has committed itself to consensual decision making and one member holds firmly to a position sharply different from that of the rest of the group, a great deal of tension is generated within the group. This "deviant" individual can be subjected to a great deal of pressure, which can have a substantial impact on the subsequent cohesion and effectiveness of the group. The typical treatment of deviant members adheres to the following identifiable pattern[5]:

1. Once divergent views have surfaced, the discussion generally begins with good will and a certain willingness to hear out the deviant view; however, the deviant member is also reminded of time and other constraints under which the group is operating.
2. Out of respect for a fellow group member, the majority typically *begins* with a commitment to reason, although often with the unspoken presumption that, after having ample time to air his or her position, the deviant member will bow to the will of the majority.
3. When reason fails to bring about agreement quickly, the next step is often to appeal to the deviant on emotional grounds, particularly those of loyalty to the group; the deviant is often accused of "putting himself before the good of the group."
4. If emotional appeals fail, the next step is often to offer a trade off or bargain of some sort; this may be jesting ("Go along on this one and we'll let you decide the next one").
5. If the deviant fails to respond to either emotional appeals or bargaining, the discussion begins to shift from the issues to the individual, and a variety of personal pressures are put on the deviant; he or she may be badgered for being stubborn for the sake of being stubborn. Gradually, such comments often shift from gentle persuasion to expressions of tension, anger, and frustration.
6. At some point, the majority typically becomes impatient and unwilling to spend further time to change the holdout's point of view and presents him or her with a choice of either going along with or leaving the group. Although this may produce a decision, it represents a clear failure to perform the group maintenance function effectively.

The maintenance of an effective problem-solving group is a delicate process, requiring a careful balancing of sensitivities, feelings, and needs of individuals with the need of the group to perform its tasks effectively and efficiently. Groups that are not sensitive to the needs of individual members and, particularly, that cannot tolerate deviant viewpoints, run the risk of losing the multiplicity of views and perspectives that is one of the major strengths of problem-solving groups.

Selecting an appropriate method of problem solving for a given task

This analysis of the essential task competence, process, and maintenance functions underscores the strengths and weaknesses of group approaches to problem solving. We may return now to the question with which we began: "When are groups likely to be more effective at problem solving than individuals"? The basic arguments are laid out in Fig. 10-1. As people responsible for problem solving, we may choose to assign a given problem to a single person, either ourselves or another, whom we feel has certain expertise. We may assign the same problem to several people, each working independently of the others, requesting each to present or develop a solution. The final solution could then be obtained either by averaging the efforts of these several people or by taking the best of their solutions. A group of individuals working independently is often called a "nominal" group. Finally, we may assign the problem to a group, of which we

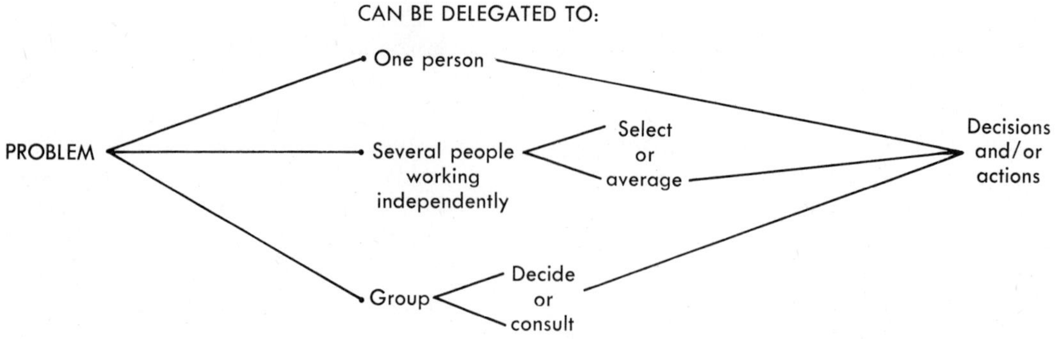

Fig. 10-1. Problem solving (alternatives) with groups or individuals.

may be a member. We may give this group authority to make decisions, or we may ask the group to serve as a consultant, providing us with options from which we may choose.

These options may be related specifically to dental practice; the dentist may treat a patient personally, he or she may refer the patient to a specialist, he or she may use a nominal group by seeking consulting opinions from several associates, or he or she may form a true group (including associates, staff, and/or patients) to analyze the situation. There are no hard and fast rules for choosing among these several options; the following guidelines are available, however:

1. For tasks involving random error such as the estimation of distances or the forecasting of random future events, nominal groups are most useful. The averaging of multiple, independent estimates will generally tend to increase accuracy. For example, public health officers often survey a large sample of practitioners in efforts to forecast the future dental needs of the population.
2. For tasks requiring creativity or recall and information, groups, either nominal or interacting, are more likely to produce a higher quality solution than any individual acting independently. It is for this reason that it is wise to seek consulting opinions from other practitioners and from researchers for patients who do not respond to normal treatment methods or who exhibit unusual combinations of symptoms. It should be noted in passing that a given individual may produce consistently better solutions than a group; the difficulty in practice is to identify that individual who is consistently better.
3. For tasks requiring duplication of effort or the division of labor, groups are consistently better than individuals. This is the basic argument for the use of hygienists, chair side assistants, and other staff auxiliaries in routine treatment procedures.
4. Interacting groups are particularly effective when successful implementation depends on the understanding, acceptance, and commitment of individuals to the solution. Thus the patient who is involved in the analysis of his or her dental problems and in the development of a program of personal dental care is more likely to implement that program effectively than is the patient who is given a set of instructions by the dentist.

• • •

In summary, groups and individuals have different strengths and weaknesses as problem-solving mechanisms. The choice of approach should be dictated more by the demand and concern of a particular problem than by any abstract commitment to one aspect or another. Each of us will frequently work in joint problem-solving situations, and it is essential to develop and sharpen our own skills in group participation as well as to understand the functions and conditions necessary for effective group behavior. The following chapters in Part two will further delineate concepts and skills helpful in functioning effectively in groups.

REFERENCES

1. Brown, R.: Social psychology. New York, 1965, The Free Press.
2. Collins, B., and Guetzkow, H.: Social psychology of group processes for decision-making, New York, 1964, John Wiley & Sons, Inc.
3. Hyman, R., and Anderson, B.: Solving problems, Sci. Technol., pp. 36-41, Sept., 1965.
4. Kolb, D. A., Rubin, I. M., and McIntyre, J. M.: Organizational psychology: an experiential approach, ed. 2, Englewood Cliffs, N.J., 1974, Prentice-Hall.
5. Leavitt, H. J.: Managerial psychology, ed. 3, Chicago, 1972, The University of Chicago Press.
6. Simon, H. A.: Administrative behavior, New York, 1957, Macmillan, Inc.

Chapter 11

CONFLICT

In the early 1950s in an action that was duplicated in hundreds of communities, the mayor of Northampton, Massachusetts, announced a plan to fluoridate the town's water supply.[4] The mayor was acting on the recommendation of a special study commission. The commission concluded that fluoridation would be a significant benefit to dental hygiene. Opposition to the plan quickly surfaced. Some researchers and scientists provided "expert opinions" that were at odds with the commission's "experts"; some community residents expressed fears about the side effects of fluoridation, whereas other residents expressed resentment about their exclusion from the policy-making process.

Pro- and antifluoridation groups coalesced through a series of public meetings and the generation of a considerable amount of statements, petitions, editorials, and pamphlets. Debates over the implications of data on the effects of fluoridation soon expanded, and the technical issues were often lost in the exchange of allegations and counterallegations. The motives, morality, and even the patriotism of individuals were challenged. Opponents of fluoridation came to see its proponents as mercenaries, serving the interests of big business, as dupes or conspirators in a Communist plot to drug the American people, or as both! Proponents were equally harsh in their view of the opponents, whom they saw as antiscientific know-nothings whose desire to resist change justified even the sacrifice of good health. Strong group loyalties were formed, and long-standing friendships were shattered as individuals took sides; even those who tried to remain neutral were criticized for their unwillingness to "stand up and be counted."

By the time the issue came up for a public referendum, the town was split into two warring camps. One's vote was cast not as a judicious conclusion reached after examination of the scientific issue but as an act of group loyalty. The referendum settled the initial issue in Northampton—fluoridation lost—but the scars of the controversy lingered on in personal animosities, in mistrust, and in "we/they" splits in the social structure.

Although present in most types of conflict, the development of personal hostility is particularly evident in intergroup or interpersonal competition that is characterized by incompatibility of goals. The consequences of interpersonal and intergroup conflict are particularly severe when the individuals or groups involved must continue to work together within a larger group or organization. It is difficult for individuals or groups to put aside emotions and convictions once an issue is settled and return to more amicable relations. This is true no matter how innocuous the issue and no matter how important cooperation is to the effectiveness of the total group. It is even more true when the loser in a pitched argument or a close vote has to participate in implementing the decision.

Winners tend to be even more cohesive and to retain their work orientations, but losers, after a period of remorse and bitterness and, perhaps, a change in leadership, tend to focus their attention on preparing for the next battle.[1] When winners and losers are members of the same family or work group, the performance of common tasks necessarily suffers as long as the effects of conflict are left unattended. When the common task involves service to a third party such as the patient caught up in conflict within the dental team, the costs of unresolved conflict can be considerable.

Conflict, whether between individuals, between groups, or between nations, is a complex process with consequences that endure beyond the initiating events. Because conflict has such important consequences and because it is an inevitability, understanding conflict and ways to manage it is the subject of this chapter.

OBJECTIVES

The objectives of this chapter are as follows:

1. To identify common sources of conflict that could occur in dentist-patient interactions
2. To practice your ability to diagnose patient's conditions in cooperation with other team members and to observe the effects of "win-lose" competition on intra- and intergroup cooperation and conflict
3. To identify means for resolving or managing interpersonal and group conflict

COMMON SOURCES OF CONFLICT

Incompatible goals or commitments

Much of the conflict between individuals and between groups can be traced to goal incompatibility. Two opposing football teams have the same goal (to win) but if one team achieves its goal, the other cannot. Conflict between individuals and groups is frequently a consequence of goal incompatibility. For example, what a group practice demands of an individual dentist in the pursuit of group practice goals such as working overtime may not be compatible with the individual's personal goals such as spending more time with the family. The group may expect 100% commitment that the individual member is not prepared to give.

Disagreement over means of achieving goals

Much intragroup conflict can be traced to differences in solutions or proposed courses of action. The conflict may stem from differences in analyses, theories, data, or experiences—but it "resides in an intellectual difference in beliefs about an issue. The issue is not emotional, but simply a difference in cognitive belief."* Even people who agree on ends or goals are likely to disagree on means.

Emotional focusing

In many conflicts objective differences in goals or means relevant to a specific issue are not apparent. Instead, an issue, often innocuous in itself, has become a lightning rod for focusing diffused, repressed, accumulated feelings of frustration, anger, and a sense of past injuries. Marriage counselors frequently deal with extremely acrimonious conflicts over objectively trivial issues; analysis usually reveals that these issues have acted as triggers for releasing long-suppressed tensions.

Even when conflict begins with rational disagreement over goals or courses of action, as in the fluoridation controversy, it is not long before emotional issues accumulate. This comes about in two ways. First, conflict is stimulating; it readily involves the emotions, generating dislike for the opposition and pride and loyalty for one's own side. Second, persons with emotional "axes to grind" are drawn to conflicts as

*From Leavitt, H. J., Dill, W. R., and Eyring, H. B.: The organizational world, New York, 1973, Harcourt Brace Jovanovich, Inc.

means of giving concrete expression to their dissatisfactions. Thus even the most rational debate can quickly be transformed into an emotionally charged conflict between persons or groups who may have lost sight of the initiating issue.

Competition for scarce resources

Our economic system is predicated on the principle of competition among participants for scarce resources such as wealth, power, and esteem. Competition is normally defined in terms of winning and losing. The profits or prizes gained by one individual or group are denied to the other. This "win-lose" atmosphere is often the norm in our society. We tend to perceive most situations in comparative terms—who is smarter, prettier, or more successful? Whose team, product, or community is better? Many people seem to feel that performance—in school, at home, or on the job—can be improved by pitting individuals or groups against each other. Thus the habit of competition is fostered by many childhood activities—striving for high grades and scholastic honors or for parental attention—and is generally maintained throughout life. Our devotion to athletics, as participants and even more so as spectators, gives testimony to the material and psychological attraction of competition.

Individuals, of course, vary in their tendency to perceive activities in competitive terms. Some people see everything in "win-lose" terms, whereas others look continually for possibilities for cooperation. Some view competition in highly personal, "we/they" terms—the competitor is the enemy—whereas others separate the competition for victory from their personal feelings about their opponents. The individual with a high need for achievement thrives on competing against self-imposed standards of excellence and feels little animosity or even conscious feeling toward other individuals in the race. Persons with a high need for power or affiliation are very much concerned with the personal and emotional aspects of competition, although perhaps in different ways.

Despite social norms and personal tendencies, however, not all situations are inherently competitive. In many cases, rewards are not limited, and cooperation may be a more effective way for individuals or groups to achieve their goals. Paradoxically, effective competition, especially at the group level, largely depends on cooperation. A football team will not be able to compete successfully if its members are more concerned with competing with each other for personal glory than with cooperating in the team effort.

What determines whether individuals or groups will treat a situation as competitive or cooperative? Certainly, adherence to some high-level goal or noble purpose is not enough. Individuals on both sides of the fluoridation controversy in Northampton felt they were acting in the best interests of the community. The conflict was in the choice of means to achieve this end. Scarce resources such as profits, a championship trophy, or a research grant elicit competition, but an abundance of resources is no guarantee of cooperation. The battle is often fought over more abstract phenomena such as ideas; religious and political values; and personal needs for power, recognition, and identity. Even when the situation is logically predisposed to cooperation, that is, conditions are such that everyone involved would be more likely to achieve their individual goals through joint effort, participants may behave competitively through force of habit, misperception, or lack of trust in the motives and awareness of others.

It becomes necessary to be able to diagnose situations as competitive or cooperative; the person who sees every situation as competitive is not likely to be effective nor is the person who sees every situation as cooperative. Problems in diagnosis arise because most situations are neither purely competitive nor purely cooperative. For example, two work groups within an organization are presumably committed to the achievement of corporate goals; they are also in competition internally for such scarce resources as budget funds, promotions, etc. Will their interactions be governed by norms of cooperation or of competition? Similarly, the members of a dental team are presumably mutually committed to providing the best possible treatment for the patient. Members of the team may also be competing for scarce resources—the auxiliaries for recognition, salary, and promotion; the hygienist for status; the dentist for power and deference. Will team behavior be competitive or cooperative?

Group conflict often seems to be an inevitable consequence of the existence of groups, as summarized in the following quote:

> Almost any mechanism that allows one group to identify itself as different from another group seems sufficient to generate conflict. And almost any group can find such a mechanism in any environment.*

*From Leavitt, H. J., Dill, W. R., and Eyring, H. B.: The organizational world, New York, 1973, Harcourt Brace Jovanovich, Inc.

A corollary to this general conclusion would be that almost any issue, idea, or event is capable of generating two or more groups holding different opinions. The fluoridation controversy exemplifies this. Similarly, as described in Chapter 10, individuals, even when they are supposedly working cooperatively in the same group, have little difficulty in finding points of conflict.

Conflict is a natural process. In the form of competition it is common in our society and valued as a motivator of performance and as an allocator of scarce resources. It is a seemingly inevitable consequence of the existence of groups and of the search for identity. It is also a focus and expression of strong emotions. In the following exercise, you will have the opportunity to experience these aspects of conflict personally.

EXPERIENCE WITH CONFLICT

This exercise focuses on the dynamics of win-lose competition. Although the competition will be among groups in this case, the patterns of conflict and cooperation that you will observe are equally common in person-to-person relations. The groups will be competing to make the best diagnosis of a particular patient. *(Treatment history will be supplied by the course instructor.)*

Forming a diagnosis (approximate time for this phase—30 minutes).* The group should be divided into problem-solving teams of five to six members. Each team should meet briefly and select one member to serve as a *judge*. The judges selected by each of the teams should then meet to form a separate judges' team.

The *task* for the problem-solving team will be to diagnose a patient's condition. Each team will be given a copy of a patient's treatment history and asked to come to a joint diagnosis and recommendation for treatment. Each team should carefully and completely write its conclusions on a sheet of paper and give it to the instructor. The instructor will distribute copies of each team's diagnosis to the judges' team and to the other teams.

*This format is based on a procedure employed by H. J. Leavitt.

Each team should select a member to represent it at a meeting with representatives of the other teams; the purpose of this meeting will be to evaluate the several diagnoses.

Selecting the best diagnosis (approximate time for this phase—30 minutes). The entire group, except for the judges' team, should reconvene when all teams have completed their diagnoses. The meeting room should be arranged so that the representatives can be seated around a table in the center of the room; the rest of the group can be seated in a circle around this table as in the following diagram.

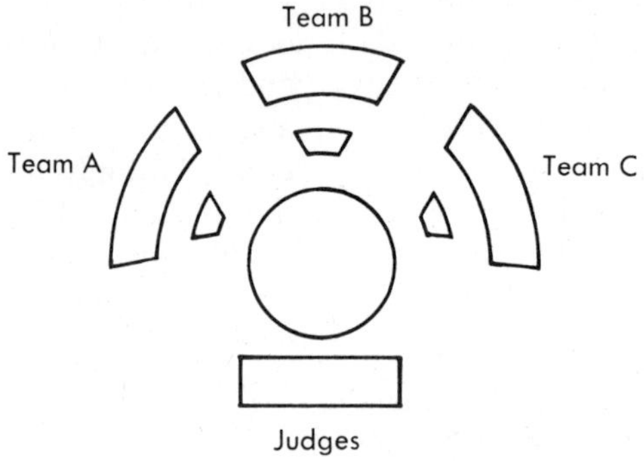

The *task* for the representatives in their meeting is to select *one* of the diagnoses submitted by the teams as the best. The following conditions should guide the discussion:

1. The choice must be made from among the diagnoses *as originally presented.* The representatives may not combine or integrate diagnoses or parts of diagnoses; they may not alter the original statements in any way nor may they form a new diagnosis.
2. The remaining team members may not take part in the discussion and should attempt to remain silent and unobtrusive; team members may, however, pass notes to their representative.

Developing criteria. While the teams are meeting to form their diagnoses, the judges' team should meet in a separate place. The judges' *task* is to develop a set of criteria for selecting the best diagnosis; the judges' task is *not* to make a separate diagnosis or to form their own opinions as to what is "correct." The criteria chosen are wholly within the discretion of the judges but should satisfy the following conditions:

1. The criteria should be explicit.
2. The criteria should be operational, that is, it should be clear how to evaluate the diagnosis in terms of each criterion.
3. It should be possible to combine the criteria to obtain an overall evaluation for each diagnosis.
4. The application of the criteria should result in a rank ordering of the diagnoses.

When the judges receive the diagnoses from the instructor, they should evaluate each in terms of the established criteria and select the best. The remaining diagnoses should be ordered in terms of acceptability.

REACTION FORM

Team ________

1. How would you now rank the efforts of each team? (1 = Best)
   Team A ______
   Team B ______
   Team C ______
   Team D ______
2. Would you like to work again with the other members of your team on a similar task?
   1 Yes, definitely
   2 Yes, probably
   3 Do not know
   4 Probably not
   5 Definitely not
3. How do you feel about the judges?

Criteria	*Fairness*
1 Very well	1 Very well
2 Well	2 Well
3 So-so	3 So-so
4 Poor	4 Poor
5 Very poor	5 Very poor

4. How do you feel your representatives did in the discussion?
   1 Very well
   2 Well
   3 So-so
   4 Poor
   5 Very poor
5. Would you choose the same person to represent the group in a similar task?
   1 Yes
   2 Do not know
   3 No

When the judges have completed their deliberations, they should return to the group discussion. The judges should remain silent until the team representatives have completed their discussion.

Reporting the decision (approximate time for this phase—15 minutes). If the representatives are unable to agree on the best diagnosis, the judges should be asked to report their decision. The judges should announce the best or winning diagnosis and explain the criteria used in reaching their decision.

The group should be allowed to question the judges. It is important that the group understand how the judges reached their decision, although it is not essential that the group agree with the decision. The discussion with the judges should not be used to renew the debate on the merits of the several diagnoses.

Group discussion (approximate time for this phase—45 minutes). The group should complete the above reaction form. While the form is being tabulated, the group should discuss the processes of competition and conflict that it has just experienced. This discussion should be used to focus on the group forces that developed during the exercise and particularly on the aspects of the exercise that tended to produce conflict. Although personal feelings about the quality of one's own team's effort and the fairness of the outcome will undoubtedly still be strong, it is important that the group try to move beyond the specific situation to generalize about the nature of the conflict. The following questions may be helpful in focusing the discussion:

- How involved did individuals become with the team task?

- Did you feel that the problem was significant and realistic?
- Did the individual members feel strongly committed to their teams? How do you feel about the quality of your team's output? How do you feel about the other teams? As diagnosticians? As individuals? How do you feel about the quality of their output?
- What are your feelings about the role of representative? What are the critical characteristics of this role? What tactics did the representatives employ, and how effective were they?
- What are your feelings about the function performed by the judges? What are the critical characteristics of this role? What was the reaction to the decision of the judges? Were they seen as equitable, rational?

When the data from the reaction form are tabulated, they should be reported to the group for discussion.

Managing conflict (approximate time for this phase—30 minutes). If time remains, the group should be broken up into new teams; this should be done so that the original teams are thoroughly mixed. The *task* for the new teams is to develop suggestions for ways to relieve whatever feelings of conflict and hostility remain from the first part of the exercise.

Group discussion (approximate time for this phase—30 minutes). The teams should report on their efforts. Some salient questions for the discussion include the following:

- How do you feel about working with your new team?
- What is necessary for the suggestions made by the team for resolving conflict to be effective?
- What can be done to avoid harmful conflict within groups? Between groups?
- Are there times or situations when conflict is desirable? Beneficial?

SUMMARY

The nature of conflict

Conflicts are often like weeds; they grow rapidly even in the most unlikely soil. Impersonal competition for a prize frequently broadens to personal antagonism and the desire for total submission of the opponent. Even when the conflict is initially a "difference in cognitive belief," it is difficult to prevent emotional issues from coloring and eventually dominating the controversy.

In an extensive study of community conflict, Coleman[2] has identified several regularly occurring phenomena in the natural history of controversy. The most noticeable aspect is the tendency for the original point of conflict to be transformed as the controversy develops. Three particular transformations follow that occur most frequently:

"Mom always liked you best": Specific issues that form the basis of the original conflict are replaced by more general issues. Debates over specific proposals or actions grow to incorporate the general policies from which the proposals derive. We have all heard (or perhaps ourselves made) the statement: "Not only do I disagree with what you propose to do in this case, but I think your entire approach is wrong." The movement from specific to general occurs most often when there are deep cleavages of values or interests or smoldering resentments of past injuries that require only a small spark to be set off. Con-

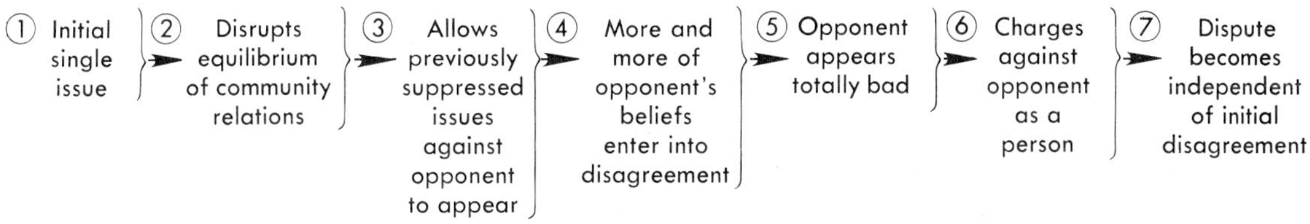

Fig. 11-1. Sequence of events from disagreement to antagonism. (From Coleman, J.: Community conflict, New York, © 1957, The Free Press.)

flicts between partners in a marriage or among members of a long-standing group are particularly prone to this transformation.

"While I'm at it, I might as well say this, too . . .": In addition to generalizing from a specific issue, new and often totally different issues are frequently attached to the bill of particulars. Issues proliferate as the conflict intensifies. These issues typically stem from the following two sources:

First, the atmosphere of conflict allows suppressed disagreements to surface. As long as things are going smoothly in a group or a personal relationship, there is a tendency to overlook or swallow irritations and disagreements in the interest of preserving the stable relationship. Once the stability has been shattered by conflict over a specific issue, "all bets are off." This sort of expansion of conflict occurs very frequently between work groups where the balance of cooperation in the pursuit of organizational goals and competition for scarce organizational resources is delicate.

The second source of expansion of issues is tactical: "a purposive move on the part of the antagonists . . . to solidify opinion and bring in new participants by providing new bases of response."* This is a form of "stripping for action," of developing and reinforcing group cohesiveness; it is typified by characterizations of the opponents as Communists, as racists, as conservatives, etc. This tactic is useful in forcing uncommitted neutrals to take one side or the other. This process of "building a base" is also a common behavior of persons in a two-person conflict.

"Not only are you wrong, but I never really liked you anyway": Emotions are never far from the surface, even in the most impersonal controversies over intellectual positions. In intergroup competition such as that occurring in the exercise for this chapter, strong antagonism toward the opponent is likely to develop and may even be fostered in order to produce more intense motivation. The shift from disagreement to antagonism is described succinctly by Coleman in the following quote:

> A dispute which began dispassionately, in a disagreement over issues, is characterized suddenly by personal slander, by rumor, by the focusing of direct hostility. . . . Once set in motion, hostility can sustain conflict unaided by disagreement about particular issues. . . . The antagonistic relationship has become direct: it no longer draws sustenance from an outside element—an issue. As in an argument between friends, a discussion which begins with *disagreement* on a point in question often ends with each *disliking* the other.*

This shift is in part material; it is easier to attack a person or to compete with a group if one feels direct, personal antagonism toward the person or group. We have all undoubtedly felt discomfort over competing with a friend and have found that discomfort reduced as we develop negative feelings toward our friend. The sequence of events in the shift from disagreement to antagonism is shown in Fig. 11-1.

Managing conflict

You have just experienced the dynamics and the aftermath of intergroup conflict. If you react like most people, you probably found yourself becoming more involved in the exercise than you expected and have developed strong feelings about

*From Coleman, J.: Community conflict, New York, © 1957, The Free Press.

*From Coleman, J.: Community conflict, New York, © 1957, The Free Press.

your group and its solution. You probably also have some very definite opinions about the choice of the winning diagnosis and how it was reached. Most importantly, you probably have had your feelings about the members of your group and of the other groups influenced by how they acted during the exercise. These new feelings will affect your ability to work with them in the future—and probably have already had some effect in the new groups formed for the last part of the exercise! Whatever the nature or strength of your present feelings, they are powerful impacts for a laboratory exercise that took only a few hours and that you knew was just that—an exercise! You can readily understand how much more severe are the consequences of conflicts over issues that matter greatly to those involved, that build up over time, and that renew the memories of other conflicts.

In the dental office, close, collaborative effort is essential, and yet the potential for conflict is high. Competent professionals can and often do disagree on matters of diagnosis and prescription. Although these disagreements are often handled by rational analysis, status relations and personalities often come into play. Any continuing relationship builds up certain tensions and irritabilities that are submerged in the interest of common goals but remain near the surface. Once conflict brings them out into the open, it is difficult to brush them aside.

Thus methods of managing and resolving conflicts are vital to the dental team. It is not enough to seek to avoid conflict; in fact, all our experience has shown us that, if conflicts are denied when they occur, they simply go underground to reemerge, in a more insidious form, in a later debate. Conflict is not only inevitable, it is healthy and constructive in reasonable doses. Conflict is a great generator of energy and can be particularly effective in bringing out new information, sharpening analysis, and stimulating innovation and creativity. The task is to contain the conflict within constructive bounds.

This is, of course, easier said than done. Conflict, once begun, is difficult to stop. The methods for coping with conflict among individuals in groups, especially extreme conflict, are similar to how individuals cope with stress and anxiety. Thus many elements of the following discussion are relevant for the problem of coping as discussed in Chapter 16. Many individuals, particularly group leaders, attempt to handle conflict either by denying its existence or by using their authority to force a solution or to smooth over tensions. The most common ways that people seek to deal with conflict and the likely consequences of these approaches include the following:

1. Avoidance and denial. Many individuals find conflict unpleasant and seek to avoid situations where conflict is likely to occur or strive to deny the existence of conflict, even if it is raging around them.

Two rather demanding conditions must be met, however, for conflict to be avoided in any group or relationship. First, there must be a high degree of common socialization within the group; all members of the group must share a common experience of social and psychological development, adhere to the same values, and subscribe to a common world view. In addition, the specific psychological contract defined for the group or the relationship must be clearly stated, fully understood, and commonly accepted, and the individuals involved must have common or wholly compatible goals. Second, the environment within which the group or relationship functions must be stable, and the activities or tasks that the group engages in must also be stable and tightly structured.

These conditions suggest an environment in which events are wholly predictable, the means of handling any particular event or situation are clearly defined, and each individual knows and accepts his or her place in the activity. This is, of course, the idealized description of the perfect bureaucracy, in which all events are anticipated and described in detail in a code of rules and regulations. Interactions among individuals are governed by procedures and, in the extreme, may become ritual. Many long-standing relationships such as marriages or dentist-patient relationships that persist over many years come to satisfy these conditions as the behavior of each party becomes wholly predictable to the other. In such cases, conflict may never occur or may become incorporated as part of the ritual and have no real meaning.

Although it is possible to conceive of relationships in which conflict is totally absent, the former conditions are seldom met or sustained for any length of time. Thus a certain level or frequency of conflict may be an inevitable consequence of human interaction. Some individuals seek to cope with the inability to avoid conflict by denying its existence when it occurs. The individual who insists that "everything is all right," that "we have no real disagreements," and that "it's all really just a matter of semantics" can be a source of considerable annoyance to others who feel that real differences in fact, value, or opinion do exist in a particular situation.

The pitfalls in denying or avoiding conflict are many. Conflict normally stems from real differences of one sort or another and typically arouses strong intellectual and emotional involvement on the part of combatants. Conflict is a powerful energizing and motivating force, and both avoidance and denial seek to bottle up this force. This can be tension producing in itself, often creating that sense of diffuse, accumulated resentment that leads to future conflicts. Also, individuals can feel manipulated and resentful if their strongly held cognitive beliefs or emotional commitments are denied expression.

A more significant aspect of the denial or avoidance of conflict is the loss of the potential positive effects of a well-managed conflict. Recalling that conflict is an energizing, motivating force that involves individuals emotionally and focuses effort and attention on a specific problem, we can see that conflict can have very positive effects on the generation of information, the stimulation of innovation, and the reaffirmation of commitments.

2. Smoothing. Many individuals who acknowledge the presence of conflict seek to deal with it by attending primarily to the emotional overtones. The desire to smooth over emerging conflict stems from the recognition that unresolved conflict can be irrevocably destructive of relationships and individuals. Smoothing can take many forms, from the withdrawal of the statement that initiated the conflict ("if I had known that it would upset you so much, I never would have said it") to the proposing of compromises that seek to satisfy everyone ("why don't we split the difference?"). Smoothing can be both a time-saving and a face-saving device: time saving in the sense that, if a middle ground can be found, the group can get on to something else, and face saving in the sense that the designation of clear winners and losers is avoided.

Although the desire to smooth over conflict may be a natural response to the discomfort caused by emotionally charged situations, this approach has many of the same pitfalls as avoidance or denial. Although hurt feelings may have been smoothed and tensions discharged, the basic issues that initiated the conflict have not been dealt with directly. The parent who resolves the argument between two children over the last apple by cutting it in half may have succeeded in smoothing over that particular situation. The basic conflict that led to the argument, which may be a struggle for dominance or parental attention, has merely been suppressed and will undoubtedly arise again in another situation, probably with greater intensity because it has been held under pressure. Thus smoothing can be effective in the short run; however, dealing primarily with the emotional tensions that accompany conflict rather than with the sources of the disagreement itself may simply delay or deflect rather than resolve the conflict.

3. Forcing. An alternative to smoothing, and one that has considerable appeal to many individuals, is to force a resolution of the issue by appeal to authority. This is the approach that most of us are tempted to use with subordinates, with children, or, perhaps, with patients. The statement that "I don't have time to argue with you, do it this way because I say so" is a very appealing method of conflict resolution if we are in the position to exercise it. Obviously, it is also a very unsatisfactory method if we are on the receiving end.

Forcing is a particularly tempting method because it avoids emotional entanglements, is clean and direct, and has at least the appearance of being rational. Not surprisingly, the pitfalls of this method are similar to those of smoothing and avoidance. Forcing avoids any resolution in terms of the initiating issue itself; "might, not right," is an apt description of a method that produces *a* solution but not necessarily *the best* solution. Further, the long-term effect of the habitual use of force is to arouse competing forces. This tends to emphasize the win-lose nature of conflict and, often, to destroy the group.

4. Confrontation. An alternative to the uses of avoidance, smoothing, or forcing in dealing with conflict is to handle the initiating issues directly, to confront them. Conflict is neither solely rational nor solely emotional. As we have seen, conflict is a complex process that can stem from many sources and that can rapidly accumulate additional dimensions and aspects as it grows and spreads. Interpersonal conflict typically reflects real and honest disagreements—over conclusions, goals, or methods—*and* strong emotional involvements, including suppressed feelings left over from earlier encounters. In order to resolve the conflict, these various pressures and tensions must be dealt with directly or they will simply emerge in other forms in the future. Thus any approach to conflict must deal with the emotional involvements and with the substantive points of disagreement if a long-term resolution is to be achieved.

In order to confront the points of disagreement directly and to seek resolutions that serve the best interests of the group or relationship, it is necessary, first, to accept the inevitability of conflict and to define the terms of the present disagreement: What are the points of disagreement, and what are the personal or emotional issues at stake? The second step is to place the conflict in the context of the larger concerns and needs of the group; this must be done by identifying a superordinate or overriding goal, one that is important to all members of the group such as providing effective service to the patient. These steps of defining the boundaries and the terms of conflict must be done explicitly if the group is to confront the issues.

By recognizing and separating the objective and subjective aspects of the situation, the group is better equipped to confront issues directly and to deal sensitively with emotional and personal involvements. At this stage, groups often find it useful to solicit the aid of a third party to keep the tension focused on central issues and to prevent the debate from expanding to a point where future cooperation is no longer possible. When a third party is used, however, the function is not that of an arbitrator who selects a winner from among the competing viewpoints but rather that of a guide and counselor who helps the competing parties to "keep on track" while they develop their own resolution. The arbitrator role, depending on its specific definition, is more properly an example of forcing or smoothing.

The benefit of confrontation is that it places the issue in terms of finding a "good" solution rather than of picking a winner and a loser. Leavitt et al. offers the following description of the value of confrontation as a means of coping with conflict:

> Confrontation . . . though it may not lead to love, often leads to understanding and reasonable accommodation. And it usually brings the tension level down . . . it will often lead to a more open discussion of all facets of the problem than will most other methods. Generally, it seems preferable . . . to confront internal conflict than to ignore it . . . but conflict must be regarded as

an expected, indeed useful, part of organizational life and not something to be feared.*

Obviously, confrontation as a method is not without its pitfalls, and there is no guarantee of conflict resolution. Most of us find it very difficult to deal openly with our own feelings, emotions, and perceptions of others in a direct face-to-face confrontation. This is a skill that, for most of us, develops slowly and with considerable practice. In Chapters 12 and 13 we will be working directly on the skills essential to effective conflict resolution, first, through a consideration of the general process of communication and, second, through the application of these insights directly to the process of interpersonal influence.

*From Leavitt, H. J., Dill, W. R., and Eyring, H. B.: The organizational world, New York, 1973, Harcourt Brace Jovanovich, Inc.

• • •

As a final note, conflict is indeed a fact of life, but not every issue or disagreement has to be seen in win-lose terms. Conflict channeled toward goals and improved service can be a useful and powerful tool.

REFERENCES

1. Blake, R. R., and Mouton, J. S.: Reactions to intergroup competition under win-lose conditions, Management Sci. **4:**1961.
2. Coleman, J.: Community conflict, New York, 1957, The Free Press.
3. Leavitt, H. J., Dill, W. R., and Eyring, H. B.: The organizational world, New York, 1973, Harcourt Brace Jovanovich, Inc.
4. Mausner, B., and Mausner, J.: A study of the antiscientific attitude, Sci. Am. **192:**35, 1955.

Chapter 12

COMMUNICATIONS AND THE HELPING RELATIONSHIP

The most memorable scene in the movie, *Cool Hand Luke,* made several years ago, presented a brutal prison guard peering down on a group of prisoners working in a ditch and saying, "What we got here is a failure to communicate." This scene characterizes analyses typically made of social and interpersonal difficulties. "Bad communication" is frequently used as an explanation for conflict and poor behavior. Moreover, effective communication is frequently preferred as a magical solution for resolving controversy. Thus campus radicals and university administrators in the early 1970s pinned considerable hope on the strategy of "keeping lines of communication open," the presumption being that open communication would clear away apparent conflict and surface more basic grounds for agreement or reconciliation. The more likely case is that improved communication (more accurate transmittal of information) serves mainly to sharpen the points of real and enduring disagreement. Although it is obvious on reflection that conflict frequently represents real differences of opinion, belief, or values, the hope that individuals, groups, or nations will reach the same conclusion if only they communicate effectively is pervasive. It is commonplace to diagnose the failures of understanding and cooperation, of marriages, and of treatment relationships as "breakdowns in communication" and to emphasize the need for people to develop communication skills.

Although a magical belief in the therapeutic powers of communication may be overly optimistic, effective communications are critical to effective interpersonal goals and relationships. In work or treatment relationships, the dentist must communicate effectively in order to achieve professional performance goals. Hansen states as follows:

> A common thread in the dental literature on human behavior and interpersonal relations is that effective communication, whether it is for enhancing efficient staff function or the doctor-patient relationship in providing care for the patient, is essential for success in the dental office.
>
> Communication and rapport, essential for understanding and trust, form the very essence of the doctor-patient relationship. However, the dentist is frequently depicted as a person carrying on a one-way conversation (including questions) with a patient whose mouth is filled with paraphernalia preventing a reply. The message is clear: dentists are not viewed as persons excelling in meaningful communication.*

Hansen has captured the essence of the concerns of this chapter. The dentist is called on to exhibit skills of "communica-

---

*From Hansen, R. G.: In Froelich, R. E., Bishop, F. M., and Dworkin, S. F.: Communication in the dental office, St. Louis, 1976, The C. V. Mosby Co.

tion and rapport" in treating patients and in influencing their subsequent behavior. Effective treatment, particularly success in influencing patients to adopt good dental practices, requires the accurate transmission of information (communication) and the establishment of a personal relationship (rapport). The utilization of these skills will lead the patient to trust and accept the dentist's efforts to help. In Part three, we will explore the specific ways in which principles of communication apply to the dentist-patient interaction.

OBJECTIVES

In this chapter, we will consider the following two aspects of the dentist's role as communicator:

1. As an effective transmitter of information
2. As a utilizer of communication skills to give and receive help in the treatment relationship

The objectives of this chapter are as follows:

1. To identify conditions enhancing attention, comprehension, and acceptance of concepts and ideas shared with others
2. To improve the effectiveness of communication by identifying typical barriers to effective communication
3. To practice communication skills for giving and receiving help
4. To identify important elements of the effective helping relationship, especially with regard to dentist-patient interactions

CONDITIONS ENHANCING EFFECTIVE COMMUNICATION

Effective communication, in which the communicator sends the message intended, where the message is received as sent, and where the intended effects on the behavior, knowledge, or beliefs of the receiver are achieved, is a complex and tenuous process. Effective communication requires that three critical stages occur: attention, comprehension, and acceptance.

Attention

First, it is necessary that the message be received, that it be seen, heard, or felt. Unless the attention of the recipient is secured, the communicator "might as well be talking to a brick wall," even though considerable information may be being sent.

Comprehension

Once the receiver's attention is secured, the message must be understood as well as heard. The mere fact that a receiver can repeat the message does not necessarily demonstrate that its meaning has been comprehended.

Acceptance

A message that is received and whose content is understood may, nevertheless, be rejected. Although communication of a sort has been achieved, it has not achieved its purpose.

• • •

Breakdowns in communication can occur at any of these three stages in the process. Failures of attention occur most often when there is a focus on sending rather than on receiving; all too often we assume that repetition will get our message across without any effort to determine if the receiver is listening. If communication is to be a two-way process and not merely an exercise in articulation for the speaker, the *focus must be on the receiver* and not on the sender.

Failures of comprehension occur most frequently when the focus is on the construction of the message rather than on the concepts represented by the message. We frequently make the mistake of thinking that rephrasing a statement explains its meaning. The phrase "Let me put it another way" indicates, first of all, that the speaker recognizes that the initial message did not get through, and second, that the speaker assumes that the failure was because of choice of words rather than clarity of ideas. Again, if the communication is to be a two-way process, the listener must be involved in describing and interpreting concepts.

Failures of acceptance often stem from a focus on the information contained in a message rather than on the attitudes and emotions the message arouses in the receiver. We often feel we have communicated effectively when a listener can repeat back to us what we have said. It is belief and acceptance, however, that are the criteria of acceptance, not mere ability to rephrase the content of a message. Thus parents who are content when their children can repeat instructions of good conduct are often disappointed when the desired behavior does not automatically follow. It is the *receiver's belief and the sender's ability to elicit evidence of acceptance of belief* that are critical to the successful completion of the process.

These three major sources of error in the communication process all stem from an emphasis on the sender's role and from the neglect of the critical role of the receiver. In the remainder of this chapter, we will be exploring these three stages of the communication process with a particular focus on understanding more fully the receiver's role in communication. We will be particularly concerned with understanding how we, as senders, can do a more effective job of attending to the needs, motives, and understandings of receivers in order to ensure that we achieve our own as well as their goals in communication. Adequate techniques in each stage of the communication are necessary to ensure that the receiver is attending to, comprehending, and accepting the message being conveyed. We will begin this examination of the communication process with a consideration of the structure of the message communicated.

IMPROVING THE EFFECTIVENESS OF COMMUNICATION

What we refer to as communication is a combination of language and gesture as well as body and facial expression. Each of these may be characterized in terms of tone, intensity, and emotional level as well as objective informational content. Much attention has been given lately to body language as a parallel channel to the familiar verbal language. We will be focusing initially on verbal language in our analysis of the formal content of communication; as we turn to a more detailed consideration of the emotional content of communication, we will consider more carefully the role of body language in the total process.

Increasing the receiver's comprehension of the message

Appropriate use of conceptualization. Our verbal language is a collection of names, ideas, concepts, and descriptions that we use to describe, organize, and share our perceptions of our thoughts and experiences with others. Most importantly, language is a collection of concepts used to describe and organize the world in order to understand it. Concepts may be thought of as the basic set of files or compartments into which we organize our experiences for understanding and for future use. Operationally, a concept consists of the following:

1. A name, a descriptor that separates a specific category from all others
2. A set of categorizing rules for choosing observable properties or cues that allow us to identify and discriminate objects belonging to one category from objects belonging to a different category
3. A set of rules of inference for inferring other, unobservable properties that are associated with a particular category
4. A set of rules of validation for validating the assignment of objects to a specific category

This set of characteristics may seem unduly complex and arcane, but it encompasses a simple process that we go through many times a day. Consider, for example, the concept of "apple." Apple is a name we apply to a particular class of objects. Among the observable properties that we use to discriminate between objects that are apples and those that are not are color, shape, aroma, and normal location (in a particular tree or in a fruit bin). Having identified an object as an apple on the basis of these observable properties, we apply a second set of rules that allows us to infer a number of things—that the apple is edible, that it will soften and rot if left in the sun too long, and many other predictions about unobservable or future characteristics. Finally, we have a third set of rules for checking our identification; we may ask an expert (the shopkeeper) or we may eat it and check the taste against past experiences. We go through a similar process many times daily, not only with physical objects, but also with actions, ideas, and feelings.

Formally, a concept may be defined as follows:

> . . . a network of time-significant inferences by which one goes beyond a set of observed criterial properties exhibited by an object or event to the class identity of the object in question, and thence to additional inferences about other unobserved properties of the object or event . . . the working definition of a concept is the network of inferences that are or may be set into play by an act of categorization.*

This formal process of conceptualization is the essence of thought and human communication. Communication is essentially the effort to share concepts with others, either for their own sake, for the satisfaction of our needs (to express our feelings), or for the purpose of altering our own or the other person's behavior. Concepts are not limited to simple physical objects such as apples. Much of our effort at communication (and much of the difficulty in effective communication) revolves around more abstract ideas and concerns. For example, the idea of freedom has captured the imagination of many writers and philosophers who have devoted lifetimes to efforts to communicate their concept of freedom to others; in so doing, they have been concerned with the value of ideas, with the need to express their own excitement and conviction, and with the desire to lead others to behave in ways consistent with their notion of freedom.

In the dentist-patient relationship, this linking together of abstract concepts (for example, good health) and specific behavioral recommendations (for example, toothbrushing) is also central to the processes of conceptualization and communication. Thus the idea of good health is an abstraction that has an emotional counterpart in the anxieties that dentists and patients may feel over future discomfort. The ability of the dentist to induce change in specific patient behaviors derives directly from the linkage made among the abstract concept of good health, the inferences regarding future health that can be made from present conditions, and the potential of recommended practices to ensure future health.

Conceptually, good health is a concept embodying certain characteristics. Given these characteristics, the patient presently is or is not enjoying good health. Further, from the present condition of the patient's mouth and from a patient's dental activities (the observable properties), the dentist may predict or infer the likely state of health of the patient's mouth at some future time. Given this prediction, the dentist is then able to recommend dental practices that will help to maintain the condition of the mouth (if the patient is presently in good health) or that will help to bring the patient to a state of good health (if the condition is presently unsatisfactory). The validity of this conceptualization may be tested directly on the patient's next visit when the dentist can correlate the condition of the patient's mouth and the practices followed during the intervening period with the predictions made initially.

This entire logical process is the essence of the message that the dentist wishes to communicate to the patient. If all these necessary components of the message are not complete, that is, if the dentist in or-

---

*From Bruner, J. S., Goodnow, J. J., and Austin, G. A.: A study of thinking, New York, 1956, John Wiley & Sons, Inc.

ganizing his or her communication to the patient does not provide a complete conceptualization (the name, categorizing rules, rules of inference, rules of validation), the communication is likely to be ineffective. Adequate structuring of information is not sufficient to effective communication, of course; the patient's attention and acceptance are also necessary. Conceptualization is, however, the part of the process most under the control of the sender and most susceptible to prior planning and organization.

Thus the study of concepts and concept formation is critical to effecting good communications. Conceptualization serves a variety of functions, as follows:

1. It reduces the complexity of the environment by grouping discrete objects, events, and ideas into easier-to-manage wholes that can be more readily retained in memory for future use.
2. It enhances psychological comfort and the willingness to take action by identifying objects and events.
3. It reduces the need for constant learning by allowing the process of recognition and, more importantly, by allowing for communication that enables us to learn from the experiences of others without sharing those experiences directly.
4. It provides direction for instrumental activities by allowing us to predict the likely consequences of action before moving to actual behavior.
5. It provides a basis for ordering and relating discrete events in order to identify underlying structures, thus providing the basis for understanding as well as identification.[1]

Validation that the receiver comprehends the message. As discussed in Chapters 7 through 9, we each come to our particular set of concepts through a lifelong process of experience, interpretation of experience, and reflection on that experience.[4] This learning process is highly individualized. We may predict with some reliability that others who have shared a particular formal education or set of courses with us will share a particular set of concepts. Thus it is not unreasonable to assume that all dentists trained in a particular school at a particular time have at least a broad, common understanding of the concept of plaque formation; even in this instance, however, these dentists probably do not have identical detailed conceptualizations of plaque formation. These detailed conceptualizations would be influenced strongly by the particular set of patients each dentist has treated, by the particular reading in the field each dentist has pursued since graduation, and by the particular ability of each dentist to absorb and assimilate information. Thus if this group had congregated a number of years after graduation to discuss plaque formation, it would be eminently sensible for them to spend some time in identifying and sharpening their understanding of the concept. It would be reasonable to predict, however, that if such a congregation should occur, little time would be spent on clarifying basic concepts and the discussion would instead proceed immediately on the assumption that the terms were understood and shared by everyone present.

This example underscores the need to validate concepts, that is, to determine in every communication instance whether or not the ideas we have sought to communicate have, in fact, been received. Anyone who has listened to politicians state whether a particular measure will increase the freedom of the individual is aware that their disagreement stems as much from the failure to define idiosyncratic concepts of freedom as it does from the likely consequences of the measure. The process of validation, of making sure that "we are both talking about the same thing," is, perhaps, the most neglected aspect of communication, and, therefore, a great potential source of ineffective communication. There are a variety of means of validations potentially available.[1]

The following example illustrates different means of validation:

Dr. Dworkin refers a patient to Dr. Giddon with the following chart entry: "Patient has an impacted third molar that needs treatment. Patient will develop extensive periodontal disease within 1 year if left untreated. Reasons: bleeding, pocket depth, and mobility. Patient is college educated and should be given extensive instructions. Patient likeable."

Dr. Giddon can check to see if he understands what Dr. Dworkin has communicated by utilizing the following means of validation:

1. *Ultimate criterion*. Dr. Giddon can see the impaction. Some events have the delightful property of being objectively real, that is, of having directly observable properties. Unfortunately, the ultimate criterion in many cases is quite dangerous; the final test for a poisonous substance is whether or not it kills on ingestion. Other ultimate criteria are available at a lower cost; the impacted tooth in the example is directly observable.

2. *Consistency*. Dr. Dworkin's statements about the likely consequences of a failure to provide treatment cannot be validated directly without letting the patient go for a year to see if periodontal disease develops. Dr. Giddon can, however, assess Dr. Dworkin's prediction by determining for himself if the observable condition of the patient's mouth corresponds with the conditions observed in other patients who subsequently developed periodontal disease or if the conditions satisfy a set of rules used to predict periodontal disease. Thus Dr. Giddon could conclude that Dr. Dworkin's prognosis is valid, since it is consistent with past experience. This is, however, less stringent than using an ultimate criterion and, thus, is an assessment of what is *likely*, but not *certain*, to happen, "all other things being equal."

3. *Consensus*. Consensus involves soliciting the agreement of a number of individuals as to the interpretation of a particular event or idea. Dr. Giddon might know that it is the consensus of many of his colleagues that college-educated patients should receive extensive instructions; he may assess the validity of Dr. Dworkin's judgment by reference to this consensus—by thinking, "Since all my colleagues agree on this point, I'll do it too."

4. *Affective congruence*. In the absence of a formal means of validation or of a pool of individuals who agree with us, we can validate our understanding of a particular concept only to the extent that it "feels good" to us. Obviously, this is a rather weak means of validation, but one to which we appeal frequently. Dr. Giddon can assess the validity of Dr. Dworkin's claim that the patient "is likeable" only by his own subjective reaction to the patient.

In communicating with patients, the dentist should be aware of the sources of validation available for the concepts that he or she is presenting. Obviously, where there is objectively definitive data or broad consistency of research in the field, there is a strong informational base available for presenting the message clearly. Even in these cases, however, information alone will not guarantee good communication. Attention and acceptance are still central to the process, and it is to these notions that we shall be returning shortly. Validation that the receiver comprehends what we are trying to communicate is a powerful tool in monitoring the effectiveness of our communication effort. If we are aware of the need to test frequently whether we are communicating concepts, we can maintain an effective check on how well the process is going. In our role as communicator, we can apply the following simple techniques to measure comprehension and sharing of concepts:

1. At the simplest level, ask the receiver to explain the message as he or she understands it; this seeking of feedback is a test of both attention (Are they listening?) and comprehension.
2. A more stringent test of comprehension is to apply the basic definition of conceptualization given previously by asking the receivers to demonstrate their grasp of the concept by drawing inferences to unobserved properties or making predictions about likely future events.

We have explored the major sources of informational difficulty (unshared concepts or different understandings of the same concepts) at some length. With this understanding of the information base of communication, we may now look at other ways to enhance effective communication.

Recognizing barriers to effective communication*

We hear what we expect to hear. All too often the communication process never really gets underway and, more importantly, never reaches the information-sharing stage. We have expectations of what others will say in given situations. We "know" that the dentist will advise us to brush and floss regularly, because dentists always give such advice! Moreover, if we do listen at all, we listen carelessly and often hear what we want to hear. A patient who is told that there is a very strong possibility of serious future problems often comes away saying, "It's not so bad. The dentist said it wasn't at all certain that I will develop periodontal trouble." Finally, in addition to filtering what is communicated through our expectations, we often fail to listen at all, and, instead, spend the time when the other individual is talking rehearsing our next remarks. The dentist who is composing his or her lecture on the seriousness of periodontal surgery may miss completely the patient's expressions of anxiety over pain or cost. Subsequent failure to incorporate responses to these concerns into the presentation of the diagnosis may well lead to rejection of the recommended treatment. It requires considerable discipline to listen carefully and attentively to what the other party is saying and not simply to focus on our own inputs.

The same statements can mean different things to different persons. We touched on carelessness in the use of language at the beginning of this chapter; there is no experience more frustrating than the patient who responds to the question, "Didn't you hear me say . . ." with the explanation, "Yes, I heard you, but I thought that it meant . . ." Even the most ordinary phrases of everyday communication are subject to multiple interpretation. The charge to "do the best you can" or to "do it whenever possible" can be interpreted in as many ways as there are listeners. Concepts and instructions should be as clear and precise as possible if communication is to have the desired effects on behavior. Thus an instruction to "brush after every meal" is much less subject to misinterpretation than to "brush whenever possible," even though the dentist may feel the two statements could be taken to mean the same thing.

We tend to ignore information that conflicts with what we already "know." The most compelling scientific data are often unable to shake long-standing beliefs, even those derived from hearsay or tradition. New information is generally filtered and tested against existing beliefs, attitudes, and behaviors. If the new information is inconsistent, it is often much easier to reject it than to reorder the existing conceptual structure. It is for this reason the dentist cannot be content with attention to and comprehension of information. In order to determine whether new information has been accepted and believed, it is generally necessary to identify preexisting beliefs and to deal with these directly when suggesting new procedures. The failure to recognize that all information is tested against prior structures leads to much wasted effort in communication.

We tend to evaluate the source as well as the content of messages. The dentist encounters tendencies to evaluate the source as well as the content of messages in several ways. His or her professional stature adds credibility to recommendations, but suggestions about good dental care may be discounted because "dentists always say those sorts of things." Similarly, many hygienists have had the experience of patients rejecting advice that would be readily accepted if from the dentist because the patient does not attribute the same status to the hygienist. The dentist must be aware of the biases and experiences of the patient in order to ensure that it is the information and not the source that is being attended to by the patient.

*This section is based on material from Strauss, G., and Sayles, L. R.: Personnel, ed. 3, Englewood Cliffs, N.J., 1972, Prentice-Hall, Inc.

We tend to ignore emotion and nonverbal communications. Just as most scientific data do not speak for themselves, communication is not an abstract, objective process of transferring information. All communication interactions are strongly controlled by the general emotional condition of the parties at the time of the interaction, by the particular emotions that each attaches to the subject of the communication, and by the relationships and feelings that may exist between the parties. The dentist is more likely to be able to communicate effectively with the patient who likes the dentist personally, who came to the office in a good mood, and who has no particular anxieties over having a tooth filled than with the patient who dislikes the dentist, who received a speeding ticket on the way to the office, and who is concerned that a needed extraction will be disfiguring. Any failure to incorporate an appreciation of the total emotional environment of the latter patient is likely to destroy any possibility for good treatment or good communication.

• • •

In the following exercise, you are offered the opportunity to test your sensitivity to these several potential barriers to communication in a situation that closely parallels that of the typical dentist-patient interaction. Most of our communication effort with others involves the giving and receiving of help. In the following exercise, you will have the opportunity both to seek help and to give help to someone else. In these situations, you will have the opportunity to experience and to observe the interplay of emotion, information, and communication skills. The experience will allow you an opportunity to identify the conditions that support attention, comprehension, and acceptance, and, more importantly, will provide you with some insight into your own communication habits and patterns.

PRACTICING COMMUNICATION SKILLS*

This exercise provides an opportunity to test communication skills in a variety of roles. During the course of the exercise, you will be asked to play the following three roles:

1. **Client.** As the client, you will be asked to seek help by presenting a problem to another member of the group for purposes of discussion.
2. **Helper.** As the helper, you will be asked to assist the client in coping with his or her problem, *not* to solve the client's problem.
3. **Observer.** As the observer, you will be asked to attend to the process of communication between the helper and the client and to provide feedback to both parties on the quality of their efforts after the problem-solving discussion has been completed; the observer does *not* participate in the problem-solving discussion.

There will be three problem-solving discussions so that each member of the group will have an opportunity to play all three roles: to be a client and seek help with the problem, to serve as helper for someone else, and to be an observer. Problems that individuals choose as the focus for their problem-solving discussions should be drawn from communication difficulties in the dentist-patient or the

*Adapted from an exercise in Kolb, D. A., Rubin, I. M., and McIntyre, J. M.: Organizational psychology: an experiential approach, ed. 2, Englewood Cliffs, N.J., 1974, Prentice-Hall, Inc.

dentist-staff relationship. After the first problem-solving interview, the entire class will gather to discuss the initial experience and, particularly, to identify observed behaviors that facilitated or interfered with the effectiveness of the communication process. The second and third problem-solving discussions will afford opportunities to test the usefulness of these observations. After completing all three problem-solving discussions, the entire class will reconvene to discuss and evaluate observations.

Premeeting preparation

Each individual should come to the class prepared to introduce and to discuss a problem, preferably in the area of communications, for which he or she would like help. The problem should deal with a meaningful situation in the individual's life and should still be current, that is, it should not be a rehashing of situations the individual has already resolved in one way or another.

Procedure for small-group meeting

The class should be divided into groups of three. If the class does not divide evenly into three-person groups, there should be one or two four-person groups, consisting of a client, a helper, and *two* observers designated for each problem-solving discussion. Four-person groups will require four problem-solving discussions in order to allow each member to experience all three roles.

Each group should designate one of its members to serve as client, another as helper, and the third as observer for the first problem-solving interview. The client should present his or her problem to the helper in whatever way they jointly decide. The observer may not participate in and must remain silent throughout the discussion. At the end of the problem-solving discussion, time should be allocated to the observer for provision of direct feedback and suggestions.

At the end of the first problem-solving interview, the entire class should reconvene to identify and discuss critical aspects of the communication process that were observed during the first problem-solving interview. The purpose of this meeting is not to discuss the specific problems raised by clients in the small-group interviews; these issues are private matters and might be embarrassing if they were brought into a larger context. The first discussion involving the entire class should, instead, focus on identifying actions or attitudes of either the client or the helper that either facilitated or hindered problem solving or effective communication. The issues of attention, comprehension, and acceptance should also be explored in the light of these interviews.

Although the discussion involving the entire class may seem disruptive and like a forced summation of the small-group discussion, the identification of useful or hindering behaviors will be helpful to all groups in experimenting with or in practicing potentially useful behaviors in the second and third problem-solving discussions.

The client can facilitate the helping process at the very beginning by specifying the type of help for which he or she is looking. To the extent that the client can identify the types of assistance that would be helpful and accepted, the chances of a useful discussion are greatly enhanced. If this strategy is effective, it would be desirable to initiate at least one of the remaining two problem-solving discussions with the statement, "I'm going to describe a problem to you; the thing you can do that will be most helpful to me would be. . . ."

After the discussion involving the entire class, the small groups should meet again and complete the second problem-solving discussion. By the end of the third discussion (or the fourth discussion in a four-person group), each person should have had the opportunity to perform each of the three roles.

After all problem-solving discussions have been completed, the entire class should reconvene for a full discussion of the process.

NOTE: Each problem-solving interview should take approximately 20 to 30 minutes, depending on class time available. In any event, the final 5 minutes of each discussion should be reserved exclusively for the observers' comments. The meeting of the entire class after the first problem-solving discussions should be limited to 30 minutes. The summary meeting of the entire class at the completion of the exercise will require approximately 35 to 40 minutes. (Naturally, these guidelines are suggestions, and the total time allocated to each step of the exercise would be a function of total classroom time available.)

Procedure for the group discussion

As previously stated, when all problem-solving discussions have been completed, the entire class should reconvene to discuss the exercise. It is important to focus primarily on the observations of the *process* of exchanging information and not simply on moving the discussion of the individual problems to a higher organizational level. It is likely that the problems observed by the clients deal with communication situations that are commonly experienced by all members of the group. In a group of 20 or 30 individuals, it is also likely that a number of the specific problems are currently of concern to more than one person. The meeting of the entire class after the third problem-solving discussion can greatly aid the process of sharing experiences about these common problems. Several broad issues that the discussion might encompass follow:

- What identification can be made of behaviors that facilitate or hinder effective communication in this exchange of information?
- What broad types of communication in the areas of dentist-patient or dentist-staff relationships were discussed, and what progress was made on understanding and dealing with them? Can the experiences that the smaller group shares with the larger group increase everyone's potential for more successful future encounters?
- How do individual members feel about being placed in situations where they are required to seek help from others? In situations where they are required to assist others?

Naturally, the decision to share a specific problem with the entire class remains solely with the client—the person who "owns the problem." Problems that are likely to be within the experience of the group members can generally be presented without going into specific details and can provide the most useful focal point for discussion. We should not forget, however, that problems that seem unique to us frequently occur in some manner for others. One of the major benefits of the discussions involving the entire class is the potential discovery that we are not alone—that our problems have been faced by others and that there are others who are willing to give us assistance.

Guidelines

Specific guideline sheets that outline the roles of client, helper, and observer more fully and that provide some useful suggestions for enhancing the effectiveness of the interchange follow.

□ *Suggestions for the client*

1. Identify a typical communication situation in which you are uncomfortable. This might be one in which you have had unpleasant experiences in the past or one you have avoided because of anticipation of difficulties. Ideally, it should be a problem that you are likely to face in the future and that is important to your effective professional performance.
2. Try to present your problem or concern as briefly and explicitly as possible so that your helper can understand not only the formal nature of the problem but also the experiences, anxieties, and uncertainties that make it particularly difficult for you.
3. After presenting your problem, give your helper the opportunity to ask questions to clarify his or her understanding of your situation. Pay careful attention to these questions and do not present your own ideas for possible solutions until the helper has had a reasonably full opportunity to sharpen his or her understanding of the problem.
4. Indicate as clearly as you can to the helper how you think he or she might best be of assistance to you in more effectively dealing with this problem.

□ *Suggestions for the helper*

1. Your task is to help the client define, or perhaps redefine, the problem in such a way that specific solutions or actions will become evident to the client. Additionally, and more importantly, your task is to help the client feel a sufficient understanding of and commitment to the potential solutions so that he or she is willing to put them into practice.
2. In listening to the client's presentation of his or her problem, it is useful to keep the following questions in mind:
   - What is the real problem being presented? Very often it is not the one being described on the surface but is, instead, a more basic difficulty of which the present situation is only a symptom.
   - How does the client see his or her role in the situation, and, more importantly, how does he or she define responsibility for effective behavior? Also, what are the client's objectives for the resolution of the situation?
   - If solutions have been tried in the past, what were their results, and what were the potential sources of ineffectiveness?
   - Are other individuals involved in the problem? What is the relationship of the client to these individuals? Where does control of the situation lie? Does the client have freedom of action, or is he or she largely restrained by the positions of others?
   - If your emerging understanding of the problem is different from that apparently held by the client, what can you do to broaden the client's understanding of the problem without directly challenging his or her statements.
3. In responding to the client and in attempting to be helpful, you should seek to avoid the following behaviors:
   - *Do not take over the problem.* Remember the problem belongs to the client and not to you. The purpose of listening to the client is to help the client in the solution of the problem, not to solve it for the client. You have been helpful only if you

leave the client better able to handle his or her future situations alone. You have not done this if you take over responsibility for the problem and solve it for the client. Avoid statements such as "The real problem seems to be . . ." or "What I would do if I were you. . . ." Try to use your questions and comments to assist the client in developing his or her own insights and ideas.

- *Do not dismiss the problem.* Even if the problem seems trivial or readily resolvable to you, remember that it must be seriously troubling the client or he or she would not have come to you for help with it. Avoid statements such as "That's no problem, it will go away if only you . . ." or "I had a problem just like that and I solved it by. . . ." Remember that the problem is both real and unique to the client and that you do *not* have full information on the situation. You can do considerable damage and greatly weaken the client's confidence in you as a helper by making too ready an identification of the client's problem with a past situation that you may have experienced.
- *Focus on what the client can or cannot do, not on moral precepts about what he or she ought to do.* Avoid the word "should" in your discussion.

□ *Suggestions for the observer*

1. Your task as observer is to listen as carefully as you can to the discussion. You should not take part in the discussion, either by verbal comment or by expressing any emotions or feelings through body language, gestures, or other signals that might distract the reaction between client and helper. When you make your remarks at the end of the discussion, remember that you are not judging the interview but are trying to help the two participants reflect more deeply on how they have behaved. It is not your function to provide yet another solution to the problem or to criticize the two parties. Try to avoid statements such as "Things would have gone much better if only you had . . ." or "If I were you, I would have asked . . ."
2. You might keep the following points in mind as you observe the discussion:
   - Keep the question "What is going on between the client and the helper?" firmly in your mind as you watch the discussion. Remember to look for emotional views and other signs of interest, attention, and involvement in addition to listening to the dialogue. Try to connect these observations with what is being said or done at the time.
   - What examples can you identify that demonstrate each of the stages of the communications process—attention, comprehension, acceptance? These specific examples will be very helpful in providing feedback to the helper and the client.
   - What barriers to effective communication seem to be operating in the discussion? You may wish to review those barriers discussed in the text or to add any additional insights of your own. For example, are the conceptual terms used clearly defined and understood by both parties? In what ways did either client or helper seek to test the validity of his or her ideas or to understand the position of the other party?

SUMMARY

For the dentist, the helping relationship is central to effective task performance. Generally, the dentist is able to capture the attention of his or her audience; the patient is, after all, generally confined in some manner to the chair when the dentist chooses to provide help. Moreover, the dentist is strongly motivated by the goal of being helpful, even to the extent of identifying problems of which the patient may not be aware. The helpful act of communicating to the patient a problem of which he or she may not even be aware requires a sensitive application of communication skills.

The exercise in which you have just participated has given you an unusual opportunity to experience and to observe the process of giving and receiving help. Before we begin to analyze the exercise, you might find it valuable to stop and think about your personal accomplishments and reactions to the experience you have just had. Before reading on, record your feelings and reactions to your experience as helper, as client, and as observer on a sheet of paper. As we analyze the communication experience, refer to your responses as data to guide your efforts to improve your own communication skills. Your reactions might touch on the following questions:

- Do you feel you received any real help with your problems? If so, what was the source of the help received—suggestions from your helper, insights that you had during the discussion, relief at being able to talk with someone about your problem? If you did not receive any help, why not? Were you able to explain your problem? Did your helper really understand it? Do you feel it is not really resolvable?
- How effective do you think you were in trying to explain your problem? Did your helper really understand it? How might the helper have improved his or her attempts to help you?
- How effective do you think you were in trying to help your client? On what evidence do you base your assessment of your effectiveness—on your client's reaction, on your belief in the validity of your suggestions, on good feedback from the observer?
- Make a list of the actions taken by helpers and clients that you observed or experienced and that you thought advanced an initial understanding of the problem and produced useful suggestions for plans of action.

Evaluating the critical stages of communication

The three major aspects of the communication process—attention, comprehension, and acceptance—demonstrated in your problem-solving discussions can now be reviewed.

Attention. The process started with a commitment on the part of the helper (and the observer) to pay attention to the problem of the client. This contract was a two-way street; the client also agreed to pay *attention* to the responses of the helper.

One way to test whether an adequate level of attention was achieved between helper and client is to judge whether the problem was identified clearly and explicitly. This is not a trivial matter. One of the major barriers we often encounter in solving our own problems is that we define the problem for ourselves in terms that block solutions. The process of seeking to explain our problem to an attentive helper requires us to be more explicit and thorough in thinking about and describing the problem than we have probably ever been with ourselves. This act of explaining our problem very often leads us to a sharper understanding of it and to a redefinition that may open up possible alternatives or solutions. Thus one of the behaviors of helpers often described as facilitating the problem-solving process is asking questions that assist the client to improve his or her identification of the problem.

A second measure of attention would be the degree to which one party interrupted the other during the discussion. Interruptions are of two types. The first is an open information-seeking question aimed at clarifying a point, for example, "Excuse me, but before you go on could you help me by telling me what you mean when you say that Dr. Jones is difficult to work with?" This type of interruption is helpful; it asks the client to further define an important aspect of the problem and often facilitates the helping process. The second type of interruption is a solution-oriented comment, for example, "I see where you are going, and I think I know what you ought to do. Let me tell you what I did in a situation similar to this." This may also be a helpful interruption, but the chances are that it is not. The person interrupting is probably reacting to some part of the speaker's presentation that triggered an association with one of his or her *own* past experiences. The person interrupting is now no longer paying attention to the other person's remarks but has "taken over the problem" and is offering solutions. By not giving the speaker a chance to finish his or her thoughts, the interrupter has probably overlooked or missed some details that might have indicated the ways in which the present situation is different from his or her past experience. Any time we interrupt another to speak of our own insights, positions, or conclusions, we indicate that our attention has wandered from what they are saying. The extreme of this is the act of rehearsing one's next remarks while the other person is speaking. If interruptions of this type occur with frequency in your problem-solving discussions, it is likely that attention was inadequate and that the effectiveness of the helping effort was reduced.

Comprehension. Comprehension is, of course, a pivotal element in the helping relationship. The helper can do very little to further the client's understanding of his or her problem or to stimulate movement toward a solution if the helper does not understand the nature of the problem adequately. The quality of the helper's comprehension can be assessed by an examination of the outputs of the conversation, that is, did the suggestions made bear directly on the problem presented? It can also be assessed by the degree to which testing for the adequacy of comprehension was part of the discussion. This is an example of the process issues that we discussed in Chapter 11. How frequently did either the helper or the client interrupt the content discussion with a consideration of process, that is, with comments such as "Before we go on, let me see if I understand what you are saying correctly"? As we noted earlier, an adequate sharing of concepts between two individuals is not achieved without considerable effort and conscious attention. Remember, however, that comprehension goes beyond simply being able to identify the surface descriptions of problems. It involves an identification of the total context of the problem, including its specific elements in the attitudes and values that shape the client's identification and presentation of the problem. In order to surface these underlying influences, the helper frequently needs to raise questions that force the client to state assumptions and interpretations. If a continual checking for comprehension were not a part of the problem-solving discussion, the potential use of this exchange was greatly limited.

Acceptance. The final stage of the process, acceptance, can be tested directly. In this case, acceptance refers to both the attitude of the helper toward the client and his or her problem and to the response of the client to the suggestions and ideas generated in the discussion.

People who seek help are often concerned about whether their problem will be seen as legitimate by others and whether they will be accepted as persons despite having this problem. The ability of the helper to convince the client that he or she is accepted as a person (without disapproval for having the problem) and that the problem is a legitimate concern is crucial to the quality of thc helping relationship. A further indicator of the quality of the exchange is whether the client appears to accept the options generated in the process as potentially useful and to make some commitment to experimenting with them. The concept of a psychological contract, discussed in Chapter 6, is relevant here. People who seek help have distinct expectations and desires about the kind of help they would like and are willing to accept. In some cases, the client really does understand his or her problem and is seeking information or suggestions for specific solutions. In such cases, the helper is effective only to the extent that he or she recognizes "where the person seeking help is really at" and responds accordingly.

Important elements of the effective helping relationship

Ensuring common understanding of the psychological contract. Even professional helpers such as therapists are not always able to interpret the psychological contract effectively. A tale is told of the therapist who utilized a nondirective interviewing technique in all his work.* In this procedure, the therapist reflects back the statements of the client without evaluating them or offering additional information. In this way, the client is led to express more and more of his or her deeper concerns and understandings of the situation and, through this self-examination, to come to personal insights leading to the resolution of the problem. One day while the therapist was reading in his office, a stranger stuck his head through the open doorway and asked, "Could you tell me where the water fountain is?" The therapist looked up from his book, fixed the stranger with a penetrating, but accepting, stare, and said, "You would like to know where the water fountain is." Frequent violations of the implied contract hinder the effectiveness of helping exchanges. Often individuals do not explain their problems very well, and time and attention should be devoted to exploration, discussion, and questioning to clarify the problem. Sometimes, however, they simply want to know where the water fountain is. The effective helper is one who can recognize the parameters of this implied contract and function within them.

Resisting the tendency to solve the client's problem. The most common mistake made in assuming the helper's role is that too many assumptions of commonality between the client's problem and past experiences of the helper are made. It is very difficult while functioning as a helper to resist the tendency to solve the client's problem. If we remember that only the client can solve his or her problem, we open the possibility of helping. Further, our efforts to help will be useful only to the extent that the client accepts them, and the client is likely to accept them only to the extent that we have fulfilled our contract as helpers. Key elements of that contract include paying attention to the client's problem, striving vigorously to comprehend the problem, and accepting the problem as legitimate and worthy of attention. These are difficult processes to accomplish effectively.

If we are successful in helping someone understand his or her problem (when we have satisfied the attention and comprehension elements of the problem), we often still feel the urge to assist in solving the problem. If the discussion does not end with a mutually agreed on and eventually successful solution, we often believe we have let the client down. We also tend to become interested in the problem in our desire to see it solved, frequently to the extent of taking it away from the other person to make it our own. We can usually see how well our solution would work if only the other person would implement it. Although internalizing the other person's problems is not consistent with the helping relationship, it is clearly understandable. Interesting problems are challenges, and most of us enjoy rising to meet challenges. Moreover, if, in fact, we have been able to suggest a reasonable solution to the other person's problem and that solution is not accepted, we have failed as helpers. We have failed in the sense that we have not completed the last phase of the communication process. Failures of acceptance are extremely frustrating to the helper, and the fear of such failure keeps many people from entering into helping relationships.

Understanding the importance of a client who can accept help. You must realize, however, that helpers, no matter how skillful they are, do not live in vacuums. The skill of receiving help is essential to a successful conclusion of the relationship. If clients do not have this skill, even the most talented helper can be defeated. Communication remains a two-way process, and the achievements of even the most effective senders are controlled by the capabilities of the receivers. In the helping process, the role of the client is frequently underestimated. Most of us are not trained to play that role well. We are generally

*Courtesy Prof. James A. F. Stoner.

not very good at asking for help. One of our problems is that we perceive seeking help as, in some sense, an admission of weakness or inadequacy. The reality, of course, is that most of us need help at one time or another and often receive it from individuals who at later times may have to seek help from us. You have had the opportunity to practice seeking help, and you might find it useful to explore your emotional reactions to being forced into this position.

In reflecting back on your experience in this exercise, you might ask yourself, and then force yourself to answer honestly, the following questions:

- How did you feel about seeking help? Most of us normally resist seeking help from other people, both because we dislike displaying our vulnerability or inadequacy and also because we often believe that our problems are so unique that no one can really understand them or help us. We often avoid seeking help until a problem has become severe; then we still resist seeking help because we fear that we will be criticized for allowing things to get so badly out of hand. It requires a conscious effort to believe that most people need help at one time or another and that seeking help is a legitimate process—even for ourselves.
- Do people normally seek help from those best qualified to help? We frequently avoid going to the expert in our problem area, particularly if the expert is a peer who might be a competitor or is someone in a superior position such as a teacher or boss. Patients often avoid seeking a dentist's help because they fear the dentist's disapproval. It is important for dentists, whose major role is to provide help, to present themselves in a nonthreatening manner to potential clients. The accepting, constructive helper's role that you have been asked to play in this exercise is one method of easing the anxieties that potential clients might have in seeking help from you.
- How do you feel about giving help? Many people find the helper's role exciting and seductive. The tendency to take over a client's problem and to control the client's actions is strong, particularly when the client is in a vulnerable position. If you find yourself falling prey to this temptation, remember that it is difficult to assess how much you have really helped and that the client, who must implement the solution, is in the controlling role of the relationship.
- How do you now feel about your role as helper, about your role as client? One of the intriguing aspects of an effective helping relationship is that both helper and client benefit from the process. Participating in an effective and productive communication process is a rare and heady experience. As client we may be grateful to the helper who has advanced our understanding of our problem and has helped to relieve our anxieties and tensions; as helper, we may be grateful to the client who has bolstered our confidence and sense of value through his or her belief in our ability to help.

Considerations in the dentist-patient communication process

Our practice with the helping relationship is an example of communication in action. It has enabled us to experience both the information exchange and the emotional interaction aspects of communication and to observe some of the typical barriers to effective communication. To summarize our examination of the communication process, we can now consider what can be done to overcome common barriers to effective communication. Some considerations in the dentist-patient communication process include the avoidance of technical jargon, the distinction between information and emotion, and the provision of feedback and maintenance of a supportive atmosphere.

Avoidance of technical jargon. The use of technical jargon emphasizes the professional distance in competence between dentist and patient. Each field or profession has a particular jargon, some of which is necessitated by the technological or scientific base of the field. Dentistry is a formal discipline involving physiological, biochemical, and psychological processes and mechanisms; dental practice is based on detailed experience and rigorous formal research. To facilitate communication within the field, special terms and special definitions of familiar terms are used to increase precision and to reduce the possibility of misunderstanding. This development of a special language is essential to the growth and development of the field and to the preparation of new members for entry into the profession. It is also generally not comprehensible to individuals outside the field. As one patient remarked, "My dentist uses such technical language in describing what is going on in my mouth that not only can I not understand him, I don't even know if he is pronouncing the words correctly!" Thus the professional value of special language is perverted when it is used in communication with nonprofessionals. Although it may be easier and require less thought from the dentist to rely on technical jargon when communicating with the patient, if time is taken to translate the technical terms into language understandable to the patient, better results may be obtained.

Of course, special language is often used deliberately with nonprofessionals as a means of demonstrating the status, importance, and power of the professional. Client populations are becoming increasingly sophisticated, however, and the emergence of consumerism has led clients to be more willing to demand explanations. Further, the aim of preventive dentistry is to improve the quality of the patient's behavior when the dentist is not present. Effective communication in the dental office is the foundation for effective dentistry, and dentists who communicate with the specialized language of their profession, either because it is easier or ego gratifying, are reinforcing a major barrier to effective communication.

Distinction between information and emotion. We have discussed the cognitive barriers to effective transmittal of information in some detail. The discussions of conceptualization and validation (the exchange and understanding of concepts) provide ample guidelines for improving the process of communication and the exchange of information. Communication would be much simpler, however, if it were primarily a matter of transmitting information.

The exchange of information generally takes place within the context of a variety of emotions, beliefs, and attitudes. Both dentist and patient are emotional as well as rational beings, and both emotions and rationality are generally present in most of our behavior. Unfortunately, although we are often consciously aware of the information we are attempting to transmit, we are much less aware of the variety of emotional and attitudinal signals that accompany the information. For example, much of the transmittal of formal information from dentist to patient takes place while the patient is still in the dental chair, quite often with the chair in the treatment position. The patient who receives a lecture on dental hygiene while strapped into a chair in a prone position with a variety of paraphernalia in the mouth is likely to receive the message through filters created by the emotional discomfort connected with the situation. Most of us, for example, find it distressing to be spoken to while we cannot speak back, and yet this is the position many patients are in when dentists choose to give them formal information.

A second example that identifies how emotional elements of the situation can interfere with subsequent informational communication is the manner in which the dentist formally encounters patients. It is not unusual for the patient to be strapped into the chair by an assistant who also places certain paraphernalia in the patient's mouth so that the dentist can immediately begin working when he or she enters the room. Contrast this initiation of the dentist-patient conversation with a situation in which the dentist greets the patient in the waiting room, escorts the patient to the treatment room, and then either prepares the patient personally or introduces the patient to an assistant who will do so. In the first case, it is fair to say that the patient is being treated essentially like a piece of meat or an automobile brought to the mechanic for repair; in the second case, the patient is being treated as an individual who has a distinct, personal identity and who happens also to be receiving dental treatment. These examples demonstrate how the dentist can introduce into the relationship emotional overtones that might help or hinder the remainder of the conversation.

Many other emotional aspects might also mediate the communication process, for example, the stress or anxiety that the patient brings to the dental office or the fatigue or impatience that the dentist may be feeling near the end of a difficult day or after a session with a particularly difficult patient. Any number of specific events during the day might allow emotion (positive or negative) on the part of either party to escalate. It is not possible to detail methods for dealing with each potential emotional situation in advance; it is essential, however, for the dentist to attempt to assess emotional states and to take these into account in initiating communication processes.

Providing feedback and maintaining a supportive atmosphere. In much of our discussion, we have characterized ineffective communication as being largely sender oriented. We have also seen that effective communication requires, initially, a receiver who is attentive, who listens, and next, interaction of both sender and receiver that produces comprehension and acceptance. The barriers to communication that we have been examining represent behaviors by the receiver that sabotage the process. Such receiver behaviors as rehearsing one's next speech while the other party is speaking, listening selectively, hearing what one expects to hear, or rejecting new information that is inconsistent with prior positions all undermine the necessary interactive character of effective communication.

Effective communication is essentially receiver oriented, and the receiver is the key to controlling the process. A sender cannot communicate well if the receiver does not listen and provide feedback. However, although we often spend considerable time and effort in acquiring sending skills through such means as public speaking courses and exercises in oral presentation, we typically devote little conscious attention, let alone practice, to the development of receiver skills. Listening is a skill that can be acquired through conscious effort and improved through practice. Good listening requires conscious effort and discipline. One means for developing good listening skills is through practicing the feedback process by using the following exercise:

- In a two-person conversation, enforce the condition that the second person cannot make contributions to the conversation before he or she feeds back the first person's last remarks to their satisfaction. Simple repetition or paraphrasing should not be sufficient; the listener should demonstrate, in his or her own words, an adequate grasp of the content and intent of the speaker's remarks. Practice in this technique will surface bad listening habits and provide practice in effective listening.

Feedback, of course, is also a two-way process. The sender can greatly increase the effectiveness of the interaction by insisting on feedback from the receiver.

This helping and consulting exercise underscores another aspect of the sender-receiver relationship: the essential value of openness. The exercise was deliberately designed to establish a supportive relationship in order to enhance the exchange of information. The barriers that we have been examining are, in part, simply bad habits, but they are also, in part, defensive behavior. The personal vulnerability emphasized in the act of giving or receiving help is present in all communication situations. As a result, individuals often have a need to protect themselves from potentially painful intimacy. When this need is coupled with a desire to sustain one's own position or with the perception that the information exchange is essentially competitive, the flow of information and the achievement of desired results are seriously impeded. Effective communication requires supportive rather than defensive behavior. Gibb[2] lists the following four qualities that are characteristic of supportive feedback:

1. *It is descriptive rather than evaluative.* Criticism, judgmental tones of voice, and remarks that imply value judgments all tend to elicit defensive responses. Descriptive feedback, which emphasizes information and is neutral in tone, tends to support and sustain the interaction. For example, the statement "Brushing in this manner will prohibit the formation of plaque," establishes a different atmosphere than the statement "If you really want to avoid decay, you must follow these instructions." The first statement is descriptive and allows for continuing discussion; the second is evaluative and calls the motivation of the receiver into question.
2. *It is problem rather than control oriented.* In the helping and consulting exercise, we have experienced the tendency to "take over" the other's problem in order to solve it. Being in control or seizing control often creates a false sense of security. A better climate for communication is established by the statement "Let's consider whether you might like to try this approach" than by the statement "Let me do it for you."
3. *It emphasizes equality rather than superiority.* The relative status of dentists and patients can present many barriers to effective communication. The dentist, clothed in professional knowledge and experience, may feel the patient should follow directions without questioning. The patient, whose status derives from his or her position in the larger society, may resent the unwillingness of the dentist to function at a peer level. The dentist who discusses rather than tells, who explains rather than demands acceptance is more likely to establish a good climate for communication.
4. *It is provisional rather than certain.* Nothing elicits a negative reaction in a receiver more rapidly than the assertion or implication that the sender is absolutely correct in his or her position. Patients are often aware of the incomplete state of knowledge in most fields and are more likely to react positively to the statement "In my best judgment, and as far as we know at the moment, this seems to have the highest probability of success" than to the statement "This is the only possible way to approach the problem, and if you do as I say, satisfaction will follow."

These characteristics are difficult to maintain in normal communication without conscious effort and practice, but the supportive, productive climate that results should more than justify the effort. These points will be applied more specifically as we delve into the dentist-patient interaction in Part three.

As sender, put yourself in the receiver's shoes—this is the oldest and most familiar piece of advice in communication and, probably, still the most important. Sensitivity to the motives and needs, knowledge, and emotions of the receiver is the most effective guide to effective sending. The demonstration of empathy, of concern and affection toward the receiver, will in itself greatly facilitate communication by establishing a supportive atmosphere. Sensitivity and empathy require, first, a genuine concern for the other person and, second, careful attention to verbal and physical cues to the motives, emotions, and comprehension of the other person.

These several methods for overcoming barriers all stress the interactive, two-way nature of effective communication. To achieve attention, comprehension, and acceptance, it is necessary for both sender and receiver to develop common conceptual understanding, listening skills, and a willingness to maintain a supportive climate.

REFERENCES

1. Bruner, J. S., Goodnow, J. J., and Austin, G. A.: A study of thinking, New York, 1956, John Wiley & Sons, Inc.
2. Gibb, J. R.: Defensive communication, J. Communication **11**(3):141, 1961.
3. Hansen, R. G.: In Froelich, R. E., Bishop, F. M., and Dworkin, S. F.: Communication in the dental office, St. Louis, 1976, The C. V. Mosby Co.
4. Kolb, D. A.: On management and the learning process. In Kolb, D. A., Rubin, I. M., and McIntyre, J. M.: Organizational psychology: A book of readings, Englewood Cliffs, N.J., 1974, Prentice-Hall, Inc.
5. Kolb, D. A., Rubin, I. M., and McIntyre, J. M.: Organizational psychology: an experiential approach, 2, Englewood Cliffs, N.J., 1974, Prentice-Hall, Inc.
6. Strauss, G., and Sayles, L. R.: Personnel, ed. 3, Englewood Cliffs, N.J., 1972, Prentice-Hall, Inc.

Chapter 13

INTERPERSONAL INFLUENCE AND THE CHANGE PROCESS

In a classic study, three separate groups of high school freshmen were presented with lectures on dental hygiene; the causes and the methods of preventing tooth decay were demonstrated with the use of slides.[6] Although all three lectures were comparable in the factual information included, the lecture to the first group was designed to arouse strong fears, using slides portraying badly decayed teeth and diseased gums. The lecture for the second group aimed for a more moderate level of fear, using slides of less vivid examples of oral pathological conditions. The lecture for the third group sought to minimize fear and employed x-ray films, diagrams of cavities, and slides of healthy rather than of diseased teeth.

The researchers reported that although each group learned as much about dental hygiene from the lectures, the "strong" fear group expressed more interest in the subject and also evidenced a greater increase in concern about their teeth. This group also had the strongest negative reactions, complaining that the slides were unpleasant and "too graphic." Thus the presentation emphasizing the dangers of dental neglect produced a marked emotional reaction. But did it result in improved personal care of teeth?

The acid test of any effort at interpersonal influence is its effect on behavior. Each of the lectures had advocated specific techniques for brushing, type of toothbrush, etc., and the students were asked to report a week later on changes in their behavior. In terms of the recommended practices, the researchers found that "the greatest amount of conformity was produced by the communication which contained the *least* amount of fear-arousing material"[6] (emphasis added). Moreover, the students in the "minimal" fear group retained their commitment even in the face of a statement attributed to a dental authority that the recommended practices "did not matter." Finally, the "minimal" fear group reported a higher number of visits to their dentist arranged as a result of the lecture. Overall, although understanding of the message was comparable in all three groups, the version that understated emotional anxieties and *stressed* information was significantly more influential in bringing about the desired changes in behavior.

Why didn't the "strong" fear message work? The students understood the message and could describe the advocated hygiene practices, but their actual behavior did not change! The researchers suggest that "the overall effectiveness of a persuasive communication will tend to be reduced by the use of a strong fear appeal, if it evokes a high degree of emotional tension without adequately satisfying the need for reassurance."[6]

The dynamics of influence—of getting other people to do what we want them to do—occupies a major portion of interpersonal behavior. The links between communication (transmittal of information), arousal of emotion and motivation, and eventual behavior are complex.[1,7,10] To stimulate new patterns of behavior in patients, dentists will have to master the fine art of interpersonal influence.

With this chapter, we begin a focus on the change process that extends over the remainder of this book, interweaving the theoretical and the practical, the general and the specific. Our intent is to call attention to the inevitable fact that when patients come to dentists, they want something changed or the dentist presumes that some change is indicated, for example, change in oral hygiene or in treatment behaviors.

OBJECTIVES

The objectives of this chapter are as follows:

1. To explore concepts and skills helpful in diagnosing the motives and need patterns of patients and colleagues
2. To practice designing influence strategies
3. To identify some appropriate strategies and their differential effects for influencing the behavior of others

STEPS IN INFLUENCING THE BEHAVIOR OF OTHERS

The following steps can be taken to influence the behavior of another person:

1. Determine the focus of the change attempt.
2. Assess motives and needs.
3. Assess the relationship with the patient.
4. Select an appropriate method of influence.
5. Organize the message.

Determine the focus of the change attempt

As discussed in earlier chapters, behavior is influenced by a number of factors: different environments, perceptual processes, learning styles, etc. It is possible to consider, then, that the manipulation of these same factors might be helpful in attempts to try to change the behavior of another person.

The clinician has a wide range of approaches to change at his or her disposal. Contained in the following are possible areas of focus (from least to most difficult) toward which the clinician could choose to direct the change attempt:

- □ Environment
- □ Skills
- □ Interests
- □ Motives
- □ Basic learning style
- □ Values

Attempting to change an individual's value system is the most difficult; additionally, it is questionable from an ethical point of view. Regardless of what focus is chosen for the change attempt, the remaining steps can be applied as the clinician continues planning and implementing the approach to the patient.

Assess motives and needs

There are two keys to influencing another person's behavior, as follows:

1. *Assess* the needs and motivations of the individual
2. *Communicate* the relation between recommended actions and those needs in terms that are understandable and persuasive to that particular individual

Each patient may require a different approach, and the approach must be carefully planned.

Assessing the patient's motives and needs can be difficult. As discussed in Chapter 7, the subject of human motivation is complex and has preoccupied psychological researchers for years. We often overlook this complexity and tend, instead, to attribute to others the same motives and concerns that presently guide our own behavior. We make our arguments in terms that would convince us and satisfy our needs. To focus on analyzing the mo-

HIERARCHY OF NEEDS*

Higher ↑	*Self-actualization:* The desire for self-fulfillment, the need to know who and what we are and to achieve our full potentials
	Ego: The need for prestige, for self-respect and the respect and admiration of others; the desire for esteem
	Social: The need for the company and the acceptance of others; the desire for affection and a feeling of belonging and of not being alone
	Safety: The need for security and order, for stability and protection from uncertainty and danger
↓ **Lower**	*Physical:* The need to satisfy the physiological conditions of survival, including control of hunger, thirst, etc.

*Based on Maslow, A.: A theory of human motivation, Psychol. Rev. **50:**370, 1943.

DOMINANT MOTIVE PATTERNS*

Need for achievement

A person with a high achievement need wants to take personal responsibility for success and failure, develops and aspires to personal standards of excellence, functions well in situations with moderate levels of risk, wants and responds well to immediate, concrete feedback on performance.

Need for affiliation

A person with a high affiliation need desires warm, friendly relations, is uncomfortable with interpersonal conflict, enjoys the company of others and wants to be liked and accepted, is sensitive to and concerned about the feelings of others.

Need for power

A person with a high power need is concerned about getting and maintaining the means of influencing others, is comfortable in situations where status relations are clear, desires to dominate and hold positions of control, wants to convince others in arguments.

Need for autonomy

A person with a high autonomy need is concerned about freedom from restriction or coercion, is comfortable acting on impulse or with disregard for convention, greatly values independence.

*Based on McClelland, D. S.: The achieving society, New York, 1961, D. Van Nostrand Co.

tives of others, two conceptions of motivation are especially useful. The first is the hierarchy of needs (above) and states that needs vary over time as the conditions of our lives change. The second is the concept of dominant needs (above) and is concerned with enduring motive patterns that persist in an individual's behavior across a wide variety of situations. Taken together, they provide a basis for selecting arguments that are most likely to influence a particular individual.

Hierarchy of needs. The essence of the notion of a hierarchy of needs is that human needs emerge in a particular developmental sequence. The so-called higher order needs (self-actualization, ego) are not likely to be aroused or to guide behavior so long as the so-called lower order needs (physical, safety, social) remain unsatisfied. When these lower order needs are reasonably well satisfied, they become less dominant (although, of course, they never disappear entirely), and higher order needs acquire a more central role. The higher order needs differ in many ways from the lower order ones—they are more cognitive than physiological, more concerned with the individual's sense of self and uniqueness, and less easily and permanently satisfied.

In our society, most people tend to have their physical and safety needs comfortably satisfied with minimal effort.[11] Moreover, although relatively few of us operate primarily at the top of the hierarchy, the demand for self-actualization—for knowledge and information, for fulfillment and challenge in our work and lives, for opportunities to develop and realize our potentials—is increasingly evident.[13] The appeal to fear—an attempt to motivate behavior through physical and safety needs—described earlier likely proved ineffective because other, higher order needs were dominant and more potent links to behavior. If satisfaction of these lower order needs is not sustained, for example, because of extended deprivation or crisis, they may become temporarily dominant. Thus a seriously ill person would likely be susceptible to attempts aimed at physical and safety needs.

Dominant needs. Individuals exhibit consistent motive patterns across situations and over time that are both observable in behavior and measurable with psychological tests. The principal needs identified by this approach—the needs for achievement, affiliation, power, and autonomy—are *acquired* through prior learning and experience and are present to some degree in everyone, although one or another is often dominant. As examples, individuals have different life histories, and the need for achievement is induced more by some histories than by others. People with strong affiliation needs behave differently across a wide range of situations than do people without such needs, but some situations will be powerful arousers of affiliation needs in most people.

The notion of dominant needs is not incompatible with the concept of a hierarchy of needs. Affiliation and autonomy exemplify social needs, whereas power and achievement are alternative expressions of the need for self-actualization.[3] Once developed, the higher order needs persist, even when an individual is operating at different *levels* in the hierarchy. Although circumstances can produce the temporary emergence of lower order needs, the high "need achievement" individual would probably seek to satisfy safety or ego needs through different behaviors and activities than would a person for whom autonomy or power needs were dominant.

The assessment of these need patterns is vital for the dentist seeking to motivate patient behavior. An effective approach to a high "need achievement" person functioning at the ego needs level would differ from an approach to a high "need affiliation" person functioning at the social needs level. For the first person, the dentist might focus on the *challenges* of adhering to a rigorous discipline of care and the admiration of others and sense of accomplishment that would follow from attaining some target condition ("no cavities"). For the second person, a more effective approach might emphasize the effects on appearance and the affection and attention from family and friends that would accompany good dental health.

The essential step is to view the attempt to influence the patient from the patient's perspective—to "stand in the patient's shoes." We can communicate effectively and achieve our purposes only when we state our message in terms that are understandable, convincing, and consistent with the present needs and persistent behavior patterns of our target—the patient.

Assess the relationship with the patient

The third step in attempting to influence behavior is to assess carefully the relationship between dentist and patient in order to aid in the selection of a method of influence that is compatible with that relationship and likely to have the desired behavioral impact. Our relations with others generally contain several aspects that might enable us to exert influence on the other person's behavior. We also normally have available several methods of influencing—alternative ways of pursuing our objectives.

The sources of influence that may be at our disposal—control over rewards and punishment, expert knowledge, official position, or affiliative relationships—are derived from our personal characteristics and positions as well as the specifics of our relationships with others.[2] The dentist normally possesses the full range of poten-

SOURCES OF SOCIAL INFLUENCE*

The principal attributes or bases that might enable one individual to influence another can be grouped in the following categories:

Reward: The ability to influence through providing desired outcomes and rewards

Coercion: The ability to influence through withholding desired outcomes or through applying punishments and sanctions

Expertise: The ability to influence through possession of specialized knowledge, competence, or information

Legitimacy: The ability to influence through status or position accorded by society or through identification with accepted social values

Affiliation: The ability to influence through appeal to existing personal relationships of friendship, affection, etc.

*Based on French, J. R. P., Jr., and Raven, B.: In Cartwright, D., ed., Studies in social power, Ann Arbor, Mich., 1959, Institute for Social Research.

tial sources of influence, although some are clearly more or less appealing than others. (See the above material on sources of social influence.) The abilities to *reward* or to *coerce* may seem limited, but praise and disapproval can be used to shape and direct behavior. The dentist also possesses considerable *expertise* and fills a socially *legitimate* role as an influencer of patient behavior. Finally, the dentist's relationships with many patients involve *affiliation;* they are friendly and highly personal. Each of these characteristics can be called on in an attempt to improve the patient's dental practices.

The dentist must assess carefully, however, the extent to which these sources are potentially influential in the relationship with each patient. A new patient may respond more positively to an impersonal approach based on expertise than to an attempt to presume on a personal relationship that has not yet been developed. Similarly, an older patient may not be swayed by reliance on disapproval.

The choice of an appropriate source of influence (reward, coercion, expertise, legitimacy, and/or affiliation) should also be guided by the dentist's assessment of the patient's needs and motives. Patients with strong achievement needs may be more responsive to influence attempts based on expert knowledge, whereas patients whose power needs are strong may be moved more by efforts grounded in legitimacy or implied punishment.

Select an appropriate method of influence

The fourth step in the development of an influence strategy is to select the method by which influence will be exerted. It is useful to conceptualize a continuum of methods—of specific behaviors that seek to influence—ordered in four broad groupings: authority, bargaining, persuasion, and intellectualization (p. 185). There is a considerable difference between attempts to influence through the exercise of **authority** (command) or **bargaining** (provision of an explicit exchange) and efforts based on **persuasion** (personal appeal) or **intellectualization** (rational argument). The methods naturally blend into each other along the continuum. It is difficult, for example, to distinguish some forms of bargaining from the exercise of authority —"Do this, and I will approve your request"—and other forms of bargaining from persuasion—"Do this, and I will be your friend." We often have more than one method potentially available. However, choice is often based not on what is most likely to produce the desired behavior, but on what suits our habits and motives or what is most convenient and easiest.

When we have authority over another person—child, employee, or patient—we are tempted to use it because authority is quick, efficient, and, for most of us, gratifying, since it satisfies our power and ego needs. Similarly, bargaining can be time saving and impersonal and often a painless way to avoid extended discussion over what

THE METHODS OF INFLUENCE

A useful classification of alternative methods of exerting influence includes the following principal approaches:

Authority: The attempt to influence through direction and command: "Do this because I order you to."

Bargaining: The attempt to influence through the provision of an explicit exchange: "Do this, and I will give you that."

Persuasion: The attempt to influence through appeal to a personal relationship: "Do this because I ask you to."

Intellectualization: The attempt to influence through rational argument: "Do this because you are convinced by evidence that you want to."

is right or wrong. These methods are economical and probably effective in the short run and may be desirable or even necessary ways to deal with individuals who are unable to absorb information-based approaches or whose behavior is dominated by lower order needs. However, these methods do not build a relationship between dentist and patient. The use of authority, in particular, often generates resentment and grudging compliance rather than an enthusiastic and enduring commitment to maximum effort.

The dentist's goals extend beyond short-run compliance. Preventive dentistry is, by definition, concerned with the quality of the patient's personal dental care practices over the long run—when the dentist is not present to observe, exhort, and correct. The primary thrust of the influence effort must be to assist the patient in establishing goals for self-directed change of hygienic practices.[8,9] *Behavioral change is most likely to occur and endure when the patient is committed to self-established goals.* The dentist's role is to provide information and feedback on the achievement of those goals. Thus the methods of persuasion and intellectualization hold forth greater potential for achieving the dentist's purposes.

Persuasion relies mainly on the personal relationship between individuals. The relationship itself is the leverage used to influence behavior. We call on the trust and confidence that exist to convince the other person that our suggestions are made from our concern for their best interests. We may derive our suggestions from our expertise, but the thrust of the influence effort is to gain acceptance and commitment through appeal to a valued personal relation. Persuasion is a particularly powerful method when the relation between dentist and patient has existed for a long time or when the patient's affiliation needs are strong. In the latter instance, both the fear of disappointing the dentist and the desire for social approval and popularity can be highly persuasive.

Intellectualization works from a different premise. It seeks to change behavior by gaining the patient's agreement that the recommended practices are inherently sound. This method requires that the dentist provide sufficient information for the patient to obtain intellectual understanding of why particular practices are being advocated. It requires, moreover, that the dentist acknowledges that the patient is capable of absorbing the scientific data and theory and can be approached on an adult-to-adult basis, rather than by appeals to superior wisdom or dire consequences.[4] The argument that "there are reasons for doing as I suggest, but they are too complicated for you, a layman, to understand" may be time saving and gratifying to the professional ego and will influence individuals with some motive patterns, but not others. Intellectualization may be an effective and probably a necessary method for influencing individuals with strong higher order needs—needs for knowledge and achievement.

Persuasion and intellectualization differ in many respects from authority and bargaining. They are more time consuming and require more attention to preparing and marshaling arguments. They are also more likely to produce higher quality and more enduring behavior—the goal of preventive dentistry. They work through higher order needs and seek to elicit a commitment, either personal or intellectual, from the patient. Finally, persuasion and intellectualization are the methods that we would most likely prefer others to use when attempting to influence us. In the exercise for this chapter, you will have the opportunity to test your ability to diagnose the motives and needs of others and to practice implementing strategies of influence.

Organize the message

Often, because we understand so well what we have to say and are convinced of its importance and validity, we give little thought to how we express our ideas to others. We forget that the patient has not had the benefit of years of dental education and practice and does not follow research developments. We also assume that the patient will be readily convinced by rational argument—by "the facts that speak for themselves"—neglecting the role of beliefs and emotions. Yet, as will be discussed in Part three, for many patients, visiting the dentist is a highly emotional event, charged with guilt over poor personal practice, anxiety, fear of pain, and personal feelings about the dentist. Any strategy designed to change or influence behavior must speak to these emotional states as well as to the objective transmittal of information.

The first hurdle in changing another's behavior is to make certain that the message is received, understood, and believed. The message that is obvious to the dentist requires careful planning of its logic and organization if it is to reach the patient. The order of presentation of ideas is particularly important if the target (the patient) has a low need to know. There is often a considerable gap between a patient's felt needs and what the dentist believes those needs *should* be; thus the ordering of arguments is critical.

First, present information that arouses need; then present information about how recommended practices will meet those needs. A demonstration of brushing techniques will have a greater impact after a discussion in which the patient's desire to enhance appearance or avoid decay has been stimulated than will a demonstration followed by warnings and promises.

First, present desirable aspects; then raise and discuss undesirable aspects. An approach focusing on pleasant issues (better appearance, feeling of well-being) will result in more attention to the message and more commitment to new behavior (more positive feelings toward the dentist) and in increased understanding of negative aspects (pain, treatment costs) than will an approach that starts with dangers and problems.

Raise and deal directly with obvious questions and objections. The dentist will be seen as credible by the patient (and thus more likely to influence later behavior) if doubts, confusions, and alternative opinions are acknowledged and evaluated.[5]

PRACTICE DESIGNING INFLUENCE STRATEGIES

This exercise provides an opportunity to practice developing strategies to influence or change the behavior of patients and colleagues. Before the class begins, each member should become familiar with the Dr. Stern case, on p. 187. In the group meeting, the class will be broken into a series of small groups, each of which will discuss one of the patients or colleagues with whom Dr. Stern interacts and will prepare a strategy for Dr. Stern to use in seeking to influence the behavior of that individual. The entire class will then reconvene to discuss and evaluate the individual strategies.

Premeeting preparation

Read the Dr. Stern case that follows carefully before class. Try to become familiar with the personal characteristics and situations of each of the four patients that Dr. Stern will be seeing today; also familiarize yourselves with the descriptions of Mrs. Carney and Dr. Jacobs. Be prepared to take the role of any of the patients or colleagues if called on to do so, and also think about how you would approach each of the individuals if you were Dr. Stern.

Dr. Stern

□ Dr. Stern, 30 years of age, has been in private practice as a general dentist for 5 years. The practice is located in a suburban community near a major city. Dr. Stern's patients typically reside in the community, where many of them also work. Dr. Stern shares the practice with Dr. William Jacobs, who has been in practice for 14 years. The two dentists employ two dental hygienists and two assistants. The receptionist, who comes in 5 days a week, also doubles as a record keeper. The two dentists send their laboratory work out to a facility located at the nearby university medical center.

A brief description follows of four patients who have appointments with Dr. Stern today. These are followed by short descriptions of Dr. Stern's relationship with Dr. Jacobs and with Mrs. Carney, one of the two hygienists.

□ John Davies is a successful business executive in his mid-40s. He was recently transferred by his company from another city to manage their sales office in a nearby town. He has seen Dr. Stern once, 4 weeks ago, for a general checkup and x-ray examination. At the first examination, it was apparent to Dr. Stern that Mr. Davies has been careless about his teeth. They were badly stained, and several small cavities were revealed by the films. There was also the suggestion of periodontal trouble that might require treatment by a specialist.

While preparing for Mr. Davies' next visit, Dr. Stern received Mr. Davies' records from his former dentist. These records tended to confirm Dr. Stern's diagnosis and showed a history of irregular visits. Mr. Davies' last visit was, apparently, 3 years ago, at which time he cancelled several follow-up appointments for treatment of minor cavities and periodontal disease. In conversation in his first visit, Mr. Davies had seen nothing particularly unusual about the long lapses between visits to the dentist and claimed that earlier visits to his former dentist had not revealed any particular problems.

Davies apparently has a very demanding work schedule, and it required considerable effort to find a convenient time to schedule the present appointment. He describes himself as follows:

I enjoy my work, but I have to keep hustling to stay on top. I don't have the fancy education some of these young folks have. I've made it on my own by working harder than anybody else and by putting in that extra bit of effort. I respect people who know what they are doing and don't get distracted. I'm valuable to my company, and they know it. They'd have trouble replacing me if I should leave.

I don't think my dental problems are serious. Mostly, they need to be cleaned up a bit here and there. I have been told before about some problems with my gums, but I don't have any pain, and I am really not concerned. I guess because I expect my kids to come—I am spending a lot of money on them and their teeth—I should set an example, but my work has to come first.

□ Robin Neuman has been a patient of Dr. Stern's for 5 years. They have talked several times about the possibility of oral surgery for removal of her wisdom teeth. She has had trouble for about 3 years but has resisted seeing a specialist. The oral surgery that Dr. Stern has suggested could be extensive, with the possibility of serious complications. Ms. Neuman seems to understand the problem but has resisted pursuing it further. In her last visit, she stated her concerns as follows:

I am at a critical point of my career, and I don't want to be away from work for any length of time. Also, my appearance is extremely important in my work, and I am afraid of any surgery that might affect my features or require a long period of recovery and adjustment. If it *really* has to be done, I want you to do it. We've been friends since we were in high school together, and I would certainly feel much safer with you. I know that you are not a specialist, but it can't be that serious, can it?

Ms. Neuman, at 28 years of age and unmarried, is an attractive woman who has built a successful career as a voice teacher and an entertainer in local theater and television. She has always adhered to a regular schedule of visits and seems to follow a conscientious program of personal care.

□ Twelve-year-old Paul Henson is a regular patient, as are his three older brothers and sisters. Paul has had a history of caries that has not abated as he has grown older. Despite regular visits and standard demonstrations of proper hygiene methods, he seems to show little improvement. His history closely resembles that of his 18-year-old sister who, despite conscientious effort, continues to have difficulties. His two older brothers, however, have had very few cavities. Dr. Stern explained to Paul the difference between his and his sister's teeth and those of his brothers and pointed out that he is simply more prone to difficulty than his brothers. He has strongly encouraged Paul to attend more carefully to his eating habits and to take good care of his teeth.

Paul is close to his brothers and has modeled himself after them in his devotion to sports and in his casual attitude toward school. He explains as follows:

My brothers eat everything they want—soda, candy, gum—and don't have any problems. I really don't see why I should either. My sister is different, all she cares about is how she looks and how skinny she is. If she is not studying and worrying about grades, she is sitting in front of the mirror looking at herself. I don't see how she has any fun. I brush all the time, just like you told me—Mom sees to that—and I come here. What else can I do?

□ Jeff O'Brien, 33 years of age, is a shop foreman in a local electrical plant. His first visit to Dr. Stern 3 weeks ago was his first trip to a dentist in over 5 years. At preliminary examination, it was apparent that his teeth had been generally neglected and, particularly, that considerable orthodontic work would be needed to avoid major future problems. He also had several cavities that needed immediate attention. However, he has postponed his second visit twice, telling Dr. Stern on the telephone:

My teeth don't bother me that much, and they brought me this far. I just can't afford having dental bills for myself now because the kids need treatment. My wife has been after me to do something about my teeth, and I came to see you to please her. You've cleaned them up, and they feel good, and she is pleased. Don't worry, I'll come back to take care of the rest when things get better.

After considerable persuasion, Mr. O'Brien agreed to his present appointment to "fix those two cavities that are hurting me." He did not agree to begin working on his orthodontic problems and seemed to dismiss their seriousness.

□ Jessica Carney, 42 years of age, is the older and more experienced of the two dental hygienists who work for Dr. Stern and Dr. Jacobs. She has been with them for 5 years and before that had spent 10 years with an older dentist who has since retired. Her two children are away at college, and she is devoted to the office, working extra hours whenever necessary.

I think there is only one way to do your work and that is right to the point, no nonsense. I see a lot of patients every day, and my job is to clean their teeth and tell them what to do to keep them clean and healthy. I'd like to take time for social chatter, but I don't have the time. I am not running a counseling office. Some of the younger hygienists think you have to be a psychologist to handle patients, but I don't—I tell them what to do and if they don't, they hear from me the next time.

Mrs. Carney is extremely efficient and technically accomplished. Both dentists acknowledge that her work is excellent. Her relations with the other dental hygienist and the rest of the staff, however, are strained. She has been critical of their methods and productivity. Several patients have also remarked that she has been curt and abrupt with them, especially in answering questions.

Dr. Jacobs remarked that "She has had some difficulty in adjusting to our clientele. Dr. Sturges (her former employer) had a much older patient group and, I think, a group with less education. They just did not make many demands. I am glad she works mainly with Dr. Stern."

□ Bill Jacobs is an outstanding dentist. I have learned a tremendous amount from him in the 5 years since we opened this practice. He can be frustrating to work with, however. I have to see many of his patients when he is out sick or off to a meeting—often without enough time to study the history carefully. I don't really mind—I am sure he'd cover for me—but he is so busy I hate to ask.

Also, although he is good with patients, he can be rough on the staff. He has been especially harsh with Jeanette Rossi, our best assistant. I am afraid we might lose her.

I know it is the pressure of his outside commitments—he is on the board of our local association and active in the Kiwanis—but it is affecting how he treats the staff.

I hate to be critical, but it may also be affecting his work. I have seen a few of his patients lately for follow-up and have found several imperfect restorations. In fact, I had to do one over completely, it was so bad—it took over an hour, yet I could not charge for it. It may have been in the way of accident, but carelessness can hurt us both.

Jacobs and Stern own their practice jointly and are incorporated as equal partners. Jacobs spent several years in research at the university before going into practice. He had done well in solo practice and had been able to provide his part of the investment in the partnership from his savings. Stern had to borrow money from the bank and from family members to supplement a small inheritance in order to match Jacobs' investment.

The task: developing a strategy

The class should be divided into six subgroups. Each subgroup should be asked to discuss in detail one of the six individuals described in the case. The task of each subgroup will be to form a strategy for Dr. Stern to apply in an effort to influence the behavior of that particular individual. Thus subgroups should place themselves in the role of Dr. Stern in preparing for a discussion with the individual assigned to them. In their discussion, the subgroups should develop clear, explicit positions on the following issues:

1. *Objectives:* What behavior or attitude change will you be seeking in your discussion with the individual?
2. *Description of the individual:* What is your understanding of the individual you will be seeking to influence? Your analysis should include, but not be limited to, the following:
   - The individual's motivation and needs, in general, with particular regard to dental hygiene and reasons for coming to you
   - The individual's general attitude toward dentistry and toward you as their personal dentist
   - The individual's distinctive personal characteristics, including age, education, and occupation as well as personality variables
3. *Nature of the relationship:* How well do you understand your relationship with the individual? Your analysis should include the following:
   - The possible sources of influence you possess with regard to this particular patient
   - The goals and objectives you have for your future relationship with this patient as well as for the accomplishment of your specific objectives in the present situation
4. *Strategy:* What is the detailed strategy or plan of action that you intend to pursue with *this* individual? Your statement should include attention to the following points:
   - The setting and timing of your influence effort: When and under what circumstances will you make your approach to the individual?
   - Specific arguments and methods of influence you will attempt to use: What kinds of information and feelings will you employ in your approach? Will you be seeking to order, to bargain, to persuade, or to instruct?
5. *Organization of the message:* How will you organize and sequence your points?

Suggestions for the discussion

The subgroups should reconvene to discuss each of the six individual cases. Each group should be given an opportunity to report the strategy it had developed. The group may find it helpful to list each of the strategies on a blackboard or easel chart for comparison.

After each group has reported, it would be useful to role-play several of the strategies, with different members taking the roles of Dr. Stern, the patients, Mrs. Carney, and Dr. Jacobs. In discussing the role plays and the strategies, attention should be given to the following questions:

- What assumptions about Dr. Stern, the patient, and their relationship have been made in developing the strategy?
- What factors—in the relationship, in Dr. Stern's presentation, in the pa-

tient's or colleague's situation—will be critical in determining whether or not Dr. Stern's efforts will succeed?

- Under what conditions is each given strategy likely to work or not work?
- With regard to the role plays, what is the probable outcome of each? What are the intentions of each of the participants in the role play, what are they communicating, and what is being received?
- For each strategy, if the initial attempt is unsuccessful, what options, if any, does Dr. Stern have for a second approach?

SUMMARY

Success in influencing others is the result of a complex, multistage process. It does not flow naturally from technical expertise and data, nor does it flow from good intentions. It is not simply a matter of common sense. The influencer must combine a sound working knowledge of motivation, communications, and influence processes with a keen sensitivity to the unique dynamics of each individual relationship.

Approaches to influencing the behavior of others

In normal behavior, there is a tendency to overlook this complexity and to rely instead on simplistic unidimensional models of human behavior. Three models that appear most frequently in efforts to influence the behaviors of others are the information approach, the action approach, and the emotional approach.

Information approach. When utilizing the information approach, the facts are allowed to "speak for themselves"; information is presented fully, explicitly, and impersonally, with the desired behavior being the only logical or rational conclusion. Unfortunately, most individuals do not operate at the level of pure, uncontaminated rationality, and even the most "objective" facts often speak in ambigous voices. Moreover, the purely informational approach often overlooks the ability of the target individual to process or to understand fully the information being offered. *Information alone may not be sufficient to stimulate the motivational or emotional energies needed to translate intellectual understanding into behavior.*

Action approach. When utilizing the action approach, appropriate behaviors are described without information as to the underlying rationale for the behavior: "Do this, and everything else will be okay—you don't have to understand why, just do as I say, and you will have no problems." This approach is particularly tempting for busy individuals who have, or feel they have, some bases for exercising authority over another person. Information-based approaches take time, often stimulate annoying questions that require even more time, and become boring when repeated frequently to individuals with similar needs and problems. Also, it is tempting and flattering to assume that others would not be able to follow the complexity of our analysis in any event. Unfortunately, *most of us require explanations for our behavior, particularly new behaviors that require changing old habits and developing new skills.* The unsupported instruction of an authority figure is generally not sufficient to sustain new behavior for any length of time.

Emotional approach. When utilizing the emotional approach, the primary focus is on feelings, and efforts are directed toward arousing the need for action. The appeal may be to negative emotions—fear of pain or of disapproval—or to positive emotions—vanity or pleasure. *Although some level of energy may be necessary for behavior to occur, there is no guarantee that a state of emotional arousal will result in desired be-*

haviors. In fact, extreme states of emotional arousal act as barriers to the effect of the processing of information that might guide the choice of actions as well as interfering with the ability to exercise skills efficiently.

Integrated approach. Each of these models is appealing in its simplicity, and yet, taken individually, each presents an obviously incomplete picture. Thoughts, feelings, and actions are mutually supportive parts of human behavior. For a patient to be motivated to use effective brushing techniques, he or she needs more than a scientific understanding of biochemical processes contributing to the formation of plaque. He or she also needs more than an understanding of the recommended procedures for brushing teeth, or more than a distaste for discolored teeth. A combination of cognitive understanding, mechanical proficiency, and emotional stimulation can be effective in initiating and sustaining a desired behavior. The problem of the dentist is to discover the balance of informational, emotional, and instructional inputs that will be most effective with each patient.

Possible responses to influence attempts

You have just experienced, either in the role of influencer or influencee, some of the dynamics of the change process. You have also been able to observe a variety of approaches designed to have maximum impact on a series of individuals with broadly differing personal characteristics and different relationships with the influencer. You probably have formed strong feelings about how successfully each of the influence attempts would have been in bringing about the desired behavioral change, particularly if you played the role of patient, of Miss Carney, or of Dr. Jacobs! When we are targets of influence attempts, our sensitivities are sharpened and our defenses aroused, particularly if we feel we are being "manipulated" in some way. If you were not persuaded by the influencer, you might find it useful to analyze carefully those aspects of his or her behavior that affected you negatively and also to try to identify arguments or actions that might have had a positive effect.

If you played the role of influencer, you might find it more difficult to introspect about the success of your approach. We generally find it more difficult to recognize the shortcomings of our efforts than we do to critique the efforts of others. In particular, we often tend to emphasize the internal logic of soundness of our presentation and to explain imperfect results in terms of the obstinacy or lack of attention of our targets. You might find it useful to have your target describe your influence strategy as he or she saw it and compare this view to the strategy you were attempting to employ.

Responses to attempts at interpersonal influence and behavioral change generally fall into four main categories: open resistance, passive resistance, identification, and internalization.

Open resistance. Open resistance is the most visible evidence of a failure of the influence strategy. The target simply refuses to "buy" what is being presented. Although this response is frustrating and disappointing, the influencer at least has clear evidence of failure and of the need to try again. Open resistance generally indicates a misunderstanding of the needs of the target or of the relationship between influencer and influencee. Thus an individual who is not overly concerned with personal appearance may resist costly treatment if its cosmetic rather than its pathological aspects are stressed. Open resistance is a clear signal that something is wrong with the strategy being used; careful probing of the sources of the resistance—understanding of the message, psychological or financial concerns, needs and motives—is essential to developing a new strategy.

Passive resistance. Kelman[7] has described the passive resistance response as "expedient conformity"; the influencee outwardly gives the appearance of agreeing with the message but remains inwardly in disagreement. Some individuals would prefer to avoid the conflict and hard feelings that often accompany open resistance and opt instead for the trappings of compliance. The dentist may not learn that the patient who sat attentively and quietly through the demonstration of brushing techniques had no intention of following the instructions until the results are observed in an examination 6 months or 1 year later. Generally, passive resistance can be identified only over a period of time, after several attempts to influence the same behavior patterns. Since passive resistance normally comes from a desire to avoid conflict or from inadequate links between motivation and behavior, a reassessment of the target's needs and a reorganization of the influence message are necessary.

Identification. The identification response presents the paradox of a successful influence attempt that is not really successful. An individual who strongly likes and admires another person will often seek to model his or her beliefs, values, and behaviors after that person and will be relatively open to influence attempts by that person. For many patients, the dentist may be an impressive figure of authority, knowledge, and confidence, and they may be motivated to comply with the dentist's instructions in order to gain approval and maintain a desired relationship. For many patients, however, this can be an effective way to induce long-term behavioral change. If the patient is responding primarily on the affiliative, or interpersonal, level, without adequate understanding of the reasons for the recommended practices and the techniques required, effective behavior may drop off sharply as the time between visits lengthens. Influence strategies that exploit the identification of the influencee with the influencer may be ultimately unsatisfactory if the initial acceptance produced by identification is not reinforced by understanding and skill.

Internalization. Internalization is the goal of every influence attempt, that is, the influencee eventually adopts the advocated new behavior because he or she understands and believes in it. When this occurs, the individual is likely to persist in the new behavior even when the influencer is no longer present. For the dentist, who sees an individual patient perhaps only once every 6 months or longer, strategies that produce internalization are essential to effective preventive dentistry.

• • •

Which of these several reactions to a particular influence attempt depends on how well the total change effort has been planned in the context of the patient's particular needs and ability to absorb information and the quality of the relationship established between dentist and patient?

Stages of the interpersonal influence process

The interaction between dentist and patient is analogous to the treatment process. Effective treatment of dental pathology depends on careful examination, analysis, and diagnosis and construction of a treatment plan that links needs to actions and implements those actions skillfully. The process of influence can be organized in similar stages: patient history, psychological contract, and selection of an influence strategy.

Patient history. In order to design an influence strategy that will have the desired impact on a given patient, the dentist must be able to assess that patient's general state of psychological or physical well-being. This requires thorough assessment of the patient's needs as well as identification of persistent motive patterns and the present level of needs. The dentist must be aware of the patient's personal, medical, dental, and psychological history and background. Sensitive questioning in conversation, accompanied by careful listening, over a period of visits can provide a deeper understanding of the patient as a whole person. Dentists who treat individual patients as anonymous collections of pathological conditions are denying themselves the necessary tools of effective treatment. A thorough understanding of patients' histories will also enable dentists to identify clearly the potential sources of influences that they might be able to draw on in seeking to alter the patients' behaviors.

Psychological contract. Dentist and patient enter the relationship with certain expectations regarding the extent and boundaries of treatment, cost, and nature of the relationship. If these expectations are not shared and reconciled at the outset, future attempts to influence and subsequent reactions are likely to be misunderstood and ineffective. A patient who is expecting only technically proficient treatment for present difficulties may respond negatively to efforts to alter his or her eating and hygiene habits. Similarly, a patient who is looking for personal attention and counseling may be disappointed by a dentist who provides only impersonal, technical treatment.

Selection of an influence strategy. The strategy must fit the treatment needs and realistic possibilities of implementation. The dental diagnoses, the patient history, and the psychological contract provide the basis for formulating an assessment of the patient's needs and motives as well as of the dentist-patient relationship. Given this information, the dentist can select a method of influence appropriate to the individual patient. The selection of a method of influence also includes constructing recommendations in a manner that will appeal most powerfully to the patient's needs and abilities to follow through on recommended practices.

Relative merits of different influence methods. As shown in the material on the sources of social influence (p. 184), the choice of a method of influence will depend on the potential sources of influence that the influencer has available. Thus one would normally not seek to influence through persuasion in the absence of an affiliative relationship. Similarly, an appeal to authority is likely to be ineffective in the absence of control over meaningful rewards and punishments. As shown in the material on the choice of a method of influence (p. 185), a number of critical factors may influence a choice of one method of influence over another. General principles that might be considered are as follows:

- *As one moves from authority to intellectualization, the time needed to implement the strategy increases.* Authority involves the direct giving of command, whereas intellectualization implies extended information sharing and conversation.
- *The long-run effect on the behavior and attitudes of the influencee will also tend to increase as one moves from authority to intellectualization.* Authority often tends to produce only immediate, superficial compliance. Intellectualization results in the influencee coming to believe that the recommended behavior is desirable. Personal belief is more likely to lead to a commitment to the behaviors that will endure over time.

EFFECTS OF METHODS OF INFLUENCE

As you move from authority → bargaining → persuasion → intellectualization, you see the following effects.

Variable	Effect
Time needed to implement influence strategy	Increases
Permanent effect on behavior or attitude change in patient*	Increases
Resentment on part of the patient	Decreases
Influencer's flexibility of available influence strategies	Increases
Quality of patient's performance	Increases
Self-motivation of patient	Increases

*"Patient" in this case means the influencee.

- *The likelihood of suppressed resentment from having one's behavior forced by another person should decrease as one moves from authority to intellectualization.* As is often evident in the behavior of children, forced compliance while under the control of the parent may lead to resentment that produces contrary behavior once the parent is absent.
- *The influencer's flexibility increases as one moves from authority to intellectualization.* It is easier and more acceptable to retreat from an intellectualization effort to appeal to reserve authority in the face of strong resistance than it is to soften or to move away from an established authority effort or pattern. We reasonably tend to distrust individuals who have traditionally sought to influence through the exercise of their authority when they appeal to friendship or reason.
- *The quality of performance tends to increase as one moves from authority to intellectualization.* Performance elicited by authority tends to be limited to the minimal level of acceptable behavior that will satisfy the authority figure; intellectualization, on the other hand, requires commitment of the individual to the new behavior and enlists his or her pride and motivation in determining the level of performance.
- *The likelihood that the desired behavior will persist in the absence of the influencer also increases as one moves from authority to intellectualization.* Intellectualization involves the transfer of control from the influencer to the influencee; its principal force is to make the advocated behavior self-motivated.

This analysis of the factors that might mediate a choice among authority, bargaining, persuasion, and intellectualization may appear to suggest that intellectualization might be the desired method under all conditions. Given the basic goals of preventive dentistry, there is a considerable element of truth to this conclusion. Certainly, in terms of the possible responses to an influence attempt, intellectualization is most likely to produce internalization. The use of authority frequently produces either open resistance (when the influencer misjudges the extent of his or her real power over the influencee) or passive resistance (expedient compliance when the potential ability to reward and punish is considerable, but the influencee is able to remove himself or herself from the surveillance of the influencer). Similarly, bargaining often produces simple compliance or minimal acceptable behavior, which persists only until the promised reward is exchanged. Persuasion relies heavily on achieving the advocated behavior change through identification with the influencer. Whether this will be a strong enough mechanism to endure over time depends on the strength of the affiliated bonds in the relationship and the amount of time between visits.

Factors influencing the choice of an appropriate influence strategy. The choice of an influence strategy is mediated by several critical factors:

- *Time available* is the most important critical factor. Under crisis conditions, when immediate compliance is necessary to prevent serious problems, appeals to authority are both effective and sensible. As the time available increases, however, it is sensible to attend to longer-range goals and needs and to move to methods that seek to transfer control of behavior to the individual. Authority and bargaining are likely to be both effective and efficient when the opportunity to observe subsequent behavior is present and when the opportunity to apply meaningful rewards and punishments continues over time. These methods are less effective when these abilities to observe and provide feedback on behavior are missing. A patient who maintains a regular schedule of visits may be more effectively influenced through the use of authority and bargaining than a patient who appears only irregularly.

- The *interaction of the personal characteristics* of the dentist and patient will strongly affect a choice of method. Intellectualization can be effective only with patients who are capable of understanding the informational inputs the dentist can provide. Very young children or individuals suffering from stress and anxiety or the difficulties of age may have to be approached in other ways, through affiliation and persuasion or through authority. Educated, informed patients may insist on extensive information and come to doubt the competence of a dentist who relies on personal charm or appeal to the mysticism of the profession.

As these examples show, the choice of an influence strategy is a complex and complicated process of analysis and planning. Time, objectives, opportunities to observe behavior, and the quality of interpersonal relationships must be weighed carefully in the choice of a method. The tendency to overlook the complexity of human behavior and to act out of habit, convenience, and our own convictions runs counter to successfully influencing the behavior of others. The time devoted to analysis and planning, to communication and counseling, and to transferring our convictions in a way that is real to others in terms of *their needs* is essential.

REFERENCES

1. Ference, T. P.: Organizational communications systems and the decision process, Management Sci. **17:**83, 1970.
2. French, J. R. P., Jr., and Raven, B.: The bases of social power. In Cartwright, D., ed.: Studies in social power, Ann Arbor, Mich., 1959, Institute for Social Research.
3. Hampton, D. R., Summer, C. E., and Webber, R. A.: Organizational behavior and the practice of management, rev. ed., Glenview, Ill., 1973, Scott, Foresman & Co.
4. Harris, T. A.: I'm o.k.—you're o.k.: A practical guide to transactional analysis, New York, 1969, Harper & Row, Publishers.
5. Hovland, C. I., et al.: The order of presentation in persuasion, New Haven, Conn., 1957, Yale University Press.
6. Janis, I. L., and Feshback, S.: Effects of fear-arousing communications, J. Abnorm. Soc. Psychol. **48:**78, 1953.
7. Kelman, H. C.: Processes of opinion change, Public Opinion Q. **25:**57, 1961.
8. Kolb, D. A., and Boyatzis, R. E.: Goal-setting and self-directed behavior change. In Kolb, D. A., Rubin, I. M., and McIntyre, J. M.: Organizational psychology: an experiential approach, Englewood Cliffs, N.J. 1971, Prentice-Hall, Inc.
9. Kolb, D. A., and Boyatzis, R. E.: On the dynamics of the helping relationship, J. Appl. Behav. Sci. 1970.
10. Leavitt, H. J.: Managerial psychology, ed. 3, Chicago, 1972, The University of Chicago Press.
11. Maslow, A. H.: A theory of human motivation, Psychol. Rev. **50:**370, 1943.
12. McClelland, D. S.: The achieving society, Princeton, N.J., 1961, Van Nostrand Co.
13. Myers, M. S.: Who are your motivated workers? Harvard Business Rev. **42:**73, 1964.

Part three

THE DRAMA

Dentist and patient interactions

The stage has been set. We have explored how the two main characters, the dentist and the patient, come to their respective roles. We have examined the setting in which dental care takes place in the United States and looked at issues such as the importance of the face and mouth as well as the objective and subjective need for dental care.

The lines have been learned. Basic psychological principles that affect the upcoming drama have been practiced. Psychological contracting, learning styles, motivation, perception, problem solving, conflict, communication, and interpersonal influence all involve different aspects that the dentist must understand to effectively play his or her role in the upcoming drama.

It is now time for the drama. Dentist and patient will meet and interact. The scene will be briefly set by looking at the dentist as a change agent. Before the curtain rises, a brief review of the timing of the lines will occur.

Then the curtain will rise. The implementation of change strategies will be explored. The plot will thicken. The aversive interactions of stress, anxiety, fear, and pain will be examined. The drama will conclude, as do many dentist-patient interactions, with the dentist and patient interacting under nonaversive conditions. The cast of characters by this time has grown, for the patient group represents the broad spectrum from young to old.

OBJECTIVES

The objectives for the chapters in Part three are as follows:

- To understand the process of behavior change in the context of the dentist-patient relationship
- To explore ways of implementing change strategies
- To better understand the aversive interactions of stress, anxiety, and fear
- To better understand the perception of pain and to explore ways the dentist might cope with the patient's pain
- To explore ways the dentist can help motivate, modify, and reinforce the patient's health behaviors
- To identify ways the dentist might better understand and work with patients of different age groups

Because our analysis of the dentist-patient interaction rests so heavily on the assumption that behavior change is necessary and is directed by specific principles, in Part three we will explore how behavior change can take place, whether it occurs under aversive or nonaversive conditions. By systematically applying the principles described in Part two to the process of behavior change, we can bring together apparently diverse problems and point to common elements of an approach to different situations.

Chapter 14

THE DENTIST AS A FACILITATOR OF CHANGE

Dentists spend a great deal of their time dealing with problems in the areas of conflict, communication, and interpersonal influence. Each of these areas of concern to the dentist implies a change process. Whenever a dentist is trying to get a crying child to hold still, resolve a fee dispute, or encourage a teenager to improve oral hygiene behavior, change is in the air.

Similarly, patients often seek greater control over the amount and type of dental treatment recommended. They may be motivated by perceived needs arising from concerns about aesthetics, pain, money, length of appointments, or less obvious personal responses to offered treatment plans. Here, too, a change process is desired, but in these instances, it is the dentist, not the patient, in whom change is sought.

One of the remarkable truisms about any change in behavior involving two or more persons is that the behavior change of one person in an interpersonal relationship, virtually by definition, compels behavior changes for others in the relationship. Dentists wishing to change patient behavior, albeit to well-intended and beneficial purposes, are modifying their own behavior in order to succeed. This is particularly evident when observing dentists who prepare and present alternative treatment plans in response to patient needs. By so doing, dentists demonstrate an understanding that the behavior change process is a reciprocal affair, and, when it works well, each person has been influenced or changed to behaviors that are personally and interpersonally acceptable.

Dental therapy as a change process

We have already seen in Chapter 13 how interpersonal influence strategies, in general, require that dentists (1) determine the focus of the change, (2) assess motives and needs, (3) assess the relationship with their patient, and (4) select a method for influencing change. The notion that dentists can and should change aspects of their patients' behavior is central to an understanding of the professional dentist-patient relationship. Indeed, to change the patient's behavior in some way or another is the prime responsibility of the dentist; and this responsibility has proved to be one of the most difficult long-term objectives for the dentist to achieve.

The significance of change and the complexity of the change process are not always self-evident to dentists or dental teachers. The excision of a palatal cyst, the replacement of a missing tooth, or the correction of a functional malocclusion are examples of changes in patients brought about by dentists through clinical activity. Dental therapy, as a matter of fact, should be thought of as a change process.

However, if the dentist had no factors to consider other than the patient's pathological condition and the choice of materials or techniques to treat it, viewing dental therapy as a change process would be of little utility. But, in fact, both patient and dentist bring to their interaction a history of objective and perceived needs: the dentist recognizes the condition, wants to treat it correctly, and wants the work to be appreciated; the patient has the condition and wants to be out of danger, but may or may not trust the dentist, appreciate the treatment, or want to return for another visit.

The dentist as a change agent

As discussed in Chapter 13, the dentist's perception of the dentist-patient interaction motivates his or her attempts to influence the patient—to "bring the patient around," so to speak—so that the patient will *understand* the required treatment, will *accept* the necessary procedures, will *appreciate* the treatment, and will *continue* to seek more treatment without undue negative or aversive behavior such as extreme anxiety reactions or avoidance of the dentist. This description of the dentist's perception and motivation is reasonably accurate when it comes to interacting with patients.

However, dental education and dental practice do not seem to adequately reinforce an equally valid and logically symmetrical concept, namely, that the process of "bringing the patient around" requires that *the dentist be a change agent who is constantly utilizing motivational and behavioral strategies to achieve desired ends.* The patient's perceptions, motivations, and behaviors change or shape how the dentist perceives and reacts. For our purposes the dentist-patient interaction can be defined as an interactive change process that seeks to accommodate the dentist's objective and subjective needs and goals with those of the patient.

In the preceding chapters, we have presented the antecedent conditions that help explain the behavior of both patient and dentist. In addition, we have laid down some principles for human behavior that operate for everyone, whether or not they are assuming roles as patients or dentists.

Behavior change definitions

Psychosocial perspective. In Part three, as in the rest of this book, dentist-patient interactions are discussed from a psychosocial perspective. By psychosocial perspective, we mean a consideration of how intrapersonal psychological factors such as anxiety, self-esteem, or concern over the body and interpersonal social factors such as being accepted by others and having needs met combine in patients and dentists to create the potential for dentist-patient relationships that range from friendly and long term to angry and abrupt.

Aversive and nonaversive conditions of interaction. For the purposes of this analysis we will assume that dentists perceive a need to shape their interactions with patients so that conditions that the patient perceives as negative, or aversive, are minimized and those the patient perceives as positive, or nonaversive, are maximized.

Conditions usually perceived as aversive that the dentist-patient interaction seeks to minimize are as follows:

1. Psychophysiological reactions
2. Stress, anxiety, and fear
3. Pain

Conditions usually perceived as nonaversive that the dentist-patient interaction seeks to maximize are as follows:

1. Communication—gathering information, identifying problems, giving information (as in case presentations)
2. Preventive oral health behavior
3. Management of exceptional patients such as the physically or emotionally disabled

Behavior. Behavior is defined, for our purposes, as a determined, purposeful unit of activity.[5] Each term in the definition needs examination, as follows:

determined The assumption that behavior is lawful and has determinants

purposeful The assumption that behavior is goal oriented, that it seeks to achieve positive and reduce negative need or motivated states.

unit of activity What a person does that can be reported or described as discrete elements.

Thus teeth do not behave, individuals do. *Observing* that a pulpal or periodontal pathological condition exists is a common behavior for the dentist. *Avoiding* the dentist, even though an objective need exists and the patient requires treatment, is a common behavior for patients. Both meet the criterion of being determined, purposeful units of human activity.

OBJECTIVES

The objectives of this chapter are as follows:

1. To explore different approaches to understanding and facilitating change, including identifying the role that the helping relationship plays in the change process
2. To explain individual differences in the ability to undertake or avoid dental treatment
3. To explore a range of inappropriate patient behaviors that might be displayed in the dental office
4. To clarify the role of the dentist in facilitating the change process

CHANGING THROUGH UNDERSTANDING VS CHANGING THROUGH DOING

When dentists want to know something about their patients' behavior, they turn primarily to psychology or psychiatry. That this is entirely reasonable can be better understood when it is further recognized that the major objective of all psychotherapy is change. Psychotherapists implicitly or explicitly seek to effect change in the emotional feelings, attitudes, and interpersonal behaviors of their patients. Without evidence of change in one or more of these areas, there can be no successful psychotherapy.

In order to evaluate whether or not any part of the psychotherapy enterprise has relevance for dentistry, it would be useful to examine some different approaches to the psychotherapy process with a view to evolving a rationale suitable for dentist-patient interactions. This examination is best begun by looking at two essentially opposing approaches for helping individuals to change their behavior. One approach follows from the work of Freud, the second from the work of Pavlov. A brief overview of the dynamics of personality as Freud conceived them follows.

The psychoanalytical (Freudian) approach to change

How change occurs. Freud[11] theorized and then claimed to demonstrate that individuals change when they *understand* their own motives and needs for behaving in a particular way. The popular expression "insight" is applicable here. A person experiencing emotional difficulty, for example, anxiety, can be relieved of the anxiety when, through the psychotherapy process, he or she gains insight into its causes.

It is the role of the psychoanalyst to facilitate the patient's insight into his or her emotional difficulties by offering to the patient a series of carefully thought-out interpretations regarding what the undesirable behaviors or feelings really mean. Psychoanalysis is one of several kinds of so-called **dynamic psychotherapies.**[8] These therapies are labeled "dynamic" because they seek to *uncover* unknown psychological dynamic (psychodynamic) factors that are responsible for the undesirable behavior. The therapist primarily uses verbal exchange to gain information about factors affecting the patient's behavior.

In psychoanalysis this is accomplished through psychoanalytical sessions that can range from two to five per week. These sessions often extend over a period of years. In these sessions the patient relates life events from far in the past to the present. The analyst, using psychoanalytical theory as a base, interprets for the patient how unpleasant life events in the present are connected to psychological problems or traumas that may have been experienced in the past. For example, an analyst might interpret a patient's present inability to tolerate receiving a "needle" as related to an incestuous sexual act forced on the patient in childhood that the patient had "forgotten."

If the analyst is successful in facilitating acceptance of such an interpretation, the patient has obtained an insight into the present dread of injections. Obtaining insight is therapeutic for the patient because it is anxiety relieving; it changes the undesirable fear from an unknown to a known, thus allowing more rational behavior to occur.

Causes of behavior. In the preceding case the causes relate to the psychological history of the person—events in his or her past that have been psychologically traumatic. These traumatic events leave a residue in the form of a predisposition to become anxious when, later in life, appropriate stimuli (real or symbolic) are encountered that have the capacity to elicit similar anxiety. For example, an emotionally painful feeding experience as an infant might predispose a child to become anxious when, later in life, persons in authority dictate how the oral cavity is to be manipulated. Similarly, middle-aged men avoiding the dentist might be interpreted as suffering castration anxiety; Freudian theory might predict that such men are avoiding the experience or anxiety elicited by the threat of tooth extraction, which for these patients might be the psychological equivalent of being castrated. Thus for persons with such histories Freud would suggest that the dentist became a stimulus to elicit the "remembered" residue of anxiety from the past.

Freud developed the theory and practice of psychoanalysis in order to help the patient change. In our example the goal of the therapy would be to relieve the patient of the experience of anxiety. Again, the prime mechanism for this change is to allow the patient, through the psychoanalytical process, to uncover the origins of his or her anxiety. Once the patient has obtained this insight, the theory is that he or she will feel less anxious and, therefore, cured. Hence the insight is held to be therapeutic. A case report by a psychoanalyst from the early psychoanalytic literature related to dentistry[12] is of interest here. In addition to revealing how long some dentists and analysts have been aware of the relationships between teeth and psychological states, the following case history demonstrates how psychoanalysis was helpful for one patient with a dental problem.

Case history*

A married woman, thirty-two years of age. Surgical pyorrhea treatment three years ago. A robust, apparently cheerful individual who, despite the splendid surgical results, stated that her teeth were "driving her crazy." She ground them day and night.

At the first visit, she described her domestic routine, which was one of extreme monotony. The health of her only child was a source of constant worry (greatly exaggerated). Her husband was very indifferent to all things connected with the home and the patient. He had the old habit of soap-boxing at the corner store with the boys, and perhaps a few rounds of the spirit which cheers. About 8 P.M. he would nonchalantly stroll in for supper. By the time he appeared, she would be in a highly nervous state, grinding her teeth and "all on edge," as she expressed it.

She was told by her dentist that she would lose all her teeth if she did not stop grinding. This thought became almost an obsession. Many times, while crossing the bay, she had a strong impulse to jump overboard; at night she dreamed of her teeth being pulled or falling out. This accumulated over a period of three years.

Subconsciously, while asleep, she was set-

*From Frohman, B.: Dental Cosmos **73**(Nov.):1117, 1931.

ting, pressing her teeth in, the thought predominating that they were coming out. Later she admitted that during the day she found herself pressing her teeth with her fingers. Voluntarily she stated that while doing this she vaguely recalled the apparition of extractions and being toothless. She preferred death to this.

Here her occlusal stress symbolized the phobia which proved to be the underlying motive.

In less than a month's time (of psychoanalysis) the mouth condition cleared up. Grinding and bruxism disappeared, and she was discharged as a very satisfactory result as far as I could determine, based upon her own enthusiasm and that of her dentist. Her first trauma was surgical; the second, psychic—when she was told she would lose all her teeth. These traumatia were with her constantly; deeply embedded in her conscious thoughts, characterized by day grinding; in her subconscious, by bruxism.

Usefulness to the dentist in the role of change agent. Does a psychoanalytical approach to behavior change have anything to do with dentists in their office? Psychoanalytical theory would suggest that, depending on the patient's past history, the contemplation of dental treatment could lead to anything from castration anxiety or dependency-authority conflicts to orality needs, body-image integrity, or narcissistic self-esteem, to name just a few possibilities.

Freud introduced several other ideas to explain how these predispositions and associations could come about. One of these concepts is extremely important; it has been labeled **unconscious motivation.** The central notion is that individuals typically do not know the motives for their own behavior. In the interests of smooth and adaptive psychological functioning, we are protected from constantly confronting the motives for our behavior. This concept of unconscious motivation is central to Freud's understanding of how individuals function in their everyday lives. Motives are kept unconscious through any one of a number of possible defenses; denial, repression, avoidance, and projection are some examples.

What this means for dentists is that persons may react to contemplating dental treatment with obscure and irrational emotions and behaviors. Freud would say that these behaviors and feelings really represent defensive operations to avoid anxiety, the threat of castration, the arousal of narcissistic concerns, etc. He would also insist that the patient's anxiety could be reduced if he or she could gain an understanding of the reasons for feeling anxious.

If man is, as Freud would have it, essentially irrational in that he behaves for reasons at best dimly understood, what hope is there for dentists confronting fearful patients? It is not reasonable nor at all appropriate for dentists to be psychoanalysts to their patients, even if they accept the psychoanalytical viewpoint. Before attempting to determine what implications this approach to behavior change would have on how the dentist might choose to interact with the patient, let us look at an opposing approach to effecting behavior change.

The behavioral (Pavlovian) approach

How change occurs. At precisely the same time Freud was developing his theories that the mind is a dark and mysterious place to which we have limited access, another equally well-known scientist, Pavlov, was also developing a theory to account for behavior. His theory required only one of the assumptions also critical to Freud's theory—the process of association. Both Freud and Pavlov assume that current behavior is associated with past events. For Freud[9] the association is complex and hidden over a long period of time. For Pavlov[18] the association between present behavior and past events is immediate and not hidden. Pavlov, working with conditioned reflexes, demonstrated that, at least in animals, desired behavior, or responses, could be elicited by certain conditions, or stimuli, and could be changed by altering environmental conditions. His work with stimulus-response conditioned reflexes in animals very rapidly was extended to human development and the prediction and control of human behavior.

The stream of therapy that followed from Pavlov has descended through the well-known American psychologists J. B. Watson and B. F. Skinner[21] under the labels **"conditioning therapy," "behavior modification,"** and **"learning therapy."** Although behavior modification (colloquially "behavior mod") is the most well-known term, the learning therapy label is the most interesting because it reveals the underlying assumption of this approach: that behavior change takes place through learning activity. For the behavior modification, or learning, therapist the main source of important data is *observable* behavior—what a person does.

To effect behavior change, the learning therapist introduces positive reinforcements when the patient exhibits desirable behaviors and delivers negative reinforcements when the patient demonstrates undesirable behaviors. Learning theory maintains that if an appropriate reinforcement schedule is used, patients may gradually be desensitized from experiencing negative emotional states such as anxiety or they may be conditioned to reduce aversive behaviors such as avoiding the dentist. Behavior therapists have been especially successful in the treatment of phobias such as an extremely irrational fear of heights or a fear of snakes. Typically the treatment time is short, often requiring only a few visits.[3] This time period might be contrasted with the time period for classical psychoanalytical treatment, which may require several years.

One example of a behavior therapy is of interest. Behavior modification approaches have been attempted with chronic psychotic patients institutionalized in "back wards" of state mental hospitals. Positive reinforcement in the form of tokens exchangeable for food preferred, self-grooming aids, etc. was provided to patients, when, for whatever reason, they exhibited some desirable behaviors such as leaving the ward to eat in the dining room. It has been demonstrated that previously recalcitrant mental patients radically change their behaviors in desired directions when the kinds and amounts of reinforcement are manipulated.[2]

Under much less strenuous circumstances, behavior modification has repeatedly proved successful in treating the recalcitrant child, the mentally retarded individual, and the extremely apprehensive patient requiring dental care. Learning therapy approaches seek to provide conditions in the environment that will enhance the elicitation of desired behaviors. In short, the environment is manipulated as a mechanism for facilitating the modification of patient behavior.

The behaviorist sees virtually no place for concepts such as insight, unconscious motivation, or defenses. With learning therapy, there is no examination of why the person feels or acts the way he or she does. As a matter of fact, Skinner himself acknowledges that his behavior modification methods are not theoretical vis-a-vis personality. He does not have, nor does he claim to need, a theory of personality.

Usefulness to the dentist in the role of change agent. Once again, it is time to ask if the behavioral approach has anything to do with dentists and their patients. Here the answer appears more obvious. Dentists do, in fact, often alter conditions to minimize their patients' feelings of anxiety and/or to encourage the acceptance of required dental treatment. Moreover, they do this apparently without benefit of in-depth inquiry into the roots of dental anxiety. When they are successful, they help patients to achieve desired behaviors and feelings in a relatively short time. So it would appear that behavior modification approaches are more effective than other approaches dentists might take to facilitate changes in patient feelings, attitudes, and behaviors.

Role of the helping relationship in the change process

Without questioning the validity of research reports that substantiate the efficacy of behavior therapy methodologies, equally valid research indicates that successful use of a behavior therapy approach does not come about solely as a function of the behavior therapy method. Other ingredients, most often overlooked by the behavior therapist, seem at least as important to the patients as the reinforcement schedule and the kinds of positive and negative reinforcers that the behavior therapist employs.[23]

These "other ingredients" that are missing from the behavior therapist's lexicon involve such variables as interpersonal relations, transference, and the psychodynamics of the rapport between patient and therapist. Although the behavior therapist largely ignores the latter factors, they unquestionably affect the extent to which the patient will allow the behavior therapist to determine the reinforcers and also the patient's degree of receptivity and ultimate acceptance of a behavior therapy schedule or program. For example, a patient who is afraid of entering an elevator might elect to see a behavior therapist, as opposed to a psychoanalyst, for the problem. The patient might believe that in-depth inquiry into personal history and early childhood experiences has absolutely no bearing on the current overwhelming fear of elevators. Such a patient would seek out an approach that would be more "objective" such as a therapy program that conditioned him or her to be unafraid of elevators. (Technically the program would seek to decondition the elevator phobia.)

But what happens when such a patient sees a behavior therapist? Usually there is a long discussion of the history of the symptoms—when they first appeared, how frequently, under what special circumstances, what reactions and feelings were experienced, etc.[26] This often involves learning about exercises or other kinds of regular behaviors the patient will undertake as part of therapy. In any event, the typical scene is one of much initial interaction, largely centered on the patient's symptoms and on methods that will be used to alleviate them.

As was implied in Chapter 12, the phenomenon of revealing one's problems to another person who is genuinely interested and who holds out the possibility of help is, in itself, known to be psychotherapeutic. Not only does the patient experience relief of at least some anxiety, but also the patient sees an intense interest on the part of another person, which has not been a typical finding for patients with phobias. In other words, an interpersonal relationship may develop, unannounced and unintended by the therapist, between the therapist and the patient. Moreover, when this interpersonal relationship is strongly positive, it meets the needs of the patient and is both future oriented and help oriented.[19]

The conviction of many workers is that the success of conditioning/deconditioning-type therapies occurs because of variables that may be operating in every type of therapy process.

> While each therapeutic orientation tends to emphasize aspects unique to that orientation as the potent or basic ingredients of psychotherapy, the common or nonspecific variables operating in each might actually be the variable accounting for much of the change secured by means of psychotherapy.[13]

In fact, critics of behavior therapy[4] claim that there are no "behavior therapies"; there are only helping relationships. Therefore behavior modification could be considered a method of allowing interpersonal relationships to be accepted by the patients.

Integrating a useful approach for dentists

Both the psychoanalytical and the behavioral approaches are useful when it comes to decisions about strategies to consider in changing patient attitudes and behavior. The psychoanalytic, or psychodynamic, view allows the dentist to understand and respond to his or her patient as a complex person, often with emotional problems that are obscure. Lengthened understanding leads to easier dentist acceptance of a broad range of patient behaviors, even if they appear strange or different from the dentist's internal set of "norms" for how persons generally, and dental patients specifically, "should" behave.

The combination of heightened understanding and easier acceptance of patient behavior gained from the dentist's awareness that psychodynamics do operate is often referred to as *sensitivity*. A "sensitive" dentist is thought to be one who attempts, uncritically and without evaluation, to allow the patient to exhibit any behaviors that facilitate accomplishing good dental care under conditions that the patient requires or at least tolerates.

On the other hand, the behaviorist's methodology provides specific mechanisms for demonstrating those sensitivities and for helping individuals to change in a manner acceptable to them. Thus the behavior therapy, or the behavior mod, method is viewed as a tool or strategy that creates the conditions and/or provides the devices allowing patients to change their behavior in desired directions to predicted degrees. However, there is more to the story.

The time has come to move toward a much sharper distinction between psychotherapy as an educational, or growth, experience on the one hand and as a technology for the achievement of behavior change on the other. The therapies extant today are typically mixtures of the two.

Psychoanalysis, for example, has tried to straddle the fence, but it has become increasingly clear that it is not impressively effective as a psychotechnology. Nevertheless, it has primarily attempted to utilize the framework of an emotionally charged interpersonal relationship to induce changes in attitudes, feelings, and behavior.

Within such a framework, psychoanalysts and behavior therapists apply the gamut of techniques that the human race has developed over the centuries for influencing and changing the behavior of its members. If it is indeed true that interpersonal dynamics are the main motivators for behavior change,[24] even in the behavior therapy setting, it is reasonable to expect the behavior therapist's effectiveness would be enhanced by training, or at the very least being sensitized to the operation of such dynamics. It would not be sufficient for a therapist to be trained simply as a technician of stimulus-response conditioning methods that he or she would then apply to people in trouble.

THEORIES EXPLAINING INDIVIDUAL DIFFERENCES IN THE ABILITY TO UNDERTAKE OR AVOID DENTAL TREATMENT

It has become apparent to many psychologically attuned observers that dentistry and the dentist-patient interaction represent a complexly interwoven cluster of cultural, social, environmental, and psychological factors that have the potential for producing emotional upset and even crisis. Although most patients demonstrate some degree of stress while contemplating or undertaking dental treatment, individual patient responses to the dental situation vary.

Various theories of personality, psychopathology, and psychotherapy explain dentistry as a psychological stressor in different ways. These theories, in addition to offering explanations of how dentistry can come to be a psychological stressor for most individuals, suggest ways that the perception of dentistry as a stressor might vary with each individual's particular history. Psychoanalytical and social learning theories provide different explanations for these questions. Let us look at how individual differences are explained from these two different perspectives.

Psychoanalytical theory

As might be expected, the "depth" psychologies and psychotherapies (psychoanalysis and its major derivatives) attach major significance to the oral cavity for the psychosexual development of the child. It is through the oral zone, initially, that the infant first learns about the world and experiences both distress and positive gratification via sucking, feeding, and early learning experiences. The importance of the mouth as the initial "erogenous" zone makes it reasonable to assume, according to psychoanalytical formulations, that subsequent activity involving the oral cavity and its related structures can acquire a significance to the individual known only to the unconscious. Thus depending on the unique psychosocial development of the infant, later dental treatment may symbolically be associated with repressed sexual or aggressive desires.

Anxiety would be the predictable consequence in a dental patient who had experienced emotional trauma (for example, conflicts over early feeding behavior) during the oral stage (from birth to 2 years of age). Anxiety in this case would be a signal[10] from the organism that there is a threat. Dental treatment might signal anxiety to organize any number of defensive operations. Defenses such as refusing to submit the oral cavity to a strong authority are "adaptive" in a patient with such an unconscious concern. Reality in the form of sharp needles and tissue damage would only lend "objective" anxiety to the situation and reinforce the neurotic anxiety that was elicited to ward off powerful repressed conflicts.

More specifically, denial is the major psychological defense aroused in situations where bodily injury and consequent blows to self-esteem are involved. Denial is an important and primitive (that is, develops early in childhood) defense used to ward off acknowledgment of narcissistic injury. It has its constructive aspects as well. For instance, temporary denial of existing injury may allow one, in a disaster such as a fire, to continue to function adaptively, helping oneself and others to escape from physical danger and death. The defense may, of course, be overdone, so that denial of bodily injury, for example, a carious tooth, leads to further bodily deterioration, for example, periapical infection. It often requires the reality of *extreme* pain and swelling to overcome strong denial mechanisms.

Generally the strength of the denial defense is determined by how much reality intrusion is required before the patient will acknowledge that something is really wrong enough to seek help. If the patient has a large swelling on the side of the face for a long time and does not have it examined, denial is working overtime as a neurotic defense mechanism.

Repression is another defense operation that serves to keep the significance of bodily states outside of awareness. Repression is distinguished from denial in that it operates on *psychological* realities such as fearful memories, whereas denial operates on *physical* realities such as infected teeth or swellings. When patients are denying or repressing excessively, they appear unassailable in their convictions that nothing is wrong and that they have no responsibility for the present problem.

Denial and repression can be thought of as a continuum of intrapsychic defensive strategies to ward off acceptance of responsibility for some coping behavior. The next (and most obvious) defensive strategy to complete the continuum is, simply, **avoidance.** Here the patient, quite consciously, decides not to do anything. Table 14-1 illustrates the different levels of awareness with which the patient responds to a problem.

The threat of actual confrontation with

Table 14-1 □ Different levels of awareness of patient response to a problem

Level of patient's acknowledgment of injury	Defense	How defense allows patient to avoid coping with bodily injuries, for example, swollen jaw	Sample patient response
Lower ↑	Denial	Filters out physical realities	"Since my teeth are fine, I don't have to go to the dentist."
	Repression	Filters out psychological realities	"Even though my jaw hurts a little, I don't need to go to the dentist—I'm certainly not afraid to go, and, besides, it's just not serious."
↓ Higher	Avoidance	Filters out both physical and psychological realities	"I don't need to go to the dentist—my teeth are fine, even if they hurt a little, and he'd hurt me if I went anyway."

body damage also elicits a series of behaviors related to another defense dimension, namely, **regression.** Because threats of bodily harm and disruption of body integrity elicit fears of abandonment and helplessness, the patient may appear childlike in his or her dependence on the dentist for help. Yet it would be a mistake to accept this childlike dependence at face value. Such regressive defenses often carry with them the childhood resentments associated with perceived and repressed memories of the deficiencies of parents at times of stress. This transference from previous to present authority figures when body integrity is at stake may lead the patient to place unrealistic expectations on the dentist. Such an occurrence may lead to conflict. Specifically, such a patient may overestimate the present authority's power or be uncertain whether the dentist is benign or malevolent.

Such a pattern of regressive behavior is seen when a patient says "Doctor, I put myself in your hands. I don't know anything about dentistry, and I don't need to or want to. You take care of everything. I know you will take good care of me, and it won't hurt, and it will last a long time." It is important to note that the dentist is not being *deliberately* "set up." Typically, the patient in this interaction is not aware of being manipulative and would be surprised to hear a wise dentist predict that when it is all over, the patient will have found that "the treatment wasn't that great," and/or "it did hurt," and/or "if only I had known what you were going to do. . . ."

Dental phobias, extremely aversive/avoidance behaviors on the part of dental patients, who stay away despite all kinds of symptoms, are said by psychoanalysts to arise from a defensive operation labeled **displacement.** In these instances the "true" source of the patient's anxiety is displaced onto dentistry, and the patient avoids having overwhelming anxiety elicited by avoiding going to the dentist. Dental phobias have been reported and have filled dental literature since antiquity.

Another popular term deriving from psychoanalysis that relates a psychological defense to dentist-patient interactions is hysteria, or more specifically, **hysterical conversion reactions.**[9] A hysterical conversion reaction is a bodily symptom for which no organic basis seems to exist and that is explained as a physiological expression of a psychological disturbance. Psychoanalytical theory explains hysterical symptoms as anxiety over repressed sexual conflicts. Symptoms that dentists have observed that have been attributed to hysterical conversion includes hysterical paralysis of the mandible (the patient apparently cannot or will not open or close the mouth) and the so-called burning tongue and burning mouth syndromes, in which painful burning reactions are present for no discernible reason.[20]

Social learning theory

Only a very brief overview statement regarding the learning theories is provided, since it should be pointed out, and indeed emphasized, that we have drawn most heavily from the social learning theorists in the discussion of learning styles, perception, and motivation in Part two. Also, the chapters on conflict, communication, and interpersonal influence are derived more from social learning perspectives than any other single school or psychological theory.

Alternative explanations have been offered for maladaptive, dentally related behaviors from the social psychological viewpoint (for example, in Adler[1]) and from the perspective of social learning theory (for example, in Mowrer[17]). These alternative explanations have not received nearly the popular attention associated with the more dramatic psychoanalytical formulations. Taken together, these groups of theories view dysfunctional dental behaviors as *learned* negative responses arising from interaction with others. Inappropriate behaviors, then, can be unlearned or changed by changing the conditions that reinforce them.

The aversive dental behaviors have the virtue of being more or less socially acceptable—after all, you have to be crazy to want to go to the dentist. At the same time these aversive behaviors serve the purpose of either denying more deeply seated fears or rewarding the manipulation of important interpersonal relationships. Thus a young child may demonstrate extreme aversive behavior during a dental visit such as moving around in the dental chair or turning the face away from the approaching dentist. This behavior might reflect a (negatively reinforcing) prior traumatic dental experience or it might reflect a positively conditioned response to previously experienced maternal anxiety about the child's visit to the dentist. It has been well established by Johnson and Baldwin[15] and others that the anxiety of the mother is accurately perceived by the child under stress. This maternal anxiety is transmitted through verbal and nonverbal behavior on the part of the mother, and it can dramatically influence her child's behavior. If, for example, the mother says "I'll give you a nice present if you only sit still for another minute," this is perceived by the child to mean "My mother is anxious for me to behave differently; now, if I don't, my mother will continue to be anxious." An association or learning experience is occurring for the child that relates the mother's anxiety and the child's undesirable behavior with the reception of dental care.

INAPPROPRIATE BEHAVIORS IN THE DENTAL OFFICE

Although conventional wisdom makes it readily apparent that dentistry elicits negative, unpleasant emotions and associations from almost everyone, it is not as readily apparent that also exhibited in a dentist's office are such maladaptive behavioral and emotional states as are seen with classic phobic behaviors, extreme anxiety neurosis, hypochondriasis, and agitated depression.[7]

General behaviors

Dentists are often puzzled when they observe behaviors of their patients that they view as inappropriate. These behaviors might include some of the following:

1. Loss of sleep
2. Loss of appetite
3. Heightened (respiration, heart rate, blood pressure, perspiration, flushing, and gastric activation) and reduced (salivation) levels of autonomic activation
4. Physical agitation, including tremors and restlessness

Localized behaviors

Both psychologists and dentists might observe a number of inappropriate signs or behaviors localized to the oral and immediately adjacent structures. Some of the following behaviors could be symptomatic of a dental-related anxiety:

1. Abnormal bruxisms (pattern of grinding or clenching the teeth and jaws)
2. Self-conscious avoidance of smiling or attempts to cover the mouth
3. Halitosis
4. Gross decay and/or periodontal disease
5. Physically unclean mouth

Often these highly specific oral signs and symptoms belie a patient unable or unwilling to contemplate dental care as a result of emotional factors not amenable to simple advice or rational explanation.

Patients influenced by strong cultural and social forces but stressed by inner conflict that is only imperfectly understood may exhibit intensely negative emotional states when contemplating dental treatment. This may lead to avoidance of dental care; uncooperative dental operatory patient behavior; failure to maintain already completed dental treatment; and paradoxical dependency behaviors, leading to apparently unnecessary dental visits.

The following case history by Wiener and Land[25] shows how emotional factors demonstrate a dental problem.

Case history*

Mrs. B was a 47-year-old woman who sought dental treatment because of extensive periodontal problems and multiple chronic ulcers of the buccal mucosa.† At each visit to her dentist (M.L.), Mrs. B would pour out her medical history. On one occasion, she said: "I don't know of very many things that haven't happened to me in a lifetime. I struck my toe and ran a knife into my left hand four years ago. I cut tendons in the palm of my hand. I wore my hand and arm in a full cast for six weeks. After the tendons were wired together and two weeks after the cast was removed, I was standing on the patio talking to a woman, and it popped just like a rubber band snapping. A tendon snapped and my hand drew up."

This operation was followed by another operation, a tendon transplant. She went on to point out where the incisions were made, how the graft was accomplished, where the wires were placed, and described a shirt button that was used to secure the graft in place. She stated that her operations had lasted four hours and went into great detail about her relationship with her physician who had taken numerous roentgenographs and photographs of her hand and arm and has used her for teaching in hospital staff conferences. When she shifted to her present history, she stated: "I am 47 years old and weigh 144 pounds. I have gained weight very fast, especially in the past three months. It seems as if I am hungry all the time now. I was never one to eat bread, but now I just crave hot bread. But then, I always seem to gain in the wintertime. It is easy to hold my weight down in the summer. When I stop to think about all the medicine, pills, injections, and glucose I've taken, it's a wonder I would like food at all." She poured out the rest of her medical history with great relish. She talked about the various accidents and physical traumata that had occurred to her. She said that she was the youngest of six siblings and was the baby of the family. Both of her parents were dead. She did not describe her relationship with her husband.

Let us evaluate this woman on the basis of her history and view it in terms of the four areas of need that were presented. In terms of her need for relatedness, it seemed quite obvious that she was hungry for a relationship. She literally pounced on the doctor verbally. She called for a dental appointment at the slightest provocation and insisted that she be maintained on a recall basis. In the area of dependence, she seemed to be eager to be cared for, especially by doctors. With regard to her need for independence and mastery she seemed to indicate that she would be a very capable person if it weren't for one or another of her many physical complaints. In the realm of physical pleasure, she made it quite evident that her desire for physical pleasure was tied closely with the infliction of pain. Her husband traveled extensively but when at home would accompany her to the dental operatory and be sympathetic to her complaints.

---

*From Weiner, M., and Land, M.: Psychosomatics **8**:308, 1967.

†In a study of recurrent aphthous stomatitis, 39 of a series of 62 patients (63%) associated exacerbations with periods of emotional stress.

THE ROLE OF THE DENTIST IN FACILITATING CHANGE

As any dentist can testify, all kinds of behaviors are demonstrated in the dental office, some of which may appear inappropriate. Dentists should, as psychotherapists do, accept the notion that the individuals who are their patients may be behaving for mysterious reasons (and this must be equally true of the dentist's behavior!). We have seen how complex the process of human motivation and perception is. Clearly, there is more to most of our behavior "than meets the eye" (or ear). The psychological, cultural, and economic conflicts that arise when most people go to the dentist result in behavior dentists see too often—avoidance of the dentist altogether or variable cooperation, both during treatment and with follow-through on preventive recommendations. These behaviors may result in poor oral or facial aesthetics and disease of the teeth and periodontium.

All the observable behaviors in the dental office have, in theory at least, an explanation or a history that is less observable. All schools of personality and psychopathology agree to that extent. We have discussed how some schools of psychology, for example, psychoanalysis, claim it useful to dwell on the "hidden" reasons for behavior. They interpret the observable behavior to be a reflection or symbol of inner psychological motivations and perceptions. We have also discussed how often psychologists, for example, behavior therapists, do not find it useful to focus on anything that cannot be readily observed. It is not necessarily that this latter group denies that such unseen motivations or perceptions exist as "explanations" for behavior, but rather that they claim greater utility in working with the observable parts of a patient's behavior.

There is sufficient evidence to recommend that dentists engage their patients with strategies that borrow the most useful aspects from each of these approaches. It is undeniable that dentist-patient interactions are enhanced—dentist and patient feel better and the dental treatment proceeds more tolerably—when dentists are armed with an awareness of the existence of inner, nonobservable patient needs.

It is also clear that behavioral approaches have provided dentists with specific strategies that the dentist might consider while working with patients. The dentist need not be a psychotherapist either to accomplish this increased awareness or to use this awareness for more effective dentist-patient interactions. Awareness, or increased sensitivity, that the patient's behavior may be the result of unknown, that is, nonobservable, factors is achieved *primarily by a willingness to listen and communicate carefully.* We have discussed at some length in Chapter 12 the principles behind the communication process. In Chapter 18 we will examine some practical strategies that the dentist might consider in enhancing his or her communication with the patient.

As far as the dentist-patient interaction goes, we are really calling attention to the *process* of being sensitized to the fact that nonobservable behavior, or inner state, of the patient is a powerful determinant of observable behavior. However, if we had to take a hard position, we would argue that being sensitized to the process by which observable behaviors come about may be more important for the dentist than establishing the specific content that underlies or explains a particular dental patient's behavior. Thus it is perfectly reasonable to urge (indeed, most behavior therapists do) that *once the dentist has established what the patient's perception of a problem is, the problem be accepted as valid, simply because the patient perceives the problem to be valid.*

The dentist need not interpret, for example, that fear of tooth extraction means fear of sexual impotence. No one would urge that dentists solve the problems either of validating that fear of sexual impotence is indeed a conflict for the patient or of "treating" that conflict. It is sufficient for dentists to acknowledge that neither the patient nor the dentist may know the "real" reason for the observable fear. Whatever the true etiology, the dentist's objective is the same—to construct patient interactions that manipulate the physical and psychological environment so that the most desirable dental treatment can be delivered within the comfort level of both patient and dentist.

The dentist's task as a facilitator of change, then, is to minimize conditions the *patient perceives* to be negative, or aversive, and maximize conditions the *patient perceives* to be positive, or nonaversive. Essentially each dentist can and should accomplish this objective in unique ways that are personally comfortable and consistent with his or her personality style and value system. Undoubtedly some dentists will emphasize physical and readily observable elements in the environment such as office decor, background music, and games to keep the kids busy; other dentists may find themselves relying more on their staff—receptionists, hygienists, and assistants—to create a welcoming and supporting dental office environment. Still others may be persuaded that their style of communication—ability to be clear, persuasive, etc.—will be the principal ingredient that shapes the environment their patients find.

Whatever uniqueness the dentist has developed as a personality, interactions with patients that lead to effective behavior change will always include the following two components: (1) a well-developed set of listening and communication skills and (2) a clear set of behavioral change (or behavior modification as opposed to psychoanalytical) strategies. Specific strategies that the dentist might consider will be discussed more fully in Chapter 15.

When to consider implementing a change strategy

Whenever the dentist-patient interaction is perceived by either party as not resulting in comfortable, efficient dental treatment, a change strategy is required. It is important to emphasize, however, that whose behavior should be changed—dentist's or patient's—depends on the circumstances at hand. Most of the time, the change strategy requires that the *dentist change some behavior first,* making or allowing the patient's behavior change to come about as a consequence of the dentist's new behavior.

For example, a patient reports intense dislike of local anesthesia: "I hate the needle, it always hurts so much going in, and I hate that numb feeling for so long afterwards. I can take the drilling, so why don't you work without giving me a shot"? The dentist, however, as a matter of routine, prefers to locally anesthetize all operative patients. By simply accepting the patient's perception about local anesthesia without further inquiry, the dentist can change routines and "begin working without giving a shot." Such a behavior change on the part of the dentist reinforces for the patient that individual needs will be perceived and acted on by the dentist. The dentist's response is consistent with the following approach to change:

1. That the dentist is a change agent in the service of creating adequate environments for tolerable dental care
2. That the dentist is sensitive to the patient's motivational and perceptual state
3. That the dentist is capable of responding to perceived patient needs by implementing behavior change strategies directed at getting the dental work done, as opposed to curing the patient's psyche

Suppose, in the preceding example, however, that shortly after drilling begins, the patient starts wincing and moving about, agitated, and quite evidently in pain. Is this not another valid perception by the dentist of the patient's receptivity to dental treatment? A conflict arises. To which should the dentist attend—the patient's stated preference for no anesthesia or the behavior while being treated? In short, is another change strategy called for? The answer is a simple *"yes!" The patient's behavior in the dental chair under actual treatment conditions takes precedence over the patient's verbalizations.* The dentist might communicate intended change on his or her part, as follows:

> I see you're moving about quite a bit. That usually means you're experiencing more discomfort than is necessary or even good for you, if the dentistry is to be done correctly. Why don't you allow me to show you how local anesthesia can, first of all, be administered almost without any pain, and then how it can help you to put up with the dental treatment while it allows me to perform the treatment according to the standards of good dentistry?

We are suggesting, by way of this example, that *dentist behavior changes come first.* The dentist can use the patient's physical behavior and verbalized statements as both criteria and reinforcers for the dentist's interventions.

Throughout the process of facilitating behavior changes, the consistent applications of the following principles of the helping relationship, discussed in Chapter 12, are applicable:

1. Establish when the patient or dentist perceives a problem with undertaking dental work.
2. Restate the problem, accepting the patient's perception of the problem.
3. Implement a change strategy appropriate to the restated problem, *not an interpretation of that problem.*

The dentist's objective should be to allow the patient to acknowledge anxiety accompanying dental treatment and then to accept the dentist's efforts to help cope with that anxiety. Patients seem best helped by empathetic dentists who demonstrate that their activities stem from concern with the patient as opposed to concern with the appointment book or the fee schedule.

SUMMARY

This chapter has attempted to summarize general behavior change rationale and strategy that dentists might consider when interacting with patients. In Chapter 15 we will explore specific change strategies the dentist can employ when, on the basis of the patient's behavior, he or she decides a change strategy is necessary.

REFERENCES

1. Adler, A.: The neurotic constitution, New York, 1917, Moffat, Yard.
2. Atthowe, J., and Krasner, L.: Preliminary report on the application of contingent reinforcement procedures (token economy) on a "chronic" psychiatric ward, J. Abnorm. Psychol. **73:**37, 1968.
3. Bandura, A.: Principles of behavior modification, New York, 1969, Holt, Rinehart & Winston, Inc.
4. Breger, L., and McGaugh, J. L.: Critique and reformulation of learning theory approaches to psychotherapy and neuroses, Psychol. Bull. **63:**338, 1965.
5. Chein, I.: The image of man, J. Soc. Issues **8:**1, 1962.
6. Dworkin, S. F.: A rationale for obtaining change in attitudes and behavior of dental patients, J. Tenn. State Dent. Assoc. **53:**147, 1973.
7. Dworkin, S. F.: Psychiatry and dentistry. In Wollman, B., ed.: International encyclopedia of neurology, psychiatry, psychoanalysis and psychology, vol. 4, New York, 1977, D. Van Nostrand Co.
8. Freedman, A., Kaplan, H., and Sadock, B.: Modern synopsis of psychiatry, Baltimore, 1972, The Williams & Wilkins Co.
9. Freud, A.: The ego and mechanism of defense, London, 1937, Hogarth Press, Ltd.
10. Freud, S.: The problem of anxiety, Co. New York, 1936, W. W. Norton & Co., Inc.
11. Freud, S.: Therapy and technique, New York, 1963, Collier Books.
12. Frohman, B.: The application of psychotherapy to dental problems, Dental Cosmos **73**(Nov.): 1117, 1931.
13. Garfield, S. L.: Basic ingredients as common factors in psychotherapy? J. Consult. Clin. Psychol. **41:**9, 1973.
14. Hunt, H. F.: Some behavioral considerations in psychiatric treatment, Paper presented at the American Academy of Psychoanalysis, San Francisco, May, 1970.
15. Johnson, R., and Baldwin, D., Jr.: Maternal anxiety and child behavior, J. Dent. Child. **36:**35, 1969.
16. Johnson, R., and Macben, J. B.: Behavior modification techniques and maternal anxiety, J. Dent. Child. **40:**272, 1973.
17. Mowrer, H. O.: Learning theory and behavior therapy. In Wolman, B., ed.: Handbook of clinical psychology, New York, 1965, McGraw-Hill Book Co.
18. Pavlov, I. P.: Conditioned reflexes, Oxford, 1927, Oxford University Press.
19. Rogers, C.: The necessary and sufficient conditions of therapeutic personality change, J. Consult. Clin. Psychol. **21:**95, 1957.

20. Scheonberg, B., Carr, A., Kutscher, A., and Zegarelli, E.: Chronic idiopathic orolingual pain, NY State J. Med. **17:**1832, 1971.
21. Skinner, B. F.: Science and human behavior, New York, 1953, Macmillan, Inc.
22. Skinner, B. F.: Beyond freedom and dignity, New York, 1971, Alfred A. Knopf, Inc.
23. Strupp, H. H.: On the basic ingredients of psychotherapy, J. Consult. Clin. Psychol. **41:**1, 1973.
24. Strupp, H. H.: The interpersonal relationship as a vehicle for therapeutic learning, J. Consult. Clin. Psychol. **41:**13, 1973.
25. Weiner, M., and Land, M.: Psychiatry, psychosomatics and dentistry, Psychosomatics **8:**308, 1967.
26. Wolpe, J., and Lazarus, A.: Behavior therapy techniques, Oxford, 1966, Pergamon Press, Ltd.

Chapter 15

IMPLEMENTATION OF CHANGE STRATEGIES

As we discussed in Chapter 14, many patients experience discomfort while contemplating or undergoing dental treatment. Moreover, in many cases the dentist may observe that the patient is exhibiting behaviors that actually inhibit the delivery of needed treatment, ranging all the way from something as obvious as a child refusing to open his or her mouth to something as subtle as a gag reflex that precludes a patient from being able to wear dentures. When the dentist determines that the patient is exhibiting behaviors that interfere with the delivery of needed treatment, some kind of change strategy is necessary.

OBJECTIVES

Once the dentist has determined that a change strategy is necessary, he or she has two options—to implement a change strategy or to refer the patient elsewhere for needed assistance. The objectives of this chapter are as follows:

1. To explore specific change strategies the dentist might use
2. To examine the use of these change strategies to remove unwanted symptoms and behaviors
3. To explore when referral is necessary, including reasons for and considerations in making referral and treatment decisions

CHANGE STRATEGIES THE DENTIST MIGHT USE

Dentistry has managed to evolve pragmatic techniques for behavior change and behavior management of the mentally retarded individual, the very young child, the older person, the terminally ill individual, and for most ambulatory, otherwise reasonably intact, dental patients exhibiting aversive dental behavior.[1] The practical exigencies of the dental treatment setting and the requirement of the dentist to focus on clinical work have predisposed dentists to develop relatively rapid methods for inducing more acceptable patient behavior. Essentially, when examined from the psychological perspective, dentists function as behavior therapists, employing behavior modification strategies that reinforce cooperative and resilient behavior. These strategies enhance the treatment by more rapid completion, a diminished experience of pain and anxiety, and a sense of positive accomplishment.

The two most widely employed behavior modification approaches to change behavior are systematic desensitization and reciprocal inhibition. Both approaches assume that "wrong" behaviors have been learned. These behaviors are maladaptive because they stand in the way of dental treatment. Both approaches employ a strategy of "going slow"[10] to substitute "better" behaviors for the maladaptive behavior. These better behaviors allow an agreed-on need—in this case, completed dental treatment—to be met.

Systematic desensitization

Procedure. Systematic desensitization requires that the dentist *identify an end* *point of patient behavior* that both the dentist and the patient wish to reach, but that is presently beyond the patient's ability. The end point should be as specific as possible; it may be a series of end points, put together in a logical sequence. End points might be intraoral injection of local anesthetic to a patient "deathly afraid of needles" or the successful completion of impression taking for an eternal "gagger" who requires a removable prosthesis.

Having identified both the end point and the present behavioral obstacles, the dentist must then elicit from the patient the *clear verbal or written understanding and agreement that the patient desires the end-product behavior*.

The systematic desensitization process, then, involves the development of a **behavior modification program,** or schedule, which consists of nothing more than (1) the series of steps the dentist will take to reach the desired end point, (2) the desired patient behavior(s) at each step, and (3) the positive (and negative, if appropriate) reinforcers to be used along the way.

Each of the dentist's actions or behaviors will be determined utilizing clinical judgment and the patient's response to the dentist's interventions. The desired patient behaviors typically consist of acceptance of a procedure without verbal or nonverbal signs of distress. The main positive reinforcers, or reward system, for the patient are the dentist's approval of how "well the patient is behaving" *and* the patient's own improved self-esteem and satisfaction that the desired end point to which he or

SYSTEMATIC DESENSITIZATION APPROACH

History

A healthy young adult with no contraindications to routine dental care presently requires extensive intracoronal restorative procedures as a result of caries. The patient has avoided the dentist because of a "fear of needles." All previous operative dentistry was done without a local anesthetic, and the patient reports that treatments were painful.

Dentist activity	Dentist and patient activity	Relationship to relevant dynamic aspects of communication, interpersonal influence, and change process*
1. Identify end-point behavior. a. Intraoral infiltration injection of 2% lidocaine, 1 : 100,000 epinephrine solution.	1. Elicit history of problem. a. Past experience with "needles" in dental and medical settings.	1. To determine focus of change attempt and assess motives and needs.
b. Patient report of lack of traumatic experience associated with intraoral injection of local anesthetic.	b. Present attitudes, concerns, and expectations about what would happen if injection were attempted.	
2. Summarize behavioral obstacles and communicate them to patient. Restate to patient an understanding and acceptance of his or her concerns and expectations regarding intraoral injection.	2. Elicit agreement of mutual dentist-patient understanding of problem and obstacles.	2. To determine conditions that enhance communication (effective transmittal of information).

*Discussed in Chapters 12 and 13.

Dentist activity	Dentist and patient activity	Relationship to relevant dynamic aspects of communication, interpersonal influence, and change process
3. State desired end-point behavior with supporting rationale. a. Objective need for local anesthetic. b. Subjective advantages to patient—increased comfort, no pain, etc. c. Objective advantages to dentist—ease of operating, etc.	3. Elicit understanding of rationale and clear agreement that patient desires end-point behaviors. a. Local anesthetic. b. Nonpainful, less anxiety-provoking experience.	3. To organize and increase received comprehension and acceptance of message.
4. Develop specific behavior modification paradigm or schedule based on systematic desensitization. a. Preliminary explanation of local anesthetic. b. Opportunity for patient to manipulate materials or observe procedures, if desired. c. Placement of local anesthetic. d. Detailed explanation of local anesthetic. (1) Drug action and method of administration. (2) Associated sensations. (3) Postoperative sensations. (4) Time course for each step in sequence. e. Inject minimal solution in place.	4. None required.	4. To determine conditions enhancing communication (effective transmittal of information) and identify considerations in communication process.
5. Implement each step of "behavior mod" schedule, that is, proceed slowly. a. Careful observation of patient. b. Repetition of rationale and explanations. c. Repeated inquiry into patient status. d. Repeated positive reinforcement *at each step:* "That's right," "You're doing well," "Now you're feeling. . . ."	5. Elicit patient understanding and acceptance at each step (called feedback by psychologists): "I'm OK," "It's just like you said," "You can continue," "I'm a little scared, but if you're sure, go ahead," "I feel the tingling now."	5. To validate that receiver is comprehending the message. To recognize barriers to effective communication. To distinguish between emotion and information.

she is committed is, in fact, being attained. The material on systematic desensitization on p. 216 will make clear how systematic desensitization operates for a specific problem.

Additional suggestions for implementation. If necessary, repeat an explanation. Give the patient sufficient time for disclosing concerns and providing feedback.

In the case of desensitization involving an injection, initially inject only a sufficient amount of the solution to elicit a subjective response so that a change in orofacial sensation is perceived. Repeat the procedure, injecting a greater quantity of the local anesthetic. If necessary, dismiss the truly phobic patient after only minimal injection.

Reinforce and elicit from the patient the nontraumatic nature of the experience. Advise that "next time will be exactly the same." Repeat the exact procedure on a subsequent visit. If patient feedback is appropriate (positive), go ahead with other procedures.

Reciprocal inhibition

Procedure. Reciprocal inhibition[10] involves the gradual extinguishing or inhibiting of an undesirable behavior while gradually increasing the appearance of a desirable behavior as a replacement. In the dentist-patient interaction, reciprocal inhibition is often applied to more general (as opposed to focal) types of undesirable dental patient behaviors such as feelings of anxiety over dentistry—"going to the dentist is the worst experience I can have."

The most common reciprocal inhibition approaches introduce relaxation as the desired behavior. Relaxation of the patient should increase as the dentist seeks to inhibit the experience of anxiety. Hypnosis, autosuggestion, progressive relaxation, transcendental meditation, biofeedback, waking sedation, and chemotherapy techniques have all been employed by dentists to help patients relax and simultaneously to diminish negative or aversive emotional states.

When utilizing the reciprocal inhibition approach, one assumes that a person cannot be relaxed and anxious at the same time! Since the approach derives from learning theory, the assumption is made that most anxiety symptoms with which dentists would be concerned are inappropriately learned behaviors. Moreover, a further assumption is made that much of what we call anxiety is a learned label applied to a particularly noxious body state—increased rapid and shallow respiration, increased heart rate, increased blood pressure, sweating, muscle tension, and gastrointestinal upset.

When utilizing this approach, one seeks to diminish or eliminate this aversive body state with the expectation that the experience of anxiety will diminish as the associated body cues disappear. Hence *relaxation* is introduced to eliminate those signs of anxiety that the patient has learned. One typically seeks to substitute relaxation for increased muscle tension and elevated noxious autonomic signs of increased heart rate and sweating. Reciprocal inhibition is similar to systematic desensitization in that the process of behavior modification is gradual, provides ample opportunities for feedback from the patient, and seeks to create a reward or reinforcement system to which the patient is committed. The material on reciprocal inhibition on p. 219 illustrates how this approach might work in a dental setting.

Additional suggestions for implementation. When used for more general types of concerns, feedback from the patient is obviously less specific than when addressing a focal problem such as "fear of needles."

Treatment initiation and/or rate should be altered relative to the dentist's expectations for patients not expressing such concerns.

Often an "education," or "training," period is involved in the hypnosis, transcendental meditation, or biofeedback treatment program. This period, as experience increases, can be relatively short (½ to 2 hours) and is more than compensated for,

RECIPROCAL INHIBITION APPROACH

History

Patient is a middle-aged man who can't bring himself to go to the dentist and doesn't know why. "It's nothing personal, doctor, but I just don't like dentists." No immediate dental emergency exists, the patient has been examined radiographically and examined clinically, and a diagnosis has been determined. The dentist decides that the most important and far-reaching first step in the treatment plan would be to employ a reciprocal inhibition approach to modify the patient's avoidance behavior and general aversive feelings about dentistry.

Dentist activity	Dentist and patient activity	Relationship to relevant dynamic aspects of communication, interpersonal influence, and change process*
1. Identify end-point behavior. a. Elimination of negative reaction to dentistry. b. Replacement with positive, but realistic, expectations that dental care is easily tolerated and that going to the dentist can even be "relaxing."	1. Elicit history of problem. a. Past experiences with dentists. b. Family experiences with dentistry. c. Present attitudes, concerns, and expectations.	1. To determine focus of change attempt and assess motives and needs.
2. Summarize behavioral obstacles and communicate them to patient. Restate to patient an understanding and acceptance of his or her concerns and expectations regarding dental care.	2. Elicit agreement of mutual dentist-patient understanding of problem and obstacles.	2. To determine conditions that enhance communication (effective transmittal of information).
3. State desired end-point behavior with supporting rationale. a. Long-term benefit gained by elimination of overriding negative behaviors. b. Short-term benefit of experiencing relaxing visit instead of anxious one. c. Objective advantages to patient—assurances of improved oral health, etc. d. Objective advantages to dentist—ease of providing care, etc.	3. Elicit understanding of rationale and clear agreement that patient desires end-point behaviors. a. Want to be able to go to the dentist and "enjoy" it. b. Want to eliminate those feelings that make me stay away.	3. To organize and increase received comprehension and acceptance of message.

*Discussed in Chapters 12 and 13.

Continued.

RECIPROCAL INHIBITION APPROACH—cont'd

Dentist activity	Dentist and patient activity	Relationship to relevant dynamic aspects of communication, interpersonal influence, and change process
4. Develop specific behavior modification paradigm or schedule based on reciprocal inhibition. a. Introduce and explain hypnosis, autosuggestion, progressive relaxation, transcendental meditation, biofeedback, waking sedation, or chemotherapy techniques.† b. Reinforce association of well-being and relaxation with technique employed. c. Suggest and reinforce inhibition of anxiety or other aversive behaviors while relaxation is increasing. d. Plan to allow relaxation experience to be positive by "titrating" timing and amount of technique employed against patient response	4. None required.	4. To determine conditions enhancing communication (effective transmittal of information) and identify considerations in communication process.
5. Implement each step of "behavior mod" schedule, that is, proceed slowly. a. Careful observation of patient. b. Repetition of rationale and explanations. c. Repeated inquiry into patient status. d. Repeated positive reinforcement *at each step:* "That's right," "You're doing well," "Now you're feeling. . . ."	5. Elicit patient understanding and acceptance at each step (called feedback by psychologists): "I'm feeling pretty good," "I didn't know anyone could relax in a dental office," "This is going to be much better."	5. To validate that receiver is comprehending message. To recognize barriers to effective communication. To distinguish between emotion and information.

†The methods named are best learned in recognized courses with qualified teachers. Many opportunities are available for interested dentists to become familiar with these techniques.

in the long run, by the creation of a dentist-patient interaction that is anxiety free, pleasant, and mutually rewarding.

USE OF CHANGE STRATEGIES TO REMOVE UNWANTED SYMPTOMS AND BEHAVIORS

"Ghost symptoms"

The dentist can be reasonably confident that behavior therapy approaches that involve systematic desensitization or reciprocal inhibition proceed quickly and rapidly with what Feather and Rhoads[2] call "ghost symptoms." In effect, a ghost symptom is an undesirable behavior whose original intra- or interpersonal need has been satisfied. The ghost symptom remains, however, simply as a "bad habit." The psychological problem that the symptom once served has been resolved. Thumb-sucking, nail-biting, and tongue-thrusting are examples of undesirable oral behaviors that may have begun in infancy or early childhood. The original need may have been for more sucking behavior, for prolonged feelings of security, or even simply for more food. As the child matured, those needs disappeared, as will happen in many instances of these types of behaviors. The behavior pattern, however, becomes a familiar and comforting one (a habit), even though it is not attached to its original need. The term "functional autonomy" has been used to describe the status of this type of behavior, wherein the symptom now seems to have a life of its own.

But if the original need is gone, there is no longer any usefulness in continuing to diagnose the undesired habit as "symptomatic." Continuing to interpret every undesired behavior pattern in every person as symptomatic of some deeper intra- or interpersonal psychological conflict is counterproductive. That practice stands in the way of providing brief, focal therapeutic assistance to help dental patients modify behaviors that interfere with normal oral functioning.

Of course, if an undesirable or phobic behavior continues to express or solve a current conflict, simple behavior therapy approaches will not be successful. But even in these instances, dentists can be more optimistic about successfully modifying patient behavior for the purposes of rendering dental care than the behavior therapy psychiatrist might be for making an important change in the patient's overall life pattern.

Behaviors with "deeper" roots

The task for the dentist is to shape all behaviors interfering with adaptive responses to dental treatment into the status of ghost problems—even if it appears obvious that an inappropriate behavior has deeper roots. For example, a markedly apprehensive, attractive young woman who cannot sleep the night before a dental visit, yet whose aesthetic facial appearance is visibly affected by decayed or missing teeth, may be assumed to have a psychological problem "deeper" than fear of an injection or of a dental drill. Nevertheless, a dentist could approach such a patient (1) with the clear understanding that he or she can accept the patient's behavior without negatively evaluating the patient as a person; (2) with an intention to meet the patient's dental needs via procedures that are relatively routine and nonpainful; (3) with the further clear understanding that whatever anxiety, personality needs, or other emotional concerns the patient has, the dentist promises to attend only to the needs of the oral cavity, not to the psyche in general; and (4) with an opportunity for the patient to undertake a few experiences designed to introduce the patient, via small steps, to the manner in which dental care is provided.

The focus of this interaction is to isolate the inappropriate behavioral symptoms of the patient so they have no relevance in the dental setting, without attacking their legitimacy for meeting the patient's other needs. Such an approach is labeled **symptom removal,** and there is no doubt that it does not provide full psychotherapeutic treatment. However, dentists need not be concerned; that is not their objective.

Some theorists assert that symptom removal is dangerous. This belief presupposes a closed-energy system so constant that eradicating one manifestation of the "psychic" energy that the symptom represents necessarily provokes a new eruption elsewhere. Although this conceptual model is clear, confirming clinical data for the claim of danger are not. Rather, case reports that supposedly support this claim may be better understood on the basis of a sequence of new symptom developments that would have occurred despite any treatment or on the basis of inept treatment intervention. Evidence that the process of symptom removal per se is harmful has not as yet been adequately established, as the subsequent, somewhat unusual case history will demonstrate.

A sensible approach to the problem is exemplified in a case history account provided by Rosenberg.[6] In the dental office he used Gestalt psychotherapy methods to modify thumb-sucking behavior. As the case history will reveal, Gestalt psychology focuses on behavior change brought about through heightened self-awareness. The underlying Gestalt concepts derive from psychoanalysis in that awareness is increased of heretofore ignored or unknown motives of the patient. Simultaneously, the therapy methods utilized in the following account are behavioral in their brevity, high degree of structure, and reliance on positive reinforcement and self-feedback. Individuals are free to judge for themselves where the "cure" comes from: Is the therapeutic success of modifying thumb-sucking a result of this particular technique of Gestalt psychotherapy or did the child stop sucking the thumb because of the unique relationship, especially for a 6-year-old child, established between dentist and child through the vehicle of the unusual therapy structure?

Case history*

The term Gestalt Psychology refers to a form of verbal and non verbal therapy developed by Frederick Perls and his associates. Its extremely effective and rapid procedures bring awareness to behavior in such a manner as to allow and encourage behavioral changes that are lasting. The technique I will be talking about is similar to role-playing but with slight variations. The following is an outline of the procedure I use.

First, it is important to attempt to relieve all pressure from parental sources upon the child and shift the responsibility for the behavior to the child and no one else. When I introduce the program of thumb therapy, I first have an appointment with one of the parents (usually the mother). I briefly explain to her that thumb sucking may be an emotional problem being expressed and that if after one or two appointments, we do not begin to get success, it is possible that I may have to refer the child to a psychologist for further consultation. I also make it clear that, in order to insure success with the therapy we are undertaking, I will need the parents' cooperation. That cooperation involves not allowing the child to shift the responsibility for thumb sucking to the parent. Thus the mother now feels she can't nag because she would be taking over responsibility; I also point out that the nagging hasn't produced any positive results. In most cases, parents are eager to have aid with the problem and cooperate willingly. I then briefly tell mother we are going to have Johnnie "Role-play" different parts of himself to help him become more aware of his behavior. In that way, we will hope to help him change his behavior.

Next step—Gestalt therapy

The next step is to start a form of Gestalt therapy with the child. Briefly the aspects of Gestalt therapy that are applicable to this procedure are the concepts of: 1) taking sides, 2) encountering, 3) bodily expression of emotion. Taking sides and merely experiencing the tendencies involved in a conflict many times is enough to precipitate a synthesis or resolution. If not, the integration of the opposites may be brought about by their "encountering." Taking sides refers to experiencing any conflict in its duality, for example, "I would like to stop sucking my thumb," and "I want to suck my thumb."

To initiate this procedure, I ask the child to come into my office where I have two chairs (should have a padded seat as we'll see later) used to represent the two aspects of the problem. The child can sit in two different chairs to see the feelings related to each aspect of the conflict.

*From Rosenberg, J.: A Gestalt approach to thumb sucking, San Rafael, Calif., 1973. (Author reprint.)

The dialogue goes something like this:

Dr.: Johnnie, which thumb, finger, wrist, etc. do you suck? (Johnnie will indicate usually by holding up his thumb.) Well, Johnnie, I want you now to put your thumb in the other chair that is facing you. (Johnnie usually looks bewildered at this point, but I explain.) Don't think about it, let's just pretend we're playing a game. (Johnnie places his thumb in the chair.) Good, Johnnic, now you can take your thumb away, but we'll pretend he's still in the other chair. Do you have anything to say to your thumb, Johnnie? (Johnnie will usually say right away that he wants the thumb to stay out of his mouth, but if this doesn't come right away, then I suggest he may want the thumb to stay out of his mouth and I tell him to tell his thumb that.)

Johnnie: Thumb, stay out of my mouth!

Dr.: Johnnie, tell the thumb why you want him to stay out of your mouth. (This approach has two aspects: 1) To further define the taking sides; 2) To find out more about the origin of the habit, and giving some clue as to the possibility of solution and possibility of success.) Johnnie's response to this "why" question may vary greatly, but in general his answers usually indicate the source of the pressure on him and how much responsibility he takes for his action. For example:

Johnnie: I want you to stay out of my mouth because—my mommy wants you to. Dr. Rosenberg wants you to. Kids tease me. You ruin my teeth. You taste bad when you're dirty. You make me feel like a baby.

Johnnie becomes his thumb

Now I have Johnnie change chairs and take the empty seat he has been addressing and "be" the thumb. In other words, he role-plays his thumb or enacts the conflict by being the thumb. The child unknowingly takes the role of that aspect of his personality that wishes to suck his thumb.

Dr.: Well, thumb, tell Johnnie why you go into his mouth.

Johnnie: I want to.

Dr.: Tell Johnnie why you want to go in Johnnie's mouth.

Johnnie: I make mommy upset. I get the teacher to shout at me. I feel better. I need to because I get lonesome. I want to be a baby. I want to make Johnnie's teeth crooked so he can have braces.

The direction the role-play goes depends, of course, on the responses that Johnnie gives and therefore it is impossible to give the exact verbal replay. But in general the approach at this point can be summarized by the doctor constantly directing the response to the concept of "whose problem is it?" If Johnnie says "Dr. Rosenberg wants you to stop coming in my mouth" I might say: "Johnnie, I don't care if you suck your thumb, and if you want to stop, I'll be here to help and that's what we're doing now, but *you're* the only one who can keep your thumb out of your mouth."

When Johnnie as the thumb is talking, I merely direct Johnnie's attention to stay with the game of being the thumb. Now we switch chairs again and Johnnie answers the thumb.

Dr.: Johnnie, how do you feel about that thumb's wanting to be in your mouth?

Johnnie: Well, I don't like it, or I don't care, or I don't know.

Dr.: Johnnie, can you tell that thumb to stay out of your mouth and really mean it?

Johnnie: Stay out of my mouth, thumb!

Dr.: Change chairs now, Johnnie. Do you believe him, thumb?

Johnnie (in thumb's chair): No.

Dr.: Doesn't sound like the thumb believes you. Now change chairs again. Johnnie, I want you to make a fist and hit that thumb and tell him to stay out of your mouth. (Usually Johnnie is more than ready by this time to express some anger, and the ferocity with which this task is undertaken is amazing. This is why we need a padded seat so the child will not hurt his hand.)

Anger releases emotion

It is not important at whom the anger is directed, but sometimes the child will tell you who else is sitting in the chair. For example: Hitting the empty chair with obvious joy, "I wish mommy or you were there," etc. The important thing is that the emotion associated with the habit be released. When this explosion calms, I again get Johnnie to tell his thumb to stay out of his mouth.

Dr. (to Johnnie in thumb's chair): Well, thumb, how do you feel now?

Johnnie: Well, I guess he means it, or I think I'll stay out of his mouth (some indication that the point got across).

Dr.: Change chairs. O.K., Johnnie, it looks to me as if you have a battle on your hands. Either you can wiggle that thumb and really tell it what to do or it will wiggle you and sneak into your mouth. I'm sure you now know that you can be boss. I'll see you in three days and we'll see how you do. Good luck.

The next appointment we again have the dialogue with the thumb, and repeat the process until the battle is over.

Thus we first enact the different aspects of Johnnie's personality, then they encounter each other. We physically express aggression that was being held and reinforce the fact that responsibility of the problem is in Johnnie's hands.

This pattern is rather typical of most of the cases I have seen with only slight variations. The therapy usually takes two appointments and possibly a third for difficult cases.

When I have had a case that goes more than two or three appointments, the pattern of the dialogue usually follows something like "I don't want to change because I don't want to grow up; I want to be a baby." When this happens, I ask the child to suck his thumb while he is sitting in the thumb's chair and be a baby. When Johnnie is asked to go into or exaggerate his infantile behavior, he becomes more in touch with his need and will then usually refuse to be a baby. I point out that there are two parts of Johnnie: A part that wants to be a baby and a part that wants to grow up. And the dialogue now takes a slightly different aspect. The fact that he will refuse to suck his thumb in front of me is useful because he can see very dramatically now that only *he* can suck his thumb and only *he* can stop; if he wants to suck or not suck, no one else can change him.

If Johnnie really gets into it when I ask him to suck his thumb and be a baby, I let him suck for a long time. Then I say "Stop, O.K., now, suck again. No, stop," etc., until he may rebel. Then we again arrive at the point where no one can make him suck or stop but himself, and it is his responsibility.

If the conflict can't be resolved in four or five appointments, I consider the possibility of referring the case for a psychological evaluation, or I reevaluate the dental problem and the need to try to change the behavior.

Again, the particular case history is presented because, although it represents one dentist's unique solution, it also represents the consistent application of a body of knowledge regarding behavior and behavior change.

The two most salient features are that (1) the behavior change is understood to come from a complex history that must be dealt with behaviorally (as opposed to talking it out) and (2) the behavior change strategy proceeds on the assumption that what is required is a carefully designed and introduced program calling for the patient's self-involvement, focusing on observable behavior as far as the patient is concerned, and providing the patient with immediate feedback by which to observe the desired behavior change.

As a matter of fact, there is some evidence that so-called symptom removal is a positive learning experience for the patient.[8] Consider the extremely frightened patient who is convinced that no dentist will ever be able to perform any dental procedures in his or her mouth or the patient in need of dentures who has an exaggerated gag reflex. Both these patients will experience, and be pleased to report, an intense sense of satisfaction once their problems have been helped to disappear. This finding is consistent with clinical dental experience and is borne out in the psychotherapy process as well. The mastery of a disabling symptom is frequently observed to generate psychological momentum that spills over into other areas of intra- and interpersonal psychological functioning.

IF REFERRAL IS NEEDED

Reasons for referral

Patients may exhibit psychiatric problems arising from dentally related concerns that cause them to seek or be referred for psychotherapy. When the dentist observes any of the following symptoms, he or she might consider expressing concern to the patient and making a referral:

1. Dentistry is perceived as a stressor of such magnitude that extreme aversive behaviors with concomitant stress or *anxiety* symptomatology are elicited. These behaviors are typically viewed by the patient as inappropriate and become maladaptive for the person's psychological or dental well-being.
2. Chronic pain states such as myofas-

cial pain dysfunction syndrome or other long-standing orofacial pain complaints yield *depression* as a major emotional symptom.

3. Disturbances in *body image* stemming from physical or treatment factors such as physical deformity or undue *narcissistic concerns*. Narcissistic behavior is inappropriate in a dental setting when anxiety, depression, or hostility over how the body looks, will look, or will be manipulated during treatment prevents dental work from being performed.

Considerations in making referral and treatment decisions

In all cases when a psychiatric evaluation and/or psychotherapy is sought (whether self-initiated or by referral from an attending dentist), decisions regarding treatment approaches and prognosis should take into account that the patient, dentist, and therapist may have different sets of outcome expectancies. The dentist will primarily be interested in helping to create a psychologically receptive dental patient who tolerates clinical dental care well and does not present the dentist with subjective symptom reports for which the dentist has no remedy; the patient may seek symptom relief, for example, anxiety or pain relief, and nothing more. The psychiatrist may discern, depending on his or her own theoretical predilections, underlying psychopathological conditions or undesirable emotional conflicts not readily resolved by attacking simply the symptoms present.

Symptom removal for dental phobias and possible conversion reactions has been quite successfully achieved with a variety of short-term therapies that include, besides more traditional forms of individual and group therapy, such therapy modalities as hypnosis,[3] biofeedback,[7] and, especially, the behavior modification therapies.[1] (Systematic desensitization and reciprocal inhibition have been widely employed.) Such approaches have also provided patients suffering from chronic orofacial pain with a more adaptive repertoire of behaviors and varying amounts of long-term relief of pain. When deciding whether or not to refer, the dentist might remember that patients who develop somatic symptoms are generally resistant to psychotherapy or even to the acknowledgment that psychotherapy is indicated. Therefore if referral is made, it must be done carefully, with heavy emphasis on the need to modify specific behaviors interfering with treatment delivery. In such cases brief therapies, especially those of the behavior modification type, seem empirically the best way to begin, since behavior therapies minimize exploration or interpretation of psychological meaning to the problem. Symptom substitution following behavior therapy is virtually never reported with these patients. Such an approach renders the patient relatively symptom free and, in most cases, a suitable candidate for routine dental care.

The clinical dentist is often somewhat skeptical of longer forms of so-called dynamic psychotherapies, especially those that rely on depth interpretation of patient motivation. Such interpretation does not seem to the dentist easily validated by observable behavior nor easily inferred from patient verbalizations.

Empirically, there is some justification of the clinical dentist's present skepticism regarding the relevance for dental treatment of such psychological constructs as castration anxiety or the symbolic sexual penetration of the oral cavity represented by a dentist's fingers and/or instruments. These constructs, drawn in this case from psychoanalytical theory, have not proved useful to the dentist in the management of the apprehensive patient.

The overwhelming burden of psychotherapy research is on the side of the dentist who structures his or her patient interactions around a sound, empathetic interpersonal relationship introducing behavior therapy strategies to modify or shape the patient's behavior away from aversive responses such as anxiety; pain; other psy-

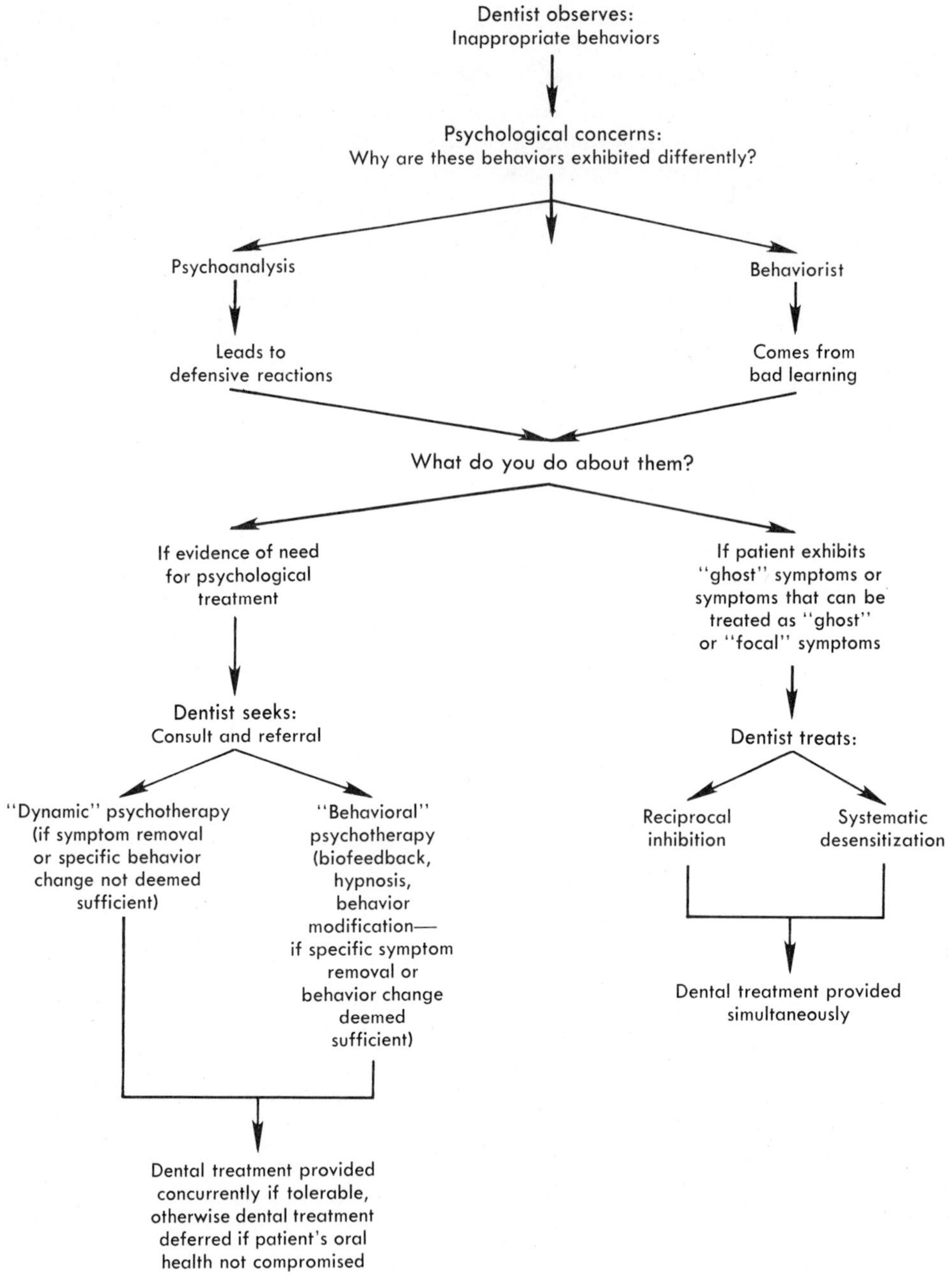

Fig. 15-1. Process of treatment and referral.

chophysiological reactions, for example, bruxism; and mistrust. Fig. 15-1 graphically summarizes how the process of treatment and referral might flow.

REFERENCES

1. Ayer, W., and Hirschman, R.: Psychology and dentistry, Springfield, Ill., 1972, Charles C Thomas, Publisher.
2. Feather, B. W., and Rhoads, J. M.: Psychodynamic behavior therapy, pt. I and II, Arch. Gen. Psychiatry **26:**496, 1972.
3. Hilgard, E. R., and Hilgard, J. R.: Hypnosis and the relief of pain, Los Altos, Calif., 1975, William Kaufman, Inc.
4. Perls, F., Hefferline, R., and Goodman, P.: Gestalt therapy, New York, 1951, Dell Publishing Co., Inc.
5. Rhoads, J. M., and Feather, B. W.: The application of psychodynamics to behavior therapy, Am. J. Psychiatry **131:**17, 1974.
6. Rosenberg, J.: A Gestalt approach to thumb sucking, San Rafael, Calif., 1973. (Author reprint.)
7. Shapiro, D., et al.: Biofeedback and self control, Chicago, 1973, Aldine Publishing Co.
8. Spiegel, H.: Is symptom removal dangerous? Am. J. Psychiatry **123:**1279, 1969.
9. Sullivan, H. S.: The interpersonal theory of psychiatry, New York, 1953, W. W. Norton & Co., Inc.
10. Wolpe, J.: Psychotherapy for reciprocal inhibition, Stanford, Calif., 1958, Stanford University Press.
11. Wolpe, J.: The systematic desensitization treatment of neuroses, J. Nerv. Ment. Dis. **132:**189, 1961.

Chapter 16

AVERSIVE INTERACTIONS—STRESS, ANXIETY, AND FEAR

There is no doubt that dentists and dentistry easily elicit negative or unpleasant emotions among patients contemplating or experiencing dental treatment. When describing how they feel about dental care, patients will often use terms such as "anxious," "afraid," or "hurts." Dentists know that dentistry is generally perceived as stressful, anxiety provoking, or threatening to the patient's physical and mental wellbeing. We have already discussed at length how the perceptual and motivational processes interact to produce patient behavior that is not "good" for the patient and often inexplicable as far as the dentist is concerned.

Dentists commonly ask psychologists for definitions of stress, anxiety, and fear. They also frequently seek increased understanding of these phenomena so they may better assess and respond to their patients' needs, making dentistry more comfortable for both patient and dentist. After all, if dentists knew their patients were "under stress," "anxious," or "afraid," they might shape dental interactions to reduce the patients' anxiety.

OBJECTIVES

The objectives of this chapter are as follows:

1. To define stress, anxiety, and fear
2. To identify major patterns of coping with stress, anxiety, and fear
3. To discuss the dental emergency as an opportunity to deal with stress, anxiety, and fear as related to the patient's perception of and the dentist's response to these phenomena
4. To examine some case histories of dental emergencies

DEFINITIONS OF STRESS, ANXIETY, AND FEAR

Stress, anxiety, and fear are terms with multiple and overlapping meanings. Defining each of the terms is complicated by the fact that stress, anxiety, and fear are words in everyone's general vocabulary. When these terms are used by behavioral scientists, medical researchers, or psychotherapists, they acquire technical connotations that are different from their usage by most persons.

The following definitions reflect a consensus of what the terms mean to many researchers and clinicians in the behavioral and social sciences and also reflect how we will use them in this book.

Similarities among stress, anxiety, and fear

Stimulus aspect. Stress, anxiety, and fear are stimuli to behavior. Generally, the behaviors resulting from these negative or unpleasant emotional stimuli are called avoidance, or aversive, behaviors, since they function to remove the person from the noxious experience. Another general tendency is for the strength of the avoidance response to be proportional to the perceived strength of the stimulus—the stress, anxiety, or fear. In extreme cases, stress, anxiety, and fear stimuli can totally disorganize the personality and lead to behaviors that are harmful to the patient. Moderately strong anxiety or fear can lead to various behaviors: cancellation of dental appointments, late arrival, apparently uncooperative treatment behaviors, and an inability to comprehend or remember postoperative instructions.

Threat appraisal aspect. Stress, anxiety, and fear stimulate an intervening behavior called threat appraisal. Threat is a psychological process by which the patient becomes ready to anticipate a harmful event. If the stress, anxiety, or fear stimulus leads to a threat appraisal that gives harmful meaning to the situation, the patient labels the experience as noxious, unpleasant, or aversive. A dentist approaching a young child may or may not induce stress, anxiety, or fear, depending on how the child interprets the dentist's approach, for example, whether it is the first treatment visit or the last prophylactic visit. Stress, anxiety, and fear as stimuli induce the patient first to appraise the threat, then to respond.

If the stimulus is perceived as very strong, the threat appraisal process does not proceed rationally. In our example, the young child would start crying and withdrawing immediately; in another instance, an older patient might experience becoming faint, even though treatment was not initiated. On the other hand, stress, anxiety, and fear that are appraised as weak to moderate often motivate the patient to more effective behavior. Under conditions of low anxiety and fear, the patient may become alerted to and constructively aware of the surroundings. Such is the case, for example, with mild forms of test stress or anxiety, which help the student "get up" for the task ahead.

Response aspect. Stress, anxiety, and fear are best known to us as responses. They are feeling-state responses that we all know very well. When individuals speak of being anxious, afraid, or under stress, they are referring to the response aspect of stress, anxiety, and fear—an unpleasant negative emotional state, full of upset, agitation, and dread. It is an obvious but pervasive concomitant of stress, anxiety, and fear that we do not like the experience, and we universally institute behaviors to remove these unpleasant emotional responses. Intuitively, most of us can tell when someone is experiencing stress, anxiety, or fear. Dentists probably tend to dismiss milder forms of these emotions they perceive in their patients as long as these signs do not interrupt scheduled or required treatment. The ways in which

Table 16-1 □ Stress, anxiety, and fear*

Behavioral component involved	Typical observable behaviors
Disturbed affect	Intensive expressions of negative emotional states such as crying or temper outbursts, even inappropriate laughter.
Changed motor behaviors	Increased muscle tension, disturbances of speech, inappropriate facial expressions, overly intense fight or flight motor behaviors.
Changed cognitive functions	Changed judgment, memory, perceptual organization, problem solving, and social interactions; failure to listen well, remember instructions or information provided. Change, per se, is the important indicator. Certain individuals undergoing certain stress responses actually improve some dimensions of their cognitive functioning; more commonly, stress induces failure of cognitive functioning.
Physiological changes	Autonomic changes, including increased cardiovascular functioning—especially increased heart rate and blood pressure—respiration, and sweat gland activity.

*Adapted from Lazarus, R.: Psychological stress and the coping process, New York, 1966, McGraw-Hill Book Co.

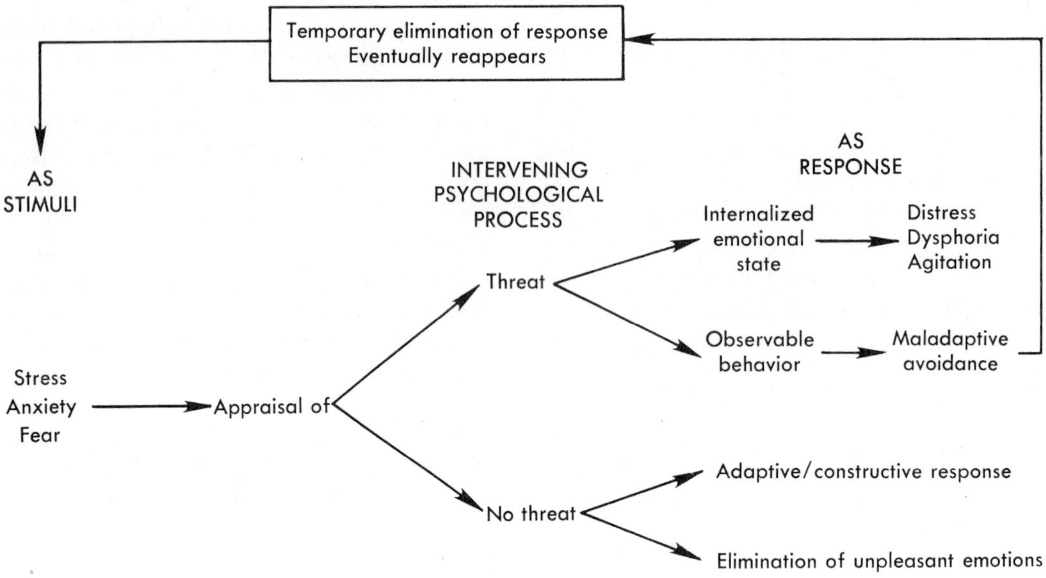

Fig. 16-1. Process of threat appraisal.

stress, anxiety, and fear typically reveal themselves are summarized in Table 16-1.

In summary, stress, anxiety, and fear are simultaneously negative, or aversive, emotional states, full of symptoms that can motivate through a process of threat appraisal (Fig. 16-1). The interaction of the intensity of emotional response with threat appraisal determines the content of the behavior that will follow—whether or not to show up at the dentist's, to submit to an injection, to accept the need for an extraction, to reject a prosthesis, etc.

Differences among stress, anxiety, and fear

Having discussed the psychological ingredients that stress, anxiety, and fear have in common, we will identify characteristics that uniquely define each term.

Stress. Stress is a term used to describe a general disturbance in psychophysiological adaptation. It implies a person who is being maladaptively influenced by more than one negative, or aversive, factor. Stress also refers to the body being overwhelmed—if stress were to continue, bodily disease and/or psychopathology would result. The term suggests the image of a person buffeted about by destructive forces and struggling to survive or flourish. Of the three terms, *stress is most associated with response aspects.*

Selye[6] defines stress solely in terms of response. In Selye's context, if dental treatment is perceived as threatening, it would be called a **stressor.**

The most important physiological stress responses relate to adrenal function during stress. Epinephrine from the adrenal medulla produces some of the autonomic changes noted in Chapter 2. The adrenal cortex, stimulated by stressors of physical or mental origin, produces steroids that can have far-ranging effects on the physiology and the psychology of the patient. Physical pain, tissue damage, and the local use of anesthetic drugs have the capacity to stimulate the release of identical quantities of free 17-hydroxycorticosteroids from the adrenal cortex. The mere anticipation of dental anesthesia also results in the *same* elevated levels of corticosteroids[3,4]; thus one cannot gauge whether this physiological stress response was induced by a clinical (the administration of local anesthetic) or by a psychological (the anticipation of an injection) effect.

Stress also seems to be a term associated with some degree of cognitive understanding and control over the elements that constitute the stress. Usually patients know they are under stress and act as if they know why. They speak of the stress of an examination or the stress of having to put up with prolonged, difficult procedures such as endodontic therapy or the removal of impacted teeth. The patient often knows what action is necessary to get over the stress.

Anxiety. *In comparison to the terms "stress" and "fear," "anxiety" seems to have greater relevance to a unique emotional state: a disturbed affect that is intensely negative and unpleasant.* Common psychophysiological indicators are trembling and increased autonomic activity—heart rate, respiration, and sweating, especially. The emphasis of the term "anxiety" is on its motivating or stimulus aspects. According to Freud, anxiety signals defensive operations. In modern behavior theory, anxiety motivates the learning of behaviors that avoid or permit escape from punishment.

Anxiety is a term with strong associations with the unknown. The relationship between anxiety and "not knowing" shows itself in two ways. One of the most common and disturbing aspects of anxiety is the inability of patients to know why they are anxious. Patients often cannot identify reasons for feeling anxious; however, they are often able to express it easily. "I don't know why, but I get so nervous when I go to the dentist. . . . I hate the feeling. . . ." The second way in which anxiety relates to the unknown is when there is no clear outcome in sight. Patients who do not know what is going to happen next or who do not know what to do next become anxious. Anxiety is always heightened when a threat appraisal is made, *but no clear behavior is possible to deal with the threat.* The behavior of anxious patients, more so than of stressed patients, can appear strange and incomprehensible to dentists. Anxious patients do not seem to behave in ways relevant to the situation. For example, patients may engage in superstitious behavior, believing that if they sit in a certain way, it will not hurt so much; they may ask to hold an assistant's hand, to have frequent drinks of water, etc.

Anxiety is understood, then, to be aroused by internal cues that are not readily observable by the dentist. This is another way of saying that it is hard to verify the source of anxiety and often the person least helpful in accounting for the anxiety is the patient.

Fear. *Fear generally refers to the anticipation of threat elicited by an external object that is generally agreed to be harmful.* An object from the real world exists of which to be afraid, and a direct, easily identifiable behavior is required to get out of harm's way. Fear is distinguished from anxiety on the basis of the person's ability to locate the threatening agent "out there" and to recognize the clear presence of a behavior that will reduce perceived danger.

Because the sources and consequences of fears are objectively verifiable, fear reduction is possible through rational explanation and prudent, reasonable behavior. It is certainly adaptive to be afraid of automobiles when crossing the street and to "cross at the green, not in between." Similarly, it is appropriate and reasonable that patients have fears concerning dental needles and drills. They are sharp, may hurt, and can do damage if handled carelessly. Such fears show themselves as reasonable questions and verbalized concerns from dental patients: "What will it feel like? How does that thing work?"

If a patient reports having such inordinate fear of the dental drill's high-pitched noise that he or she does not know what to do, we can now understand the patient is using the term "fear" colloquially. The patient has not been able to identify an external source that is realistically associated with a clear behavioral alternative that would reduce the fear. We would not deny the patient's unpleasant state nor would we be surprised to see negative, or aversive, behaviors. Technically, however, we would prefer to describe the patient as highly anxious.

PATTERNS OF COPING WITH STRESS, ANXIETY, AND FEAR

The manner in which these aversive states are managed when patient and dentist interact is one key element in maintaining successful, long-term dentist-patient relationships. Coping mechanisms and strategies need to be understood as well as our current knowledge allows.

A formulation offered by Lazarus has been modified to summarize in useful fashion the following three main kinds of coping reaction patterns to stress, anxiety, and fear: attack or avoidance, defensive reappraisal, and anxiety reaction patterns.

Attack or avoidance

A course of action may be chosen that includes either attack or avoidance components. The individual's perception of all the circumstances surrounding a threat helps to determine whether an attack or an avoidance pattern is chosen. Circumstances that might affect a person's perception of threat include the following:

1. Nature of possible harm
2. Resources at the person's command
3. Situational constraints against certain actions
4. Internal values that restrict the person's actions

Attack or avoidance actions include the following:

1. *Directly expressed attack or avoidance with anger*. Physical assault on or total withdrawal from the harm-producing agent—an early developmental form of reaction
2. *Anger without attack or avoidance*. Inhibition of overt behavior as a result of situational or developmental constraints—a "grin and bear it, but I hate you" situation
3. *Attack without anger or avoidance without fear*. A goal-oriented behavior where there is no anticipation of being thwarted

The main determination of whether an attack or an avoidance coping pattern will be employed resides in the patient's appraisal of the threat. If the harmful agent is appraised as dangerous, avoidance instead of attack is likely.

Defensive reappraisal

The patient reappraises the threatening aspect of the situation because no direct coping behavior seems possible; this may be because the stress, anxiety, or fear reaction is based on some intra- or interpersonal conflict that the patient cannot or will not talk about. *The patient becomes defensive, externalizing the blame, or scapegoating, instead of either accepting responsibility or "telling it like it is." If the threat is perceived as great, defensive behavior is more likely*. The greater the threat, the more likely denial as a defense will also appear. One method of estimating how severely the patient feels threatened is to evaluate the degree of "insight" or "reality testing" the patient is exhibiting. For example, a patient has just been informed that he or she will require extensive and expensive restorative dentistry to replace an existing prosthesis that is failing. The patient might respond with a defensive reappraisal if the dentist is perceived as blaming the patient for the failure, for example, the dentist castigates the patient for having a "filthy mouth." The patient, not being able to accept the responsibility, denies there is anything wrong and accuses the dentist of "building an expensive case."

Anxiety

Anxiety becomes a coping mechanism when no clear coping behavior, that is, attack or avoidance, can be instituted. This typically occurs when the threat is appraised as ambiguous. In this situation there is an impulse to avoid something unknown or to flee, but it is not undertaken because of situational or social constraints.

Avoidance and anxiety reaction patterns are the coping mechanisms most frequently seen when dentists and patients confront each other. Attack reaction patterns are much less frequent, probably because of the social sanctions against them rather than because the patient or the dentist does not often "feel that way."

THE DENTAL EMERGENCY—AN OPPORTUNITY TO DEAL WITH STRESS, ANXIETY, AND FEAR*

It is only reasonable to expect that many dental situations will contain a number of the ingredients for eliciting stress, anxiety, and fear. The dental emergency situation is an especially useful one to examine from the psychological and interpersonal perspective. Many of the elements that we have been discussing about how stress, anxiety, and fear come about and are dealt with can be clearly seen in dental emergency situations.

Deciding when a situation is an emergency

Dentists expect emergencies. By objective criteria of reality, some emergencies are extremely serious, whereas others appear to have less of a reality base for the dentist to take too seriously. The patient, of course, often feels otherwise. To begin with, we present some typical emergency cases that dentists routinely confront.

CASE HISTORIES*

Case 1: something wrong . . . but really?

A harried call to the dentist. While brushing his teeth, the patient noticed an area of the upper gum that looked and felt "different." It coincided with the area of the mouth where the dentist had worked only 2 days ago. The patient tells the dentist that there must be something wrong . . . an infection or something left in the mouth that should have been removed. The dentist finds a slightly irritated area in the upper canine region. He observes that the area of the mouth he treated was, in fact, in the lower jaw and several teeth posterior to the upper "gum area" that the patient is certain was the locus of the last treatment.

*This section is excerpted with slight modification from Dworkin, S. F.: Dent. Clin. North Am. **19:**403, 1973.

Case 2: pain . . . but why?

An infrequent patient appears at the dental office. Unable to sleep soundly all night because of extreme pain, he awoke to notice that his face was swollen, his eye was partially closed, and he felt slightly sick. Further questioning revealed that he had been to the office last about 4 years ago; he reports intermittent pain over the last 2 months. Some pain and a vague feeling "that there was something there" had been felt in the upper jaw for about 2 weeks. About 2 weeks ago, he also felt something break and thought it might have been "a piece of tooth or a piece of filling that came out."

Case 3: damage . . . but whose?

Just as the dentist is ready to leave for the day, there is a flurry of activity in the waiting room. An upset mother, near tears, has hurriedly entered the office carrying a frightened child, who has obviously been crying but is now quiet. She informs the dentist that her 4-year-old daughter has fallen from a tricycle, slamming her teeth into the handle bars and then landing on her face. The mother reports bleeding and loose and broken front teeth. Without waiting to be asked, nor pausing to hear responses, the mother informs the dentist that something must be done immediately. She insists that the child is in immediate danger from loss of blood and that pain from the broken teeth must be prevented. She is also extremely agitated over the present appearance of the child's face and mouth and the future consequences of this accident for the permanent teeth. The child has not been to the dentist before. As far as the dentist can determine in the waiting room, there is a swelling of the upper lip, no visible bleeding, and no obvious pain.

Case 4: loss . . . but what?

An attractive career woman in her midthirties who is undergoing treatment for anterior fixed prosthetic dentistry called earlier in the day to inform the receptionist that an anterior temporary jacket had fallen off and that she was on her way to the office. She enters the office looking very agitated, with an angry expression on her face and her hand held, she hopes not too obviously, so as to obscure a clear view of her mouth. She expects to be treated immediately!

Clearly, these emergency situations differ as to how quickly and to what extent the dentist must modify his or her own routines. Most dentists would agree that a different sense of priority would be elicited in dentists for each of these typical emergency situations. What these hypothetical cases have in common, however, is the *sense of urgency in the patient*. In each instance, it is reasonable to assume that the patient is threatened, either by pain, its subjective analogue anxiety, or the consequences to the body of disregarding currently perceived symptoms.

Dental emergencies typically precipitate a dental visit because of pain, damage, loss, and change. The emergency may arise from a directly discernible pathological condition or trauma. The emergency may also arise from factors less visible or obvious such as anxiety over future consequences. Concerns over the future as a result of present pain and swelling following damage to a tooth are the rule rather than the exception (for example, case 2).

It is important to accept the notion that for management purposes, any emergency situation implies two loci from which behavior will originate. Both the patient "having" the emergency and the dentist responding to the emergency will have their respective behaviors influenced by previous learning, cognitive decisions based on available information, and emotional factors that are less amenable to observation.

The dentist may, for instance, decide that no true emergency exists. Criteria for such a decision could be the fact that the patient's life is not in danger nor is the patient's oral or systemic well-being in any way threatened by the present situation. The dentist may, therefore, be inclined to dismiss other aspects of the "emergency" situation and deny that the patient needs any response at all. Then he or she will see patient responses that are almost assuredly negative. The patient will "put the dentist down" and relegate him or her to that collective realm of unconcerned practitioners who only treat *teeth* and who are not interested enough in a person's well-being to go beyond minimal expenditures of effort in order to really find out if something is wrong.

In effect, then, every dental emergency is composed of two parts: a **clinical emergency** and a **psychological emergency.** For decisions relating to clinical aspects, dentists rely on their clinical training and experience and the best treatment plan for the clinical aspects of a dental emergency. For the psychological aspects of the emergency, dentists rely on their knowledge, intuition, and experience regarding how persons who are stressed, anxious, or afraid behave.

Unfortunately, a paucity of information exists about the specifics of psychological emergency states stemming from dental problems. Most of the information we can present stems from the controlled observations of behavioral scientists looking at how individuals respond to general surgery, both pre- and postoperatively. What has been gleaned from these careful reports can be combined with laboratory research on psychological stress and the coping process we have already presented as well as observations of the dental emergency situation to yield generalizations and guidelines for the dentist confronted with a patient labeled "emergency."

As we would expect, as soon as we must consider the psychological reactions of the patient (and the dentist, too!), defining dental emergencies becomes almost impossible. For instance, studies of persons about to undergo both major and minor general surgery in the hospital indicate that they are experiencing the same quantity of fear as are persons about to be treated for routine dental decay! The strength of the fear an hour before surgery or before dental treatment shows no statistical difference between the hospitalized group and the dental group. However, major differences were found in the time courses for fear within each group. Patients contemplating routine dentistry experienced far less fear the day before and 1 hour after treatment. Hospitalized surgery patients experience a sustained fear days before the surgery and lasting days after.

So even routine dental patients at the time of treatment are often highly fearful! This finding comes as no surprise to any dentist at all attuned to his or her patients. But it does reinforce the problem of defining a dental emergency. At least as far as the psychological component is concerned, the dental emergency, as gauged by its emotional impact on individuals, *must be defined in terms of the patient's responses, not the dentist's.*

The similarity here to the problem of defining "pain" will become apparent. To paraphrase the most accepted definition of pain, making it applicable to dental emergencies, we could define a dental emergency as *the set of signs and symptoms that the individual decides requires emergency attention.*

The major apparent difference between emergency patients and routine dental patients would seem to be priority for immediate treatment. Unquestionably, bleeding must be stopped, and pain must be relieved as soon as possible. Our case reports, however, indicate that patients can be seized with an emergency psychology, perhaps better labeled a crisis psychology, even in the absence of any requirement for clear-cut and immediate clinical intervention (for example, case 1 and perhaps case 3). Does this mean that the crisis patient is assigned a low priority for immediate treatment, or does it mean that the patient is given an equally high priority for treatment, but that the treatment is "different?" Clearly, only the latter approach will help the *crisis* aspect of the emergency, as defined by the patient.

Intuitively, most of us can tell when patients are under stress. It is probably fair to say that we dismiss most verbal and nonverbal manifestations of stress when they are exhibited by patients appearing for routine treatment. As long as signs of stress do not interrupt scheduled dental treatment, dentists do not usually consider them too important. But we have implied earlier that this may be a mistake. The major difference between stress emergency problems and stress as a result of many routine visits seems to be the intensity of the patient's stress reaction. Specific ways of knowing the patient is under psychological stress have already been listed (Table 16-1) but now can be expanded on.

Disturbed affect as indicating stress. Intensive expressions of negative emotional states are generally taken as indicators of stress. Reactions of *fear, anger, depression, guilt,* and certainly *anxiety* reveal a stressed individual. Manifestations of these negative affects, in themselves, are usually insufficient for labeling the "real" cause of the stress. In the case of the mother with the hurt child (case 3), expressions of fear and anxiety may arise both from anxiety over the child's physical damage and from guilt feelings for not being a careful enough mother.

Fear, as we have seen, is usually distinguished from anxiety in terms of its relationship to a real and imminent threat requiring a realistic appraisal of harm. Stress responses of the patient before an injection or drilling contain large elements of fear. Stress responses of the patient contemplating an injection or drilling some time in the distant future are most appropriately labeled anxiety.

Motor behaviors indicating stress. Whereas increased muscle tension, disturbances of speech (especially facial expressions accompanying speech), the directionality of behavior (whether fight or flight), and the intensity of behavior are motor clues of stress response, the potential for similarity between emergency and many routine dental patients is apparent. The dentist should be sensitive to these nonverbal dimensions of the psychological state of his or her patients.

Cognitive functioning indicating stress. The more important cognitive functions affected by stress are judgment, memory, perceptual organization, problem solving, and social interactions. Patients in emergency situations do not listen well, often do not remember instructions, and seem unable or unwilling to make intelligent use of what they are being told. The implications of these findings for the dentist will be discussed more fully later.

The physiological changes associated with stress, anxiety, and fear are well known and often readily observed. Evidence is accumulating that stress, anxiety, and fear can be differentiated physiologically by measurement of adrenal corticosteroid output, cardiac acceleration patterns, and autonomic profiles of arousal. However, we are using the terms "stress," "anxiety," and "fear" in the context of dentist-patient interactions. In this context, where stress, anxiety, and fear are sometimes understood as stimuli to behavior and sometimes as responses, the physiological differences between stress, anxiety, and fear are not of great relevance to the dentist, even if they could be readily measured and distinguished in the dental setting.

While the four indicators of stress—affect, motor behavior, cognitive functioning, and physiological change—are the most important parameters of psychological stress, one additional point must be made. **Psychological stress** is not equivalent to the definition of **stress** ordinarily used to denote changes in bodily functioning. *Psychological stress includes the critical intervening variable of threat or the anticipation of a harmful event.* Threat is a psychological process occurring obviously in advance of the harmful stimulus. **Threat** can be defined as an appraisal process. Factors in the stimulus interact with psychological structures to yield decisions regarding which behaviors will most effectively reduce the threat.

The anticipatory aspect of the threat appraisal process is probably the single most important determinant of the stress response in terms of which behaviors will ensue—whether or not to allow the dentist to see anger, fear, or anxiety; whether or not to clutch the chair and brace the body for the worst.

• • •

In summary, patients undergo stress responses by experiencing negative affect and changes in motor behavior, cognitive functioning, and autonomic physiological processes. These stress responses are induced by the psychological process of threat appraisal. The stress responses have observable behavior components, some of which are very obvious. The four case reports reveal how stress responses arising from different appraisals lead to different psychological states and different observable behaviors.

Understanding the patient and the dentist in an emergency situation

Patient response parameters

Conflict. The psychological stress that a dental emergency represents is essentially the psychology of *conflict*. Defensive operations that have operated over time to allow the emergency to develop must be reappraised in anticipation of the treatment process and in anticipation of the consequences of treatment. Emergency behaviors can be viewed as those behaviors that resolve the conflict between allowing the present emergency state to continue and submitting oneself to treatment and its consequences.

This problem-solving process involves cognitive structures such as learning, memory, thought, and judgment. Other psychological processes are also assumed to be involved. These are generally referred to as the defensive operations that we discussed in Chapter 14. Patients may defend against the real personal significance of the emergency situation by behaviors that appear irrational and inappropriate to the dentist. Patients, however, often view these behaviors as quite appropriate, providing ready rationalizations of their denial, avoidance, or repression behaviors. They may, for example, say they did not have the time or nothing bothered them.

Threat of bodily harm. The intra- and interpersonal significance of threatened or actual body damage and disruption of body integrity is probably the overwhelming psychological concern of persons labeled "dental emergencies." In their extremes, these concerns may represent excessive narcissism, hypochondriasis, or neurotic anxiety over body integrity.

Other important psychological concerns represented in the threat of a dental emergency include passive-dependent feelings and the relationship to authority figures. Again, reference to our case history sketches reveals examples of patient behavior that can reasonably be interpreted as holding an authority figure personally responsible for the trouble and its resolution. In case 1, for example, the patient might act as if he knew the dentist caused the trouble despite adequate reality factors that leave the dentist blameless; case 4 may involve narcissistic and passive-dependent conflicts.

Dentists should be sensitized to these powerful psychological forces. Concerns over the body and over submitting oneself to the care of another apparently have the capacity for tapping a wide range of unconscious defensive maneuvers so that the patient need never acknowledge that the focus of the threat of a dental emergency revolves around these conflict areas.

Dentist response parameters. As sparse as the literature is concerning the psychodynamics of patient responses to dental emergencies, it is voluminous relative to the reports of how dentists respond to these emergencies. The classical assumption is that the health professional is a perfectly objective observer, who by virtue of his or her professional training and experience is beyond personal interaction with the stresses of his or her patients. Indeed, the argument has traditionally been made, in medical training especially, that it is necessary to postulate a physician who is personally neutral and noninteracting. Interaction of the physician's feelings with the stress of the patient would lead, it has been feared, to a contamination of the diagnostic and evaluative process. The physician would not be able to tell objectively if the patient response he or she observed was a drug treatment effect or simply the effect on the patient of personal attributes of the physician.

This classical model of the health professional as a neutral and noninteracting observer has been demonstrated repeatedly to be fallacious. Studies of placebo effects, suggestion, and psychosomatic phenomena indicate the inevitable and powerful interactions healers have on sick persons. If the picture we have presented has any validity, that is to say, that individuals respond to crisis in complex and obscure ways, it can reasonably be argued that crisis situations in others represent a possible source of conflict and threat for at least some dentists. There is no reason to assume that certain dental emergencies will not be interpreted by the dentist as partially his or her fault depending on the dentist's security needs and strength of self-esteem. Suppression of guilt and repression or denial of blows to self-esteem could easily be imagined to elicit defensive behaviors on the part of the dentist that are not always constructive and patient oriented.

Further, it must be recognized that many persons chose dentistry because of a desire to avoid extreme emergency situations. We have, however, alluded to the possibility that the definition of an emergency is largely determined by individuals as a function of their appraisal of past experience, present danger, and future threat. Confronting a patient with pain, swelling, and a closed eye may become, for some dentists, a personally stressful emergency. Similarly, dealing with an hysterical mother making unreasonable demands or an angry woman holding one responsible for extreme embarrassment may be as much of an emergency for some dentists as for their patients (cases 2 and 3, respectively). There is evidence, for instance, that dentists experience patterns of physiological stress response that parallel their patient's responses (for example, increased heart rate, sweating) when injecting local anesthetic or performing other dental procedures under conditions of patient anxiety.

Not to belabor the point any longer, it is sufficient to point out that dentists are people first! Therefore they are susceptible to the same psychodynamic variability as the general population. Dentists need to give more thought and study to their own reactions. If anxious and apprehensive patients, for example, elicit negative affect, tension, and physiological distress in the dentist, should he or she not be sufficiently open to acknowledge these stress responses and to take appropriate therapeutic steps? Denial and avoidance of such problem areas are not consistent with professional ideals and, more importantly, are not consistent with patients' expectations of a health practitioner.

Managing the "psychological emergency"

When discussing emergencies and stress responses, it seems inevitable to dwell on negative considerations—negative affects, threats to body integrity, denial, and avoidance. Dentists do, however, perform positive and constructive acts on behalf of their emergency patients, providing relief from discomfort and restoration of function and aesthetics. But in those same clinical procedures undertaken to meet the dental emergency are also the ingredients for making the patient feel better in a sense broader than relieving pain. Guidelines and preferred modes of conduct on the part of the dentist can be suggested that reduce patient stress, elicit cooperation, and allow the dental emergency visit to end optimistically and in a future-oriented way.

Cognitive responses of the dentist to emergency patients. Independent of the precipitating cause, whether it be trauma or a pathological condition, the dentist confronted with an emergency patient quickly engages in a decision-making process. He or she *evaluates* the objective reality of the emergency in terms of the levels of real and imminent threat to the physical well-being of the patient as a whole or of major parts of the body; the clinical procedures necessary to eliminate or reduce such a threat to acceptable levels; the psychological state of the patient and the dentist's readiness; and the probability of effectiveness of the clinical treatment, given the nature of the emergency and the psychological state of the patient.

This cognitive process calls on the learning, memory, and judgment of dentists as they assign priorities to their responses according to the balance between real, objective threats—the clinical emergency—and anxiety or stress responses—the psychological emergency. Entering directly into this evaluative process should be the following factors:

- How the dentist acts and talks may at least in part be determined by his or her own need to label certain emergency situations as highly perilous and to deny that any danger exists in other emergency situations.
- Understanding and acceptance of atypical behaviors precipitated by the emergency are expected of the dentist if he or she is to be of help to the stressed patient. Atypical behaviors at times of stress include irrational attitudes, disordered emotions, and negative or hostile responses.
- The intensity of anxiety over the dental emergency is likely to be exaggerated in relation to the objective seriousness of the clinical emergency (cases 1 and 3).
- Body damage or its perceived threat often elicits regression, bringing a fear of abandonment, feelings of helplessness, and the need for reassurance, affection, and protection.
- Stress induces cognitive blocks and perceptual confusions, yielding misconceptions about the nature and implications of the emergency. These cognitive blocks and misperceptions are generally the result of denial, repression, and suppression. They may render the patient resistant to rational

explanation and prone to forget postoperative instructions.

- The typical dental crisis situation is self-limiting in time. Usually it will be over shortly, for both dentist and patient.

Interpersonal responses of the dentist to emergency patients

We have already presented a model for behavior change that is equally applicable here. However, certain features of the emergency situation need special emphasis.

It is especially important in any kind of crisis situation requiring psychological management to begin by staying with the patient's presenting complaint. Initial responses should indicate that the dentist understands the patient's major concerns and will promptly deal with them. One can rapidly obtain a clue as to the degree of reality distortion by listening to the patient's complaint and contrasting it to the dentist's determination of what is really wrong (cases 1 and 3).

Initial responses to anxious individuals should obviously be warm, empathic, and reassuring. If denial (or repression) is operating to such an extent that the emergency patient has no real grasp of what is happening or what could happen, it is the dentist's function to sensitively "titrate" denial with reality, striving to make the patient's painful reality less threatening.

Dentists may become aware, as they provide support and clarification in appropriate doses, that their efforts are to no avail. The denial and repression defenses are so effective that nothing seems to be getting through. This is an indication that the psychological aspects of the emergency treatment scene are predominant. Although the impact of the emergency may be overwhelming and dentists may see its disorganizing effects in terms of confusion, ineffective functioning, and intense upset, they should not be dissuaded from their therapeutic efforts on the patient's behalf. If it appears, despite patient protestations, that the patient does not want to know what is going on or even want sympathy, continued patient-oriented support is still warranted. Afterwards, patients often comment appreciatively that the dentist's attitude and desire to explain was most helpful during those very times when the patient verbally and behaviorally denied that the dentist's approach was a helpful one.

If dentists have been successful in diminishing anxiety and countering denial, their clinical procedures are generally easier to accomplish. The vast body of psychosomatic literature makes it evident that drug efficacy, postoperative course, and reliability of patient follow-up can be functions of interpersonal dynamics between dentist and patient. One study, for example, found that morphine was not significantly different from a placebo in its ability to relieve pain when the attending physician was "supportive" and provided the patient with full information. By contrast, when the attending physician was "cold" and objective, morphine was found to have a significantly greater effect than a placebo on pain in hospitalized patients.

But there are more benefits to be gained from rendering the emergency patient relatively anxiety free and informed. In appropriate situations, the dentist may profitably spend some time, immediately after the emergency has been resolved, to educate and motivate the patient toward better oral health behavior (cases 2 and 3). A patient who is psychologically capable of hearing such a message now leaves the dentist not only feeling physically better, but oriented toward the future care of the mouth.

Summary

In summary, it is not too much to expect that dentists strive for a therapeutic alliance with their stressed emergency patients. Such an alliance begins with dentists acknowledging their own needs. They must then be able to listen and observe, nonjudgmentally, in order to evaluate the personal and interpersonal needs of patients at a difficult time. The beneficial effects on pain and discomfort of a few well-chosen words have long been known. More will be said on this subject in Chapter 18. Similarly, undue anxiety and inappropriate defensive reactions elicited by perceived threats to the body can be greatly resolved, as every psychotherapist knows, by interventions on the part of a healer–authority figure. These interventions are therapeutic in relation to how able and willing dentists are to be supportive and understanding of their patients' current state of distress and confusion.

Writing for psychotherapists, Haley has commented on the art of being a failure as a psychotherapist. Some of his obviously tongue-in-cheek comments on guaranteeing such failure have been liberally paraphrased for their applicability to present concerns. In busy dental practices, the untimely appearance of a dental emergency has at one time or another surely precipitated one or more of the following:

> Insist that the problem which brings the patient is not important. Dismiss it as merely a "symptom" and shift the conversation elsewhere.
>
> Refuse to directly treat the presenting problem. Offer some rationale of your own, such as the idea that symptoms are "mental" to avoid treating the problem the patient is paying his money to recover from.
>
> It is particularly important to confuse diagnosis and therapy. A therapist can sound expert and be scientific without ever risking a success with treatment if he uses a diagnostic language which makes it impossible for him to think of therapeutic operations.
>
> Put the emphasis upon a single approach to people, no matter how diverse the problems which enter the office. Patients who won't behave properly according to the approach should be defined as untreatable and abandoned.
>
> Perhaps the most important rule is to ignore the real world that patients live in.
>
> Avoid the poor because they will insist upon results and cannot be distracted with insightful conversation.*

Finally, Haley offers the following suggestions entitled "Five B's Which Guarantee Dynamic Failure":

Be passive.
Be inactive.
Be reflective.
Be silent.
Beware.

Clearly, our preference would be to end on a positive note. For handling dental emergencies with their inevitable patient distress, we would add:

Be active.
Be supporting.
Be sensitive.
Be thorough.
Be rewarded.

---

*From Haley, J.: In Barten, H. H., ed.: Brief therapies, New York, 1971, Behavioral Publications, Inc.

REFERENCES

1. Dworkin, S. F.: Psychodynamics of dental emergencies, Dent. Clin. North Am. **17:**403, 1973.
2. Haley, J.: The art of being a failure as a therapist. In Barten, H. H., ed.: Brief therapies, New York, 1971, Behavioral Publications, Inc.
3. Janis, I.: Psychological stress, New York, 1958, John Wiley & Sons, Inc.
4. Kupperman, A.: Stress and the general adaptation syndrome, J. Dent. Med. **11:**53, 1956.
5. Lazarus, R.: Psychological stress and the coping process, New York, 1966, McGraw-Hill Book Co.
6. Selye, H.: The stress of life, New York, 1956, McGraw-Hill Book Co.
7. Spielberger, C.: Anxiety and behavior, New York, 1966, Academic Press, Inc.
8. Spielberger, C., and Sarason, I.: Stress and anxiety, New York, 1975, John Wiley & Sons, Inc.

Chapter 17

AVERSIVE INTERACTIONS—PAIN

Pain, or, more precisely, pain management, is one of the few sources of positive reinforcement and gratification that patients willingly supply to dentists. Pain should be the outstanding instance that everyone can understand where objective need, perceived need, and the psychology of interpersonal relationships all come together, bringing the patient to the dentist for relief and gentle handling. The potential for the dentist to relieve the terrible pain associated with dental disease provides a major rationale for the high level of prestige associated with the dental profession in our society. However, there are a variety of pains that dental patients suffer or anticipate they may suffer; causes of these pains are sometimes obvious, sometimes obscure; the remedies available for the dentist to use are marvelously effective for specific types of pain in certain settings. However, pain relief often eludes the patient, especially when it becomes chronic pain as a result of etiologies that are difficult to ascertain. Much has been written about pain as an inevitable human condition and also about pain remedies. There is probably no greater evidence of the need for dentists to understand this complex phenomenon than the existence of a vast body of scientific and popular writing on the subject, for if the answers to pain problems were simple, the preoccupation with pain would not be so universally compelling nor the literature so rich and varied.

OBJECTIVES

The objectives of this chapter are as follows:

1. To discuss the complexities of defining pain
2. To identify factors that affect why an individual labels a situation as painful
3. To explore different pain control strategies

DEFINING PAIN

Problems of definition

Pain is an enigma. It occurs when it is not expected and is absent when there is apparent cause. Dental and medical clinicians, probably by virtue of training and scientific orientation, tend to view pain as a unitary phenomenon. Clinically, pain seems to be understood as a physiological sensation elicited in response to a "condition" (that is, a stimulus or cause) that induces body damage, tissue destruction, or disordered functioning. The clinician assumes that for every pain the following hold: (1) there must be a discernible cause; (2) the cause can be eliminated by mechanical/surgical or pharmacological intervention (treatment of pathological conditions involving hard and/or soft tissue; adjustment of a prosthesis; prescription of analgesics, anesthetics, anti-inflammatory agents, or antibiotics); and (3) when the cause is eliminated, the complaint of pain will cease.[4,14]

Etiology of pain is not always clear. In reality, of all the symptoms of patients, pain more than any other complaint requires careful analysis and then, most of the time, a response directed toward the *person in pain* rather than a response simply directed toward the *pain*. However, because we have less than complete understanding of pain phenomena and want to do something to help the patient, our universal impulse is to act—to treat the pain.

Responses to pain vary with the individual. Each of us knows the meaning of pain—we *know* when we hurt. Yet pain is a profoundly personal, psychological experience that has defied adequate definition, either in psychological or in physiological terms. Everyday observation allows us to accept the notion that responses to pain are varied, highly personalized, and modifiable. Consider, for instance, responses to dental treatment. One patient can sit placidly during treatment, feeling almost no pain, and tolerating the whole affair as a necessary annoyance. Another dental patient, receiving the same treatment under ostensibly the same conditions, finds the situation almost unbearable and reacts with deeply felt pain.

It turns out there is limited usefulness in viewing pain as merely a physiological process initiated by objective or observable stimuli and mediated by a nervous system whose functioning follows predictable laws of biology. On the contrary, *pain is best understood as a uniquely determined individual perception, giving rise to uniquely determined motivational states and behaviors*.

Almost universally, researchers and clinicians are trying to better understand the subjective experience that patients in pain are having. Melzack puts it in the following way:

> The psychological evidence strongly supports the view of pain as a *perceptual* experience whose quality and intensity is influenced by the past history of the individual, by the meaning he gives to the pain-producing situation, and by his "state of mind" at the moment. . . . [in this way] pain becomes a function of the whole individual, including his present thoughts and fears, as well as his hopes for the future.*

Without disputing the intimate relationship between pain responsivity and well-known facts of neurophysiology, no one seriously believes that diverse responses to pain are explicable solely in terms of the physiology of sensation. As Buytendijk[4] affirms, ". . . neither the results of research nor of common experience are compatible with a purely physiologic explanation of pain." Similarly, Zbrowski[33] states ". . . the physiology of pain does not explain the acceptance of intense pain in torture as part of primitive initiation rites . . . nor the anxiety of some people to the slightest sting of the hypodermic needle."

Operational definitions

Because etiological factors in pain are often elusive and because pain behavior is so varied, an adequate definition of pain is still not available. Anticipating the discussion that follows, two definitions are offered that are reasonably adequate as working definitions for the clinician, although they fall short of many biological scientists' need for more exact operational precision.

One definition comes from Mersky and Spear[24]: **Pain** is "an unpleasant experience which we primarily associate with tissue damage or describe in terms of tissue damage or both." This definition is useful because it connotes that the presence of pain means a *person* is having a *negative* (aversive) experience that is related to *body damage* or is *perceived* as being related to body damage.

An even broader definition is as follows: **Pain** is "that which the *individual decides hurts*."[10] Our discussion of pain throughout this book implies this definition. The key terms in the definition are as follows:

the individual Connoting long-term developmental, personality, or characterological *traits* of the patient that contribute to current pain behavior

---

*From Melzack, R.: Sci. Am. **204:**41, 1961.

decides Connoting momentary, more immediate factors in the environment that determine the current psychological *state* of the patient, leading to a decision to either report or not report pain

hurts Connoting the quality and quantity of the sensation perceived and responded to as pain, including the intensity, duration, location, and nature of the pain

Before distinguishing between the different ways individuals report pain, it is necessary to point out the source of much of our information about pain and to isolate the different classes of pain that dentists confront.

The source of much of our information about pain

Most of the information available about how individuals react to pain comes from reports gathered within the framework of the psychological laboratory. In this setting, it has been demonstrated that individuals shift their subjective evaluation of the intensity of the *same* physical stimulus when the experimenter manipulates such factors as the perceived origin or importance of the pain. *As more information is supplied about when and how much pain is to be expected, tolerance for pain increases.* Many studies support a hypothesis of Melzack,[21] coauthor of the well-known "gate control" theory of pain, that as laboratory subjects are given increasing control over onset and duration of the painful stimulus, pain tolerance increases. Other laboratory studies[2,3,7,12,32] adequately demonstrate that pain tolerance is influenced by psychological "set," motivation, varying instructions for responding, and other factors.

Again, it should be noted that these investigations of pain responsivity were all conducted in the psychological laboratory. Taken together, they did not demonstrate the modifiability of *all* pain parameters. Quite notably, *pain threshold was shown to be resistant to change, whereas pain tolerance was proved to be readily modifiable.*

Pain threshold is defined as the onset of pain. It is generally discussed in terms of the amount of stimulation or trauma required before the patient first reports (usually verbally) feeling pain.

Pain tolerance is defined as the most intensive level of pain the patient is willing or able to take. Pain tolerance is usually discussed in terms of the amount of stimulation or trauma required before the patient (again, usually verbally) reports not being able to take any more. At the pain tolerance level in the laboratory, the patient or subject will ask for the pain to stop, whereas in clinical situations, the patient will demand analgesics and/or sedatives.

Different classes of pain the dentist confronts

Laboratory vs clinical, or "real," pain. Studies of the type just described do not allow for the distinction to be made between what Kessen and Mandler[15] call "cognitive pain" and the "distress" or anxiety that accompany that pain. **Cognitive pain** is defined as the subjective report of the individual that he or she is experiencing pain. They define **distress** as the *anxiety component* that accompanies pain and modulates the reaction to a painful stimulus.

As we shall see, depending on the type and duration of the pain, the patient's anxiety *and* depression are the most important reasons for responding to the patient as opposed to the pain per se. Anxiety especially plays a major role in almost all the aversive dentist-patient interactions. *Anxiety is an especially important variable in pain phenomenology associated with dental treatment; it is the antecedent condition for appraising the meaning of pain.*

Most laboratory studies of pain threshold and pain tolerance have limited generality, however, because they do not involve the "real-life" meaning of pain experience, that is, they do not engage anxiety attendant on the pain. Beecher,[13] a most important reviewer in the field of pain and analgesics, puts it this way: "The casual discomfort of laboratory pain does not compare to pain implying disease or perhaps death." Pain experienced in a laboratory study is different qualitatively and quantitatively from pain experienced as a result of a pathological condition of the body. The element of stress is missing in laboratory pain. The patient with clinical or "real" pain as a result of a pathological condition is obviously concerned about the *potential consequences* of his or her pain in contrast to the typically casual attitude of the laboratory subject. Strong evidence on this point comes from the clinical evaluation of analgesics. Dosages of analgesics, especially potent narcotic analgesics that have been found effective in the laboratory, cannot be usefully carried over to "real-life" pain situations.

An extreme view is reflected by Szasz,[29] who is most caustic on this point. He doubts whether any laboratory subject has ever experienced anything he would call pain. For him, pain experiences in a laboratory experiment have no real significance for individuals. The subjects know the pain will end soon, and they know no permanent damage is implied. Szasz concludes that the laboratory setup is hardly a useful place to examine pain responsivity, since it is impossible to arouse anxiety in that setting—specifically, anxiety as a signal of threat to the ego. Individuals see no greater threat to their bodies or to themselves, as it were, than that of a momentary discomfort for which they are usually paid.

Unfortunately, very few controlled studies have been undertaken that examine whether individuals modify their pain reactions when they experience "real" pain in contrast to laboratory-induced pain. One area in which such work has been done involves the efficacy of analgesics in alleviating pain. Where attempts have been made to introduce anxiety into laboratory drug research, increases in drug level are observed that begin to approximate those found in "real-life" circumstances. Otherwise, laboratory studies of analgesics have not been found to yield dosage levels for pain relief related to the dosage levels required for pathological pain encountered clinically.

Iatrogenic vs pathogenic pain. In addition to the environmental context within which pain behavior is observed, it is critical for clinicians to consider the perceived source of pain. For the most part, when dentists interact with patients in pain, they are dealing with iatrogenic pain—actual pain that the dentist causes or the threatening appraisal that pain may be anticipated with dental treatment. Thus most pain-related behavior of dental patients is really an interaction of the process of threat appraisal with the ongoing experience. Because dentists must interact with pain the patient is not yet experiencing, the control of anxiety plays a potent role in managing iatrogenic pain.

Patients presenting with pain in acute emergency situations involving active infection, other disease, or traumatic consequences of prior dental care are infrequently seen by the average dentist. Specialists (oral surgeons, endodontists, and, to a lesser degree, periodontists) probably see a much greater proportion of patients who report pathogenic pain—pain as a result of a pathological condition present from the beginning of the interaction. The interaction of the dentist with the patient will be markedly different if the dentist is managing anxiety mostly attendant on the threat of pain as contrasted to managing anxiety associated with the implications of pathological pain.

In summary, the pain of dental patients is perceived to arise from two sources: either externally—from the dentist and his other treatments—or internally—from the body. In a later section of this chapter we will deal with pain control as it applies to iatrogenic pain. Additionally, we will distinguish that aspect of pain control from the management of patients with pathogenic pain.

Acute vs chronic pain. Still another crucial distinction required when encountering pain behavior and evaluating dentist-patient interactions is the duration of the

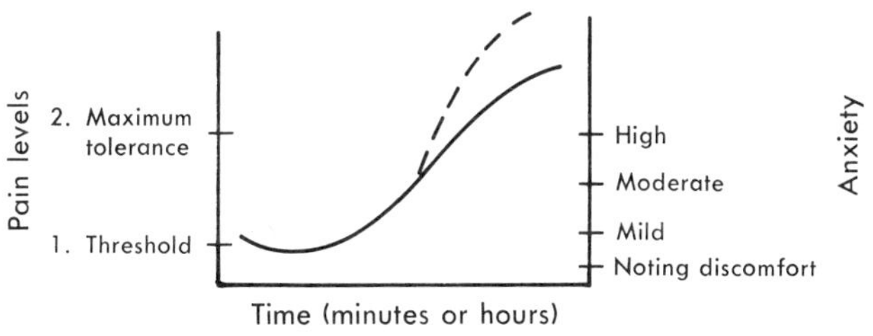

Fig. 17-1. Reaction to acute pain. (From Sternbach, R.: Pain: a psychophysiologic analysis, New York, 1968, Academic Press, Inc.)

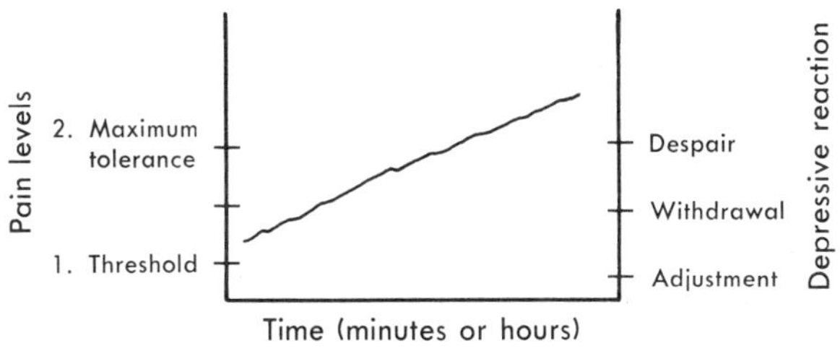

Fig. 17-2. Reaction to chronic pain. (From Sternbach, R.: Pain: a psychophysiologic analysis, New York, 1968, Academic Press, Inc.)

pain episode. Both a time and a psychological reaction dimension are relevant.

Acute pain is the kind of pain we have in mind when we think of going to the dentist. Simply put, we are referring to the pain of a toothache, abscess, injection, or drill. Whether iatrogenic or pathogenic, the time scale is in terms of minutes, hours, or sometimes days, for example, when the dentist is playing golf. It is perceived that the pain will end at some point in the near future. The pain is often pronounced in intensity, has a palpable quality of sharpness or throbbing, and is relatively localizable.

The amount of anxiety experienced by patients in pain decreases to the extent the patient perceives a cause; understands the implications or meaning of the pain (for example, does it indicate a local or systemic problem?); and understands and perceives the therapy as nonthreatening (for example, the patient knows what will be done and when the treatment will be over).

Chronic pain involves an expanded time frame and a completely different set of psychological reactions. In chronic pain the time frame is weeks, months, and years (most typically, months and years). The most common, indeed, almost universal psychological concomitant to chronic pain is depression. **Depression** is characterized by a marked decrease in activity, a withdrawal from interpersonal and social contacts, and a negative affect or emotional tone that is described as being sad and despondent with loss of pleasure.

Reactions to acute vs chronic pain have been schematically represented by Sternbach.[27] As Figs. 17-1 and 17-2 illustrate, *anxiety is usually associated with acute pain and depression with chronic pain.*

Patients with chronic pain tend to describe their pain as having a dull, aching, or gnawing quality; a relatively constant duration or predictable occurrence (for example, it hurts every morning or it never hurts during the day; often chronic pains are worst at night); a poor capacity to localize; and a generally *unilateral* location in the orofacial region.

Behavioral consequences reported with chronic pain are loss of sleep, extreme worry about the cause of pain (Is it cancer?), and concern about it never disappearing (Will I ever be rid of it?). Especially significant is the tremendous amount of professional help chronic pain patients have received and continue to seek. Probably the best discussion of chronic pain patients to date is presented by Sternbach in his book entitled *Pain Patients: Traits and Treatments.*[28] Several hospital admissions or comprehensive diagnostic workups are common for these patients. Additionally, they have been involved with numerous surgical, medical, and pharmacological treatment regimes. Patients with chronic pain seem always to be going to the physician for something, and—physicians please note—typically something is always being done by the physician in an attempt to respond to requests for relief.

Some of the more common chronic pain complaints with which dentists are confronted include *myofascial pain dysfunction (MPD), syndromes*[16,20] *of burning tongue or palate,*[26] and *neuralgias and neuritises*[1] of the second and third divisions of the trigeminal nerve. General practicing dentists will rarely see true cases of tic doloureux or chronic pain of vascular origin around the mouth. Because chronic pain is often so elusive of clear diagnosis, it has been popular in the past to lump together any kind of unusual pain complaint for which no cause can be uncovered. Labels such as atypical facial pain have been used for those pains that are mysterious to dentists. However, newer classification systems discourage such catchall labels.

Psychogenic vs somatogenic, or "true," pain. Dentists and other medical clinicians seem most of all to be mystified and skeptical about those pains for which there appears to be no discernible pathological condition. Apparently because of our deeply rooted Western tradition of scientific skepticism, it is hard for the "objectively" oriented dentist (or physician or paraprofessional) to accept the notion that a person is "really" in pain when no clinical evidence substantiates the claim. In the absence of body or tissue damage or dysfunction, we tend to dismiss such pain reports lightly, perhaps saying (to ourselves or to the patient), "Don't worry, it's all in your mind" or "There's nothing wrong, you must be upset or neurotic."

The term "psychogenic" is currently used to identify those pain reports that are not accompanied by or do not appear to have reference to discernible body damage. In psychogenic pain the prime etiological factors are to be found in the psychological, as opposed to the physical, state of the patient. The most useful way to understand such pain complaints is to view them as expressions of pain in the language of psychology instead of the language of physiology.

Psychogenic pain is a "real" pain for the patient. The patient experiences the same qualities of pain (burning, stabbing, piercing, etc.) with the same intensities (dull, severe, excruciating, etc.) as does the patient reporting a "true" pain, that is, a pain we can better explain because the patient can point to where it hurts *and* the clinician can see why.

The prevalent view in the field at this time is to abandon trying to force patients with pain onto a single continuum of pain response that has somatogenic components (for example, a pathological condition or trauma) at one end and psychological components at the other. Such an either/or dichotomy (Fig. 17-3) reflects an old-fashioned mind/body dualism that is not consistent with our present knowledge of psychophysiology.

Instead of this either/or approach, most clinical pain researchers, especially where chronic pain is involved, now conceive of at least two relatively independent dimensions; the patient's pain is now understood as always being determined by both a somatogenic *and* a psychological component (Fig. 17-4).

In reality, there are many psychogenic factors, including anxiety, depression, concern over the future, and relationship to the dentist. Similarly, the somatogenic factors

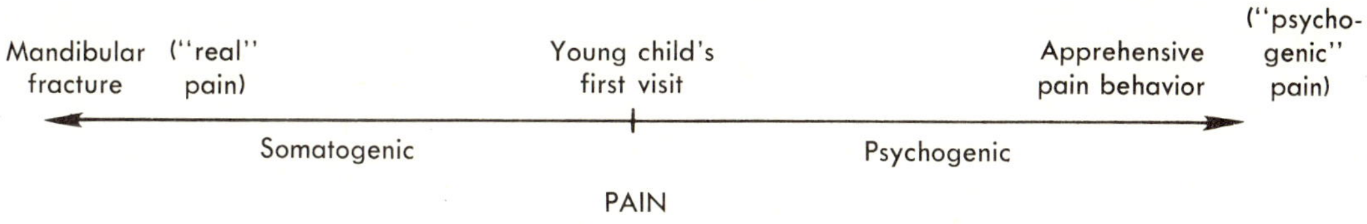

Fig. 17-3. Pain response: a single-continuum model.

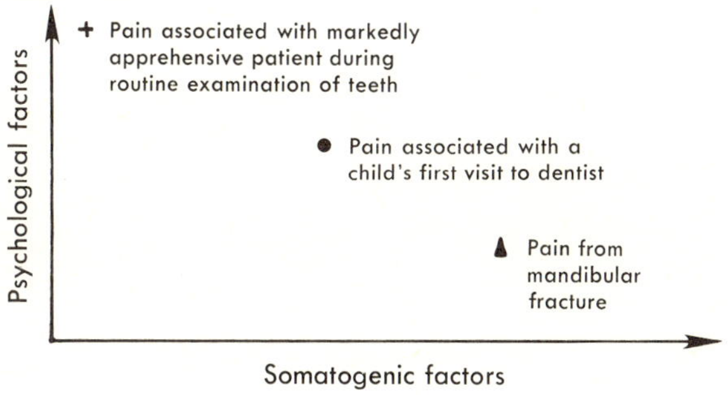

Fig. 17-4. Pain responses: a two-continuum model separating pain complaints into somatogenic ("real") and psychogenic factors.

Table 17-1 □ Summary of different classes of pain dentists confront

Class of pain	Definition of each type of pain	Distinction to be made
Laboratory	Operationally defined by laboratory scientists	Situational context in which pain behavior observed
Clinical or real	Individual decides hurt in a non-laboratory situation	
Iatrogenic	Associated with anticipation of current treatment and its consequences	Perceived and objective source of pain
Pathogenic	Associated with disease, dysfunction, or trauma prior to beginning of treatment	
Acute	Of shorter duration—measured in terms of minutes, hours, days	Duration of pain episode and previous treatment history
Chronic	Of longer duration—measured in terms of weeks, months, or years	
Psychogenic	No discernible pathological condition* consistent with pain report	Source of prime etiological factors and previous treatment history
"True" or somatogenic	Discernible pathological consistent with pain report	

*Psychogenic pain reports may be difficult to distinguish from hypochondriasis. Hypochondriasis is defined as an undue preoccupation with the body and its processes. Hypochondriacal pain reports can often be distinguished because they are made by patients who continually report disturbances in more than one organ system (for example, "My back hurts, and I get these headaches, and don't you think I need a GI series . . .").

could include objective general health status, extent of body damage or disease, and types of treatment required.

Since psychogenic pain patients are understood to be expressing pain in the language of psychology rather than in the language of physiology, it is not easy for the dentist to determine exactly what is hurting the patient. Psychiatrists and psychologists to whom these patients are frequently referred (often against the patient's better judgment) have demonstrated that such patients have neurotic tendencies, at least as measured by conventional psychological means such as the Minnesota Multiphasic Personality Index,[5] the Eysenck Personality Inventory,[19] and psychiatric interviews.[25] As a group, these patients demonstrate depression, hypochondriasis, and psychosomatic symptoms to a greater extent than appropriate control groups that have been studied.

Since, as was pointed out earlier, these patients have a history of repeatedly seeking and accepting the widest variety of medical and surgical therapies, the dentist must remain skeptical about the ability of dental treatment to relieve psychogenic pain. In fact, such patients are probably better treated conservatively until the underlying psychogenic disturbance can be at least evaluated. Supportive reassurance is important for these patients. Unfortunately, however, the collective clinical experience of dentists with this type of patient is not particularly gratifying.

• • •

Table 17-1 may be helpful as a summary of the different classes of pain dentists confront.

FACTORS AFFECTING AN INDIVIDUAL'S PERCEPTION OF PAIN

Individuals, whether they are in pain or not, bring more than their present concerns to the dental setting. They bring their past experiences—their predispositions to respond in particular ways to stress, anxiety, body damage, interpersonal dealings with authority, and a host of other innumerable intrapsychic and interpersonal considerations. When all these experiences are taken together, they add up to the whole person.

When a person enters the dental setting about to take on, once more, the role of patient, all these considerations are resolved into a general set of factors that we could call personality. Some of these personality factors—the enduring characteristics or "traits" of the patient—interact with pain or its threat to yield observable pain behaviors.

Long-term factors affecting the individual's pain behavior

We have discussed different classes of pain dentists confront. Now we turn to those different aspects among individuals that lead to a variety of pain reports. Differences among individuals in pain reaction have been attributed to cultural influences in their upbringing, psychiatric status, learning influences, and age and sex influences.

Cultural factors. Fascinating research and clinical findings lend real credence to the notion that patient reaction to pain is connected to cultural and ethnic background. In a book entitled *People in Pain,* Zbrowski[33] reported the attitudes and pain behavior of different cultural groups. He found that Jews and Italians were vocal about their pain, tending to complain loudly and often, but for different reasons. Jews were more concerned about the meaning of their pain: How long would it last? Did the pain mean they were seriously ill and not getting better? Italians were less concerned about the future significance of their pain. They complained with about the same intensity but were more often willing to accept analgesics for symptom relief than were Jews. Irish and "old Americans" (at least third-generation Protestant Americans) kept the pain experience to themselves. Irish patients seemed more inclined to suffer but quietly; old American patients were stoic and accepting of their pain but also tended to be concerned about its future meaning.

Using psychophysiological measures as well as attitudinal and behavioral indices, Tursky and Sternbach[30] found similar cultural influences when they described the "typical" reaction to pain of Jews, Italians, Irish, and "old Americans."

Individuals from different ethnic and racial groups also tend to be more like each other, on the average, when reacting to pain. In clinical dental settings, it has been observed that Puerto Ricans exhibit more anxiety than blacks or whites when asked about their pain. Blacks tended to deny or avoid dealing with the pain to a lesser extent than Puerto Ricans, but to a greater extent than whites.[31]

Psychiatric status. Besides the impact of cultural norms, other long-acting aspects of personality affect how individuals might respond to pain. Psychiatric diagnosis is one such consideration. Patients who have been institutionalized for marked emotional disturbances demonstrate wide differences in pain tolerance, depending on the nature of the mental illness. Mental patients with the greatest tolerance for pain seem to be those labeled psychopathic or sociopathic personalities. Their emotional disturbance shows itself as chronic, destructive antisocial behavior. These patients have very low levels of emotional response in general and specifically appear to exhibit little anxiety. Another group of psychiatric patients, labeled as schizophrenic, also shows such apparent pain tolerance as to be able to mutilate parts of their own bodies, even amputating fingers and toes, with no apparent painful reaction.

Learning influences. Although it has not been carefully documented with pain patients, there is evidence that large portions of our pain reactions are learned behavior. We have all seen the young child who, while playing with friends, falls and scrapes a knee. If the mother is around and the conditions are appropriate, the child may begin to cry and run to the mother, seeking comfort. The reassuring look, kiss, and affection reinforce that everything is all right.

The child also learns that pain can be used as a communication to elicit desired behaviors from others. This inevitable learned-response component to pain was demonstrated clearly by Melzack and Scott[23] in a study involving puppies reared in complete isolation. Young puppies raised out of sight and sound of other dogs do not ordinarily avoid painful stimuli to the same extent as do litter mates reared normally. In contrast to "normal" puppies, they will repeatedly stick their paws into a flame or fail to withdraw from sharp stimuli; they seem driven by curiosity. For some breeds, only when severe tissue damage has occurred does the puppy act as if it "learned" anything about pain.

Age and sex influences. It seems fair to say that the data concerning how age and sex are related to pain are, at the least, incomplete.[8,9] Some clinicians believe that older persons (for example, those above 60 years of age) complain more about the same amount of painful stimulation than do younger individuals. Other researchers believe that "true" changes in threshold and tolerance take place with age and that the pain behavior of older patients is not simply a function of increased complaining. It is not uncommon for middle-aged dental patients to report that when they were younger, they "never needed anything" (for example, local anesthetic or sedation) for dental treatment, but now they absolutely "must have a shot of Novocain." Again, it is not clear how much of this change is a shift in response bias—the tendency to call something painful sooner or to "not want to take it"—as opposed to a change in physiological functioning. In patients approaching middle age and beyond with intact nervous system functioning, the weight of the evidence seems to favor an increasing response bias to report acute pain sooner.

Sex differences and pain reaction reveal a similarly unclear pattern of relationships.

Some researchers report lower pain threshold and tolerance among women than men; others claim these differences, when they exist, reflect a response bias on the part of women to report pain sooner than men. Generally, our culture supports the notion that women are freer to verbalize complaints. Men experience cultural and peer pressures to be "manly" or stoic about their pain and other bodily symptoms.

Dentists should not be misled into equating "silence" with "no pain" when their younger and/or male patients are receiving dental treatment. Often even the most casual inquiry will reveal that such patients are experiencing pain but are reluctant to report it to the dentist or their peers.

Situational factors affecting the individual's pain behavior

There are many momentary or current factors that contribute to a patient's decision about whether or not pain is present. The most important of these factors is the presence and appraisal of *anxiety* (Chapter 16). Factors contributing to the perception of anxiety include the presence of *uncertainty* and the *lack of clear information* and *control.* The *interpersonal relationship* between the dentist and patient also affects the patient's perception of anxiety.

These situational factors are, in fact, so powerful in determining the patient's momentary decision to label a situation as painful that they often override predisposing cultural, racial, or ethnic long-term conditioning factors. In other words, when the patient's anxiety is high as a result of lack of information about procedures or uncertainty over outcomes, pain responses are heightened in patients from almost every sociocultural background. As we shall see, *there is probably no greater force for changing patient pain behavior than how the dentist relates to the patient's concerns over pain.*

Amount of perceived anxiety about the treatment. Anxiety is the most common emotional response accompanying pain behavior. Anxiety acts as an intervening variable, as we have discussed, between the painful stimulus and the behavioral response. When anxiety is aroused over or during treatment, patients will markedly lower their pain threshold and their pain tolerance levels and restrict the pain sensitivity range (the difference between pain threshold and pain tolerance levels). This inverse, easy-to-understand relationship between anxiety and pain is one of the most consistent facts of life about patient pain behavior: *the higher the anxiety, the less pain the patient will tolerate.*

State anxiety, or **acute anxiety,** refers to a current acute anxiety experience (or state) of the patient. The same type of anxiety-pain behavior relationship is found in persons suffering chronic anxiety. When anxiety exists over a long period of time and characterizes one aspect of the patient's personality, however, it is called **trait anxiety.** Patients who exhibit trait anxiety are similarly predisposed toward significantly lower pain threshold and pain tolerance levels.

Important contributors to the level of a patient's perceived anxiety are under the dentist's control. In the dentist-patient interaction, when the patient is appraising the threat of pain, the dentist can do much to modify the patient's perceptions of anxiety. The patient actually labels the situation as painful. Hence *the more the dentist can respond to the anxiety, the less pain the patient will perceive.* It seems fair to conclude, then, that for most dental treatment situations, dental patients are "more scared than hurt."[9]

Level of cognitive clarity about the treatment. Several elements that contribute in part to dental patient anxiety are related to the uncertainty of what is to be done, when it has to be done, and what the outcome will be. Dentists can provide a "map" of the treatment situation, informing the patient of the following:

1. The rationale for the treatment
2. What the various steps will be and what some of the instruments do

3. How long it will take
4. A description, as accurate as possible, of what the treatment will feel like
5. What the patient will look and/or feel like during and after treatment

This process is called providing cognitive clarity for the patient, and psychologists call the "map" provided a "cognitive map." The information and explanations reduce uncertainty and ambiguity that, when heightened, always elevate anxiety. It has been demonstrated repeatedly in the clinic and the research laboratory that ensuring a clear cognitive map leads to a more comfortable and less apprehensive patient.

One of the virtues of providing information about treatments and outcomes is that it helps the patient to know the source of his or her symptoms. "Yes, I felt a little sting, just like you said." "It was tender for a few days, but you told me that was because of the newness of the bridge."

The act of being able to attribute a bodily symptom to something known is very anxiety relieving for patients. In a study involving medical students, Schachter[25a] administered intravenous epinephrine, with and without explanation of its effects, to two groups. Intense emotional outbursts of uncontrollable anxiety were experienced by those subjects to whom he did not explain that the pounding heart and the generally "uptight" feeling were results of the action of epinephrine they had just received. Other subjects, receiving exactly the same doses, maintained their equanimity because they could attribute their symptoms to the explanation they received that epinephrine was the responsible factor.

Dental patients are often concerned about similar mysterious symptoms such as pounding heart or flushing reactions, which sometimes accompany the administration of local dental anesthetics. The easily visible anxiety of such patients can be tremendously reduced by the dentist with a simple explanation that "those feelings are very brief and a result of the injection's temporary effect on you. It is a common reaction and will last less than a minute."

Amount of control over treatment. *Anxiety is reduced and pain behavior modified when the patient is given as much control as practical over the onset, duration, and intensity of stimuli appraised as threatening or painful.* It is frequently not practical or efficient for the dentist to relinquish some kinds of control (over, say, how long the drill is turned on). Although some kinds of control are admittedly impractical, experience with certain types of patients indicates that the *perception* of control is what they need—the knowledge that they could control the stimulus if they so chose (for example, turn the drill off). Such patients, in fact, rarely use the control. A commonly used instruction from the dentist who wishes to give the patient some control is to suggest that "you raise your hand when you want me to stop . . . for any reason." It is frequently observed that given this degree of control over the onset and duration of the treatment, the patient proceeds to relax and does not experience the need to exercise the ability to control dental procedures.

Control of treatment can be provided in a variety of ways besides mechanical intervention into specific procedures. Aspects of treatment that a patient might control include length and frequency of appointments; rate of treatment; choice of materials, aesthetics, or alternative treatment plans; or permission to be accompanied into the treatment room. All these are relatively easy strategies for dentists to employ with those patients who evidence the need to control what is happening to them.

Patient's perception of his or her relationship with the dentist. The power of interpersonal relationships to influence what the body does has been known for a long time. Miracle workers, shamans, and witch doctors offer ample evidence, for example, that one person's behavior can modify another's healing processes. Postoperative patients could not tell the difference between morphine and a placebo when both were administered by a physician perceived as warm, empathetic, and supporting. On the other hand, morphine was readily distinguished from a placebo in its ability to relieve postoperative pain when administered by a physician perceived as cold, nonempathetic, and objective.

Closer to our own concerns, the interpersonal relationship is viewed as the most important vehicle by which long-term patient satisfaction is maintained. We have already made reference to that viewpoint when discussing strategies for behavior change. In the context of changing dental patients' pain behavior, the process of establishing and maintaining effective interpersonal relationships with patients is conducted through the strategy of reducing anxiety by providing cognitive clarity—reduce uncertainty and ambiguity, give information, and allow the patient control—and then by carrying through behaviors consistent with the explanations. In other words, say what is going to happen and then be certain of exactly that happening. Such activity on the part of the dentist reinforces that he or she will be perceived as empathetic, credible, supportive, and patient oriented. "Imagine, he took the time to tell me it might hurt. Usually, the dentist says everything's fine, and then he kills you." Interpersonal influences are most effective when the dentist is perceived as patient-oriented as opposed to self-oriented and when the behaviors of the dentist are consistent with what the patient has been led to expect.

CONTINUUM OF PAIN CONTROL METHODS

Decreasing need to invoke psychological factors ↓	Hypnosis
	Behavior modification
	Biofeedback
	Acupuncture
	Preoperative oral sedation
	Waking sedation
	Local anesthetic
	General anesthetic

PAIN CONTROL STRATEGIES AND THE DENTIST-PATIENT INTERACTION

A wide array of pain control strategies are now available for dentists. If these were arranged on the above continuum, at one end would be proved chemoanesthetic agents and at the other would be equally profound interpersonal or nonchemotherapeutic methods such as hypnosis and acupuncture. Dispersed along the continuum would be less profound drugs than general anesthetics, especially local anesthetics and the relatively newer waking sedation drugs such as nitrous oxide in low concentrations and sedative-narcotic combinations given intravenously. Each of these pain control modalities is appropriate and safe for general or specialized applications in dentistry, provided the correct clinical diagnosis is made, the clinician is appropriately trained, the setting is correct (including supportive personnel and apparatus), and the need states of the patient all have been taken into account.

Selection of appropriate pain control strategy

The previous discussion about long-term and situational, or momentary, factors that influence pain behavior should have a direct bearing on the pain control strategy chosen for most dental procedures. It seems very fair to conclude that the time spent with patients in changing their pain behavior through some of the nondrug approaches mentioned earlier results in a less anxious patient who requires less chemoanesthetic and whose postoperative course can be expected to be smoother. In fact, reports of healing following surgery done under hypnosis and acupuncture consistently showed relatively uneventful postoperative experiences. Hypnosis and perhaps acupuncture seem to be extreme examples that lend credence to the notion that the dentist, through the utilization of interpersonal change strategies, can significantly modify patients' pain behavior.

When evaluating which type of pain control strategy might be most appropriate, attention must be paid to the obvious fact that combinations of approaches are, in fact, what happens most of the time. Some dentists attempt anxiety reduction prior to the use of any chemical agent. This is especially true with the waking sedation methods. Nitrous oxide is more effective in low concentrations (up to 40% nitrous oxide, 60% oxygen) when preceded by ample explanation of the apparatus and the subjective experiences that can be expected. There is some evidence that as the amount of time spent in patient education decreases, on the average, the dosage of nitrous oxide required *increases*.

Finally, when evaluating an appropriate pain control strategy from the psychological perspective, attention should be directed to the type of pain behavior being modified. Specifically, consideration should be given to the following:

1. Source of the pain: iatrogenic or pathogenic
2. Duration of the pain: acute or chronic
3. Attribution of the pain: psychogenic or somatogenic

Iatrogenic pain lends itself to modification by psychological interventions of anxiety reduction and the establishment of effective interpersonal relationships, followed, for routine dental treatment, by local anesthetics and waking sedation approaches. In contrast, the acute pain of an inflammatory process (for example, a "hot abscess") requires more immediate clinical intervention and, often, drug routes other than injections of local anesthetic agents.

Suggestions for preventive control of acute pain

Most general practicing dentists are concerned with modifying treatment pain. Table 17-2 presents a brief paradigm of preventive pain control that is consistent with the "empathetic" behavior modification strategy explained earlier. We refer to such an approach in this context as preventive pain control because we assume pain and anxiety are possible results of almost every dental treatment, *unless some care is taken by the dentist before treatment begins*.

Before every dental procedure, dentists should initiate the steps in Table 17-2 either superficially or in detail, according to the behavioral response of the patient. Typically, this paradigm requires the dentist to go through a mental rehearsal of the key elements in preventing pain behavior to ensure that the important components will be covered when he or she meets the patient.

In general, seek to provide labels for everything you anticipate will happen or will be experienced. Then observe the patient for cues about impact on level of cognitive clarity, level of muscle tension, and expressions of psychological state.

Suggestions for dealing with chronic pain—an example

Chronic pain states are not frequently seen by a general practicing dentist. One exception might be myofascial pain dysfunction (MPD) syndrome. MPD, formerly thought of exclusively as a temporomandibular joint disturbance, has received attention in the dental literature[11,18] because of its elusive etiology and its apparent resistance to cure. We will discuss MPD at some length as an important instance of how intra- and interpersonal factors influence pain behavior and should influence dentist-patient relationships.

MPD is a functional disorder of the masticatory system. Symptoms are usually unilateral, with the most important being dull chronic pain in the preauricular area, masseter muscle, and temporal areas of the face and head. Additional symptoms include clicking or other noises and limited movement in one or both temporomandibular joints. Most clinicians view the etiology as a combination of physical factors related to muscle function and/or occlusion with psychological factors or personality. Thus MPD would qualify as a psycho-

Table 17-2 □ Preventive pain control

Stage	Key element	Amplification
1	Assess patient's entry behavior.	Previous history with dental treatment. Previous experience with present dentist. Patient's expectations with regard to (1) rate of treatment, (2) nature of treatment, (3) type of chemoanesthetic, and (4) duration of treatment and drug effects. Observed anxiety, depression. Is pain present now? Is patient male, female, old, young?
2	Seek clarity.	Ask patient to specify his or her concerns, if any, regarding needles, drills, clamps, mask, bleeding, or cancer. Is anxiety and/or pain control required? Assess patient's clarity level with regard to what he or she will understand and how much information is required.
3	Provide information.	Explain why. Explain what. Explain how long. Explain reactions, including physiological—numbness, etc.—and psychological—OK to be anxious.
4	Ensure support.	Reaffirm frequently that patient is OK. Allow patient to question, challenge. Touch patient. When appropriate, physical contact is reassuring—laying on of of hands; touching of shoulder, arm, cheek; etc.
5	Relinquish control.	Seek decisions where you can allow the patient some control. Distinguish between patient behavior and technical or health requirements that cannot be relaxed. Provide a communication method—hand signals, etc.
6	Observe behavior.	Extremely important when any drugs are being used. Check if anxiety is, in fact, being reduced: Patient appears calm, relaxed, positive, no agitation; speech and respiration patterns normal; etc. Is patient receiving you clearly? Listen to the patient's pain vocabulary: Are words employed such as cruel, terrified vs annoying, noisy, tired of sitting, etc.?

physiological disorder, that is, a physiological expression of a psychological disturbance.

A consistent psychodynamic constellation has been confirmed in MPD patients by many researchers.[11,20] It includes depression, isolation, denial, and passive-aggressive conflict. These feelings and defensive modes lead to disruption of interpersonal relations. The patients see themselves as unable to control and cope with life situations filled with conflict. They want to remain dependent while struggling with the need to aggressively assert themselves. The MPD symptoms serve the patient through the mechanism of secondary gain. They gain advantages such as attention, sympathy, and the opportunity to manipulate others. Further, the symptoms provide a constant justification for feelings of depression, desire for isolation, and need to be dependent. However, these symptoms are not readily visible to others, so the defensive system in itself elicits conflict, since credibility is perceived as hard to maintain.

Finally, the expectations of clinicians that symptoms can be eliminated is seen to run counter to the current needs of the patient. We interpret that the clinicians' well-intended desire to relieve the symptoms by mechanosurgical procedures apparently is perceived by the patient as irrelevant. The patient's persistent search for alternative mechanosurgical treatments may be a maneuver to give the illusion of seeking a cure. To the extent that these maneuvers are successful, the patient is not compelled to deal with underlying psychodynamic conflicts.[20] Our view is that the chronic MPD patient is best served by supportive, palliative, reversible treatment until the patient is ready to resolve the basic underlying conflicts. Newer forms of behavioral methods such as those advanced by Fordyce, especially, hold promise for helping many of these patients.[11]

The following question naturally arises: How does the dentist know when the patient is ready to resolve underlying basic conflicts? At least a partial answer can be provided by making reference to our earlier discussion of so-called ghost symptoms and the patient's readiness to abandon behaviors that are not adaptive.

It seems safe to conclude that the patient has not resolved such conflicts *if* there is a continued search for esoteric or complex and irreversible surgical or medical treatment *and* a simultaneous rejection of simpler, reversible, nonsurgical approaches to pain resolution. Reversible approaches could include hypnosis, acupuncture, biofeedback, behavior modification, and/or brief individual or group psychotherapy.

The dentist who is confident that clinical findings and review of the patient's history do not warrant further irreversible procedures may suggest to the patient that "Until we find out more about any organic damage or pathological condition, it is best not to remove any more teeth, do more endodontics, perform extensive occlusal splinting, and so forth. Instead, it seems more judicious to pursue a conservative course and explore alternative approaches that have been developed to help individuals like yourself who suffer chronically from pain that eludes the physician's understanding. I'm speaking of such things as biofeedback or other methods of modifying your pain behavior so that you learn to get along better, do more, and even, perhaps, require less pain medication."

SUMMARY

We have seen that the pain dentists observe in their patients can arise from two sources, either from treatment (iatrogenic pain) or from a pathological condition (pathogenic pain). Different strategies are applicable for the management of each kind of pain. As pain becomes chronic, one-time remedies such as surgical intervention that are perhaps appropriate for acute pain often lose their effectiveness.

It is unquestionably valid that dentists seeking to manage pain problems comprehensively be required to evaluate, for every patient, the physiological *and* the psychological dimensions of the pain problem. The notion that pain is either physiological or psychological, that is, "it's in your mind if it's not in your body," is simply no longer a useful concept for any health practitioner. All pain simultaneously involves the patient's bodily processes and perceptions, needs, and anticipations for the future.

REFERENCES

1. Alling, C.: Facial pain, New York, 1975, Lea & Febiger.
2. Barber, T. Y.: Pain and hypnosis, Psychosom. Med. **25:**303, 1963.
3. Beecher, H.: The measurement of subjective responses, New York, 1959, Oxford University Press, Inc.
4. Buytendijk, F.: Pain, Chicago, 1943, The University of Chicago Press.
5. Carr, J., Brownsberger, C., and Rutherford, R.: Characteristics of symptom-matched psychogenic and real pain patients on MMPI, Proc. Am. Psychol. Assoc. 1967.
6. Chapman, C. R., Gehrig, J. D., and Wilson, M. W.: Acupuncture compared with 33 percent nitrous oxide for dental analgesia, Anesthesiology **42:**532, 1975.
7. Clark, J., and Bindra, D.: Individual differences in pain threshold, Can. J. Psychol. **10:**69, 1956.
8. Clark, W. C., and Hunt, H.: Pain. In Downey, J. A., and Darling, R. C.: Physiological basis of rehabilitation medicine, New York, 1971, W. B. Saunders Co.
9. Corah, N.: Development of a dental anxiety scale, J. Dent. Res. **47:**154, 1968.

10. Dworkin, S. F.: Pain responsivity and its relationship to situational context and body-concept, Dissert. Abstr. **31:**3, 1970.
11. Fordyce, W. E.: Behavioral methods for chronic pain and illness, St. Louis, 1976, The C. V. Mosby Co.
12. Gelfand, S., Ullman, L., and Krasner, L.: Placebo responses—an experimental approach, J. Nerv. Ment. Dis. **136:**379, 1963.
13. Green, R., and Reyer, J.: Pain tolerance in hypnotic analysis and imagination states, J. Abnorm. Psychol. **1:**29, 1972.
14. Keele, K.: Anatomies of pain, Springfield, Ill., 1957, Charles C Thomas, Publisher.
15. Kessen, W., and Mandler, G.: Anxiety, pain and inhibition of distress, Psychol. Rev. **68:**396, 1961.
16. Laskin, D.: Etiology of the pain-dysfunction syndrome, J. Am. Dent. Assoc. **79:**148, 1969.
17. Lipton, J., and Dworkin, S. F.: Psychosocial considerations in MPD patients, Abstr. Int. Assoc. Dent. Res. March, 1974.
18. Lupton, D. E.: Psychological aspects of temporomandibular joint dysfunction, J. Am. Dent. Assoc. **79:**131, 1969.
19. Lynn, R., and Eysenck, H.: Tolerance for pain and extroversion and neuroticism, Percept. Mot. Skills **12:**161, 1961.
20. Marbach, J., and Dworkin, S. F.: Chronic MPD, group psychotherapy and psychodynamics, J. Am. Dent. Assoc. **90:**827, 1975.
21. Melzack, R.: Perception of pain, Sci. Am. **204:**41, 1961.
22. Melzack, R.: The puzzle of pain, New York, 1973, Basic Books, Inc., Publishers.
23. Melzack, R., and Scott, T.: The effects of early experience on the response to pain, J. Comp. Physiol. Psychol. **50:**155, 1957.
24. Merskey, H., and Spear, F. G.: Pain: psychological and psychiatric aspects, Baltimore, 1967, The Williams & Wilkins Co.
25. Moulton, R.: Emotional factors in non-organic temperomandibular joint pain, Dent. Clin. North Am. **2:**609, 1966.
25a. Schachter, S.: The interaction of cognitive and physiological determinants of emotional state. In Berkowitz, L., ed.: Advances in experimental social psychology, vol. 1, New York, 1964, Academic Press, Inc.
26. Schoenberg, B., and Senescu, R.: Group psychotherapy for patients with chronic multiple somatic complaints, J. Chronic Dis. **19:**649, 1966.
27. Sternbach, R.: Pain: a psychophysiologic analysis, New York, 1968, Academic Press, Inc.
28. Sternbach, R.: Pain patients: traits and treatments, New York, 1974, Academic Press, Inc.
29. Szasz, T.: Pain and pleasure, New York, 1957, Basic Books, Inc., Publishers.
30. Tursky, B., and Sternbach, R.: Further physiological correlates of ethnic differences in response to shock, Psychophysiology **4:**67, 1967.
31. Weisenberg, M., ed.: Pain: clinical and experimental perspectives, St. Louis, 1975, The C. V. Mosby Co.
32. Wolff, B. B.: Quantitative measure of deep somatic pain—use of hypertonic saline, Clin. Sci. Mol. Med. **28:**43, 1965.
33. Zbrowski, M.: People in pain, San Francisco, 1969, Jossey-Bass, Inc., Publishers.

Chapter 18

INTERACTIONS WITH PATIENTS UNDER NONAVERSIVE CONDITIONS

It is probably fair to say that unpleasant emotional states are present in most dentist-patient interactions at one time or another. The intensity of the unpleasant experience is compelling and certainly colors patients' associations with dentists. However, if many dentist-patient interactions were to be observed over a period of time and in a variety of settings—in general and specialty practices as well as in clinics—one would be impressed with the amount of time dentists and patients spend with each other where negative or unpleasant emotional states are totally absent or present in only minor degrees.

For most patients, going to the dentist is a well-tolerated experience. By and large dentists report patient behaviors that are appropriate to the relatively transient and weak noxious stimuli that accompany the routine dental care most patients require. The interaction between dentist and patient, *when aversive factors are perceived to be minimal,* represents an opportunity for the dentist to modify patient behavior by motivating, modifying, or reinforcing desirable health-related behaviors. By doing so in a positive manner, lasting dentist-patient relationships are frequently established and maintained so that patients respond to recall appointments, accept required dental treatment, become sources of referral, and make the practice of dentistry more rewarding for the dentist.

OBJECTIVES

The objectives of this chapter are as follows:

1. To explore ways the dentist can help motivate, modify, and reinforce patients' desirable health behaviors
2. To discuss different aspects of the issue of prevention in dentistry

WAYS THE DENTIST CAN HELP MOTIVATE, MODIFY, AND REINFORCE PATIENTS' HEALTHY BEHAVIORS

We have already considered the psychological factors involved when individuals need to communicate with clarity and effectiveness. In this chapter we look at the communication process as it might be applied by dentists seeking to modify their patients' behavior toward increased prevention of dental disease.

Establishment of a therapeutic contract

The communication process in dentistry is the vehicle by which the **therapeutic contract**[13] is established between dentist and patient. This therapeutic contract is similar to the **psychological contract** discussed earlier. The therapeutic contract has the following three components.

The dentist and patient agree:

1. *To relate:* Dentist and patient will assume and act out their respective roles.

2. *To exchange information:* The patient will communicate what is wrong, and the dentist will explain how it will be remedied.
3. *To give and receive treatment:* The patient will submit to therapy provided by the dentist, who is presumed to be knowledgeable and competent.

Utilization of a reciprocal listening/verbalizing/performing network

The communication process by which the therapeutic contract is developed and fulfilled involves the dentist and the patient in a reciprocal listening/verbalizing/performing network. The dentist, in addition, must be informed and have developed the necessary clinical skills. A communication model that contains the essential ingredients—knowledge and performance skills for modifying desirable behaviors of the dental patient is outlined in Fig. 18-1.

Knowledge

Cognitive domain. In the cognitive domain, effective communication requires that the dentist be knowledgeable about the scientific and clinical basis for preventive dental health programs—how and why they work. In other words, the dentist must possess adequate *clinical information* to know what to say and do and also know the appropriate and necessary *clinical skills* to deliver a preventive program so that the patient can observe the resulting positive changes. For example, the dentist must know when plaque has been removed. This cognitive or intellectual aspect of knowledge should extend from competency in problem identification, diagnosis, and treatment planning to knowledge about the pathology of plaque, relevant nutritional information, and up-to-date information regarding advances in newer materials or techniques such as sealants and anticaries agents.

Affective domain. In the affective, or "emotional," domain, the dentist has the responsibility to be knowledgeable about the cultural, racial, or ethnic factors that might determine how different individuals feel about health, the care of the body in general, and the oral cavity in particular (Chapter 4). The dentist's knowledge of the affective domain is additionally enhanced by his or her awareness of effective interpersonal skills.

Observing/listening. Observing/listening skills significantly affect the dentist's ability to know the patient.

Active listening. Active listening involves attention to the *content, organization, emotional quality, rate,* and *idiosyncracies* of the patient's speech that allow the dentist to *understand what the patient is communicating.*

Furthermore, the *context* in which the communication occurs adds to the verbal and nonverbal behaviors additional mean-

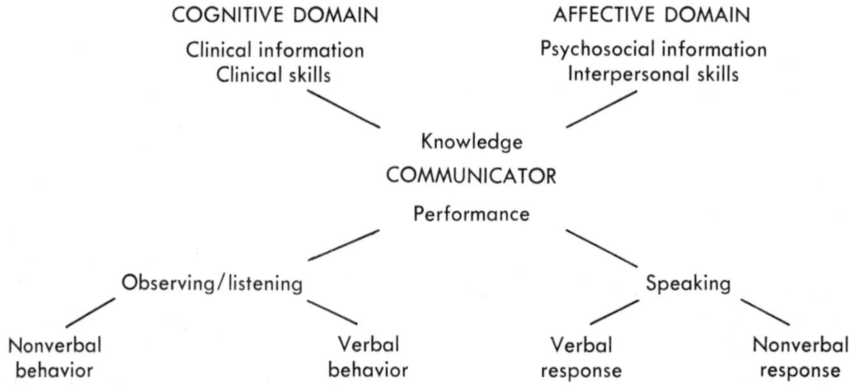

Fig. 18-1. Ingredients in an effective communication model.

ings that help both the patient and the dentist understand each other better. The too frequently heard comment ". . . took my words out of context" reveals that a perceived misunderstanding occurred.[2,21]

Listening for the proper context is critical to true understanding. When the patient says, "I am glad you are finished," is that comment to be interpreted within the context of a just completed difficult technical task (for example, "wow, that was hard for me" or "wow, that was hard for you") or in the context of an explanation about plaque control and the benefits of prevention (for example, "how much is all this time costing me" or "thank you, now I understand")? As discussed in Chapter 12 understanding the context is enhanced if the dentist, in addition to attending to the content, organization, emotional quality, rate, and idiosyncracies of speech, is also aware of the following ingredients that contribute to the enhancement of communication:

- Social genesis. Are the patient's verbalizations standard for his or her culture, the culture of the dentist, and/or the culture of the dentist-patient relationship?
- Discernible pathological conditions. Do the patient's verbalizations contain internal inconsistencies, undue intensity, frequent tripping over words? Is the content appropriate? ("Why is the patient talking about her children when I'm talking about dental floss?")
- Range of activity. Are the patient's verbalizations restricted appropriately to the topics at hand or are they too restricted?
- Adaptational influences. Does the patient show acceptance or resistance to the dentist's communication influences?

Consider the following case histories to determine how these factors can give communications different meanings and how different responses might be indicated on the part of the dentist.

Case histories

Case 1. A "successful" male business executive comes to the dental office for the first time. He requests a "checkup, just to make sure everything is all right. I don't really have much time to go to the dentist, but I hope he (the dentist) will find everything all right so I won't have to spend much time here."

Several alternative interpretations seem possible for the dentist hearing these statements. First, perhaps the range of activity of the patient is too constricted—the patient only wants to talk about what he wants to talk about, that is, there are not going to be any problems. Similarly, the patient may exhibit resistance to the dentist's verbalizations that are not consistent with the patient's self-perception of why he came to the dentist. On hearing, for example, that another visit is necessary to complete the diagnosis and treatment planning phase, the patient may believe he has come to the wrong office.

By being alert to the context surrounding what the patient says, the dentist may wish to modify his or her own communicating behavior. For example, he or she might decide to talk less and/or to find out if the patient has underlying anxiety concerning dental treatment.

Case 2. A male adolescent enters the operatory and says "Hiya doc, what's new; who's the cute chick that answers the telephone, I really dig her; well, what are you going to do today; say did you hear that the Yankees traded Smith for a million dollars; well, wash your hands and start drilling, I've got it all together today and won't give you a hard time at all."

If the stream of chatter is reasonably paced and relaxed in tone, perhaps the idiosyncracies and vernacular speech reflect a "nice, loose kid" who "has it all together." The dentist might respond in kind, with pleasant banter while proceeding with dispatch to initiate treatment. Suppose, however, the dentist knows that the young man comes from a religious family, does not get along with his father, has run away from home, has rebelled against school authority, shows a history of poor oral hygiene and undependability in keeping dental appointments, and has caused your receptionist to talk to you about his disruptive waiting room behavior. Under the latter circumstances, the dentist's behavior would probably be markedly different, recognizing and perhaps believing that the patient's verbalizations reflect "disrespect" and belligerence. Instead of pleasant banter, perhaps the dentist in the latter context would be more guarded. In such a case, the dentist might choose to respond only to the need to perform dental work and to lead the patient to understand that the rest of his statements will not be rewarded or responded to positively.

Observing nonverbal behavior. Regarding the dentist-patient communication interaction for nonverbal behaviors,[13,15] the dentist can examine the following:

1. Voice inflection, tone, and volume
2. Gestures—hand and body
3. Posture
4. Touching behaviors
5. Physical distance assumed
6. Skin responses—blushing, pallor, etc.
7. Facial expressions of emotion—anger, anxiety, calm, etc.
8. Appointment-related behaviors—punctuality, dependability, etc.

Nonverbal behaviors are important in the communication process because they lend a *context* to the patient's words. The value for the dentist of attending to nonverbal patient behavior has been found to include the following:

1. More accurate understanding of what the patient *means*
2. Instantaneous additional information: a sort of multimedia effect of combining sight and sound in the communication process
3. Understanding of the emotional flavor behind the patient's words: Did you just hear an angry "no!" or a questioning "no?"
4. Positive feedback to the patient that

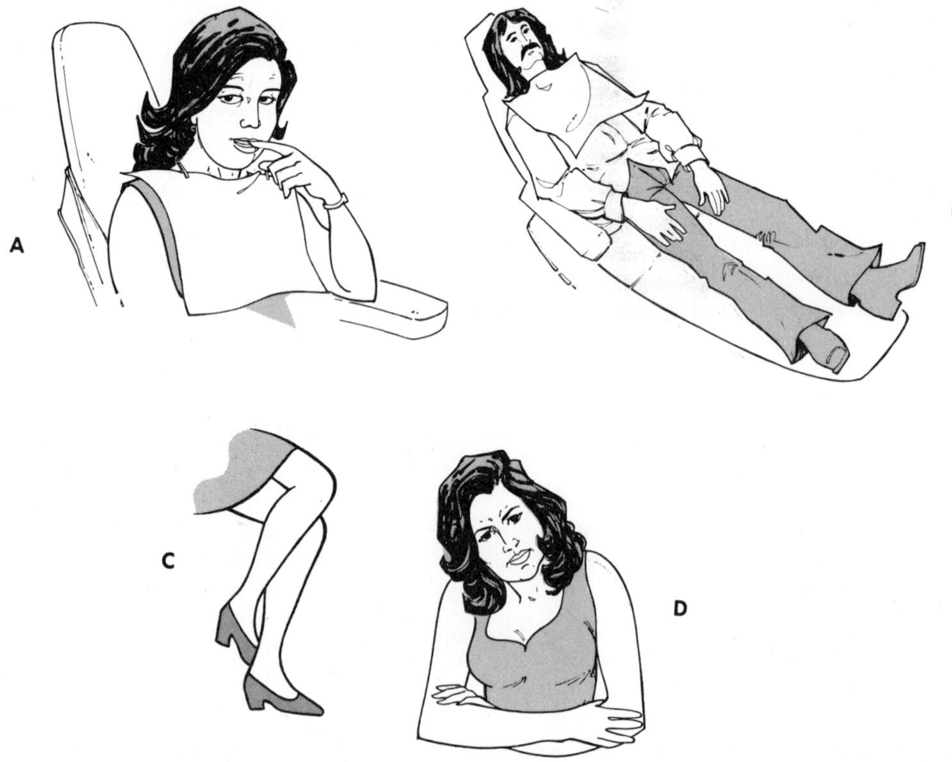

Fig. 18-2. A and **B,** Nonverbal behaviors that are clues to openness for new ideas and creative patient listening. **C** and **D,** Postures that imply being closed to new thoughts or being preoccupied. (From Froelich, R. E., Bishop, F. M., and Dworkin, S. F.: Communication in the dental office, St. Louis, 1976, The C. V. Mosby Co.)

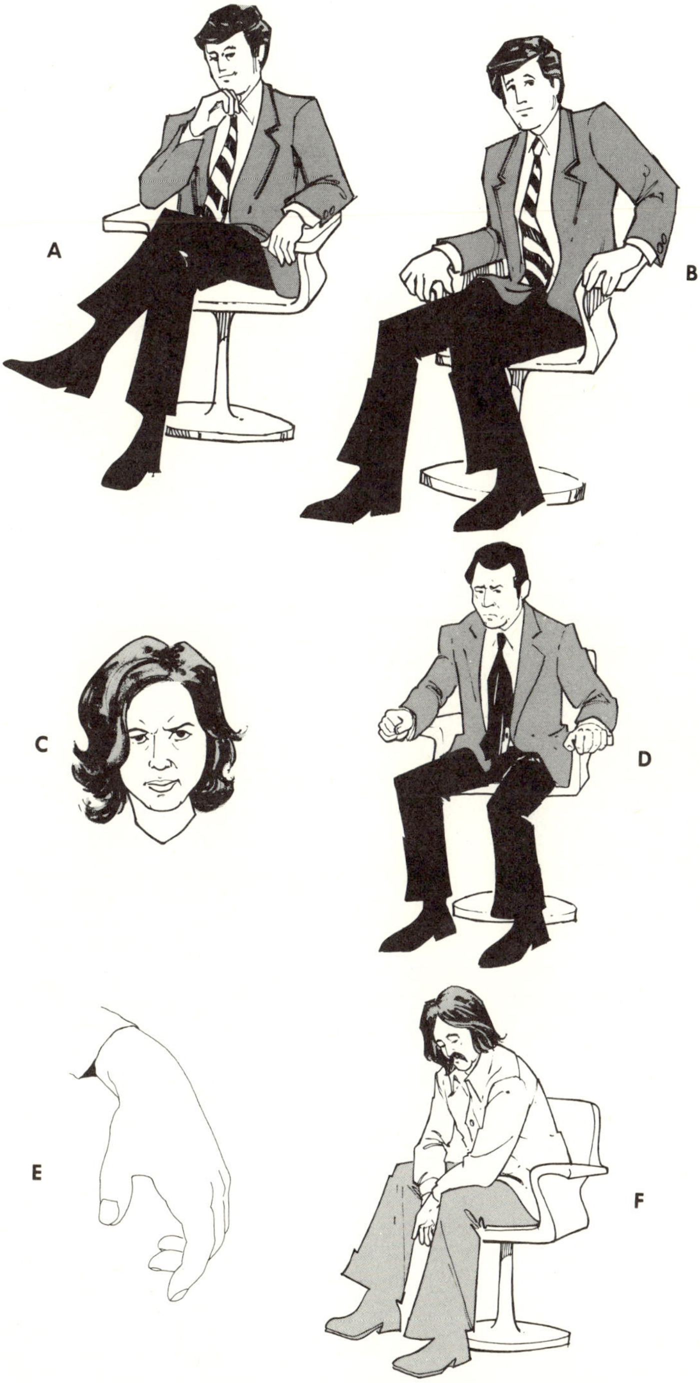

Fig. 18-3. A and **B,** Nonverbal clues to anxiety. **C** and **D,** Nonverbal expressions of anger. **E** and **F,** Nonverbal depiction of depression. (From Froelich, R. E., Bishop, F. M., and Dworkin, S. F.: Communication in the dental office, St. Louis, 1976, The C. V. Mosby Co.)

the dentist is an interested and attentive listener

5. Availability of the only communication channel (as when the patient's mouth is occupied by the dental treatment)
6. Certainty that at least a nonverbal communication link exists, which is reassuring to the patient and evidences a concerned dentist

Some instances of interpreting nonverbal clues that seem to find agreement among many communications experts are depicted in Figs. 18-2 and 18-3.

Nonverbal behaviors have been organized by Froelich, Bishop, and Dworkin[13] into a framework within which meaning can be given them. Some examples of how nonverbal behaviors can serve as clues to communication are contained in their book entitled *Communication in the Dental Office.*[13]

OPEN VERSUS CLOSED NONVERBAL BEHAVIOR. Whether or not the patient is receptive to new ideas and thoughts can be partially evaluated by the patient's nonverbal behavior. Open and closed nonverbal behaviors serve as clues to the degree of attentive listening the patient is exhibiting, as depicted in Fig. 18-2.

AFFECTIVE NONVERBAL BEHAVIORS. Positive and negative affect, emotion, or attitude that can often be evaluated from the patient's nonverbal behavior includes anxiety, anger, and depression. Nonverbal clues to anxiety are revealed by the behaviors illustrated in Fig. 18-3, *A* and *B,* and are often interpreted as having a "ready to take off" look. Nonverbal expressions of anger are revealed by behaviors that look like "holding back" and frustration, as seen in Fig. 18-3, *C* and *D*. Nonverbal depictions of depression are portrayed in Fig. 18-3, *E* and *F*, and are often described as facial and body musculature that has lost "interest" even in merely supporting themselves.

Speaking and related behaviors. The dentist communicates when he or she makes verbal and nonverbal responses to the patient. Although we generally think of communication as primarily a speaking process, speaking should come last in the actual chain of communication between dentist and patient. In terms of sequence, initially the dentist should be armed with *knowledge,* to know what to say. Next he or she must possess *observational powers,* to speak at the right time and in the correct context. One cannot speak effectively unless one has observed the situation.

In the role of communicator, the dentist's responsibility is to elicit or to provide information and/or support.[11] When engaged in speaking, these objectives are accomplished by verbal and nonverbal communicator behaviors.

Verbal communicator behaviors. The verbal communication behaviors are as follows:

Asking questions

facilitating questions Questions that encourage the patient to say more, without specifying an area or topic: "How are you"?

open-ended questions Questions that request information in the patient's own words and specify a general content area: "How are you doing with your brushing and flossing"?

direct questions Questions that ask the patient for a specific bit of information: "Is it easier to hold the brush this way"?

probing questions Questions that ask for more specific information than the patient offers spontaneously: "What else did you notice about your gums"?

laundry list questions Questions that ask the patient to respond from among a list of alternative adjectives or descriptions provided: "Is the pain burning, aching, dull, or sharp"?

Supporting the patient's narrative

reassurance Response that tends to elicit a sense of self-reliance in the patient: "You'll be able to handle your new dentures just fine."

empathy Response that recognizes and accepts the patient's emotional states or feelings without evaluation: "You feel like none of this toothbrushing makes any difference anyway."

support Response that demonstrates interest or concern for the patient: "I'm worried about your gums in this area, so I'll attend to that today, making sure you leave here OK."

Providing a narrative

organization Sequence and logic of ideas presented to the patient.
clarity Sequence of words spoken to the patient.
level Choice of words spoken to the patient.
affect Emotional pattern and timing of ideas presented to the patient.

Nonverbal communicator behaviors. Nonverbal communicator behaviors include the dentist's posture, movement, and emphasis, in other words, the same set of nonverbal factors identified for the patient. For the dentist, however, these nonverbal behaviors include how the dental work is performed: Is the dentist gentle, thorough, clean, etc.?

When the dentist is listening to the patient, his or her physical characteristics deserve attention. The listener behaviors of positive concentration, facial expression, and eye gaze all contribute positively or negatively to a communication exchange. For the patient doing the talking, these listener behaviors are what the patient observes as the nonverbal behaviors of the dentist. Posture should be relaxed, whether sitting or standing. It is also helpful to face the patient as directly as is possible or natural, depending on the particular physical arrangements of the setting.

The dentist should obviously transmit the impression of concentrating on what is being said.[21] Distracting noises, interruptions, changes in posture away from the patient, and excessive body movements (nail biting, waving a dangling crossed leg, hair combing, etc.) should be reduced to an absolute minimum.

Facial expression should be neutral, friendly, and interested. Eyes should be directed toward the patient and engage the patient's eyes as frequently as is comfortable for talker and listener.

For most dentist-patient exchanges, it is probably best if the dentist, nonverbally as well as verbally, refrains from revealing personal judgments or evaluations about the patient. When the patient says "I haven't been to a dentist in 6 years," "You dentists sure like to charge," or "Oh, we're not married, we've just been living together," it is probably best if the dentist does not reveal, through his or her nonverbal behaviors, a personal judgment concerning the worth of the patient or the value of the patient's personal views. The dentist may, instead, reflect interest in learning something new about the patient and encourage the patient to continue to be open and communicative, for example, "That's probably true for a lot of people, thanks for letting me know."

Some of the most essential behaviors in communicating effectively are listed here.

SOME SPECIFIC DO'S AND DON'TS

Do	Don't
Describe	Evaluate
Be specific	Be general
Be responsive	Be evasive
Time appropriately	Be premature or too deep
Pay attention	Be inattentive or wander

Use feedback from the other's verbal and nonverbal behavior to determine if these criteria are achieved.

ISSUE OF PREVENTION IN DENTISTRY

Our discussion assumes that encouraging the patient toward health-related or preventive behavior is desirable. We will now step back a bit to look at the whole issue of prevention in dentistry.

Why the preventive dentistry movement is important to dentists

It is instructive to examine the preventive dentistry movement for the following reasons:

1. Because the goal of disease prevention is *the* driving force behind the health professions
2. Because it has invoked so much psychology, both in the area of motivat-

ing individuals to modify their behavior and in the area of communicating to increase the patient's level of accurate information

For the goal of prevention to be de-emphasized as a result of unrealistic expectations would be a tragic error. If, as many investigators now believe, dentists have "turned off" preventive programs because patients will not follow them, it may be fair to conclude that we have learned more about the dentist's behavior than about the patient's. Specifically, we may be confirming that dentists are relatively unsophisticated students of human behavior and are especially naive regarding the psychosocial aspects of health- and illness-related behaviors.

Background of the preventive dentistry movement

In recent years there have been strenuous attempts to bring motivational and communication psychology to bear on the field of preventive dentistry.* Many strategies and programs have been developed to motivate the patient to adopt better preventive health practices, or, more specifically, to accept plaque control programs. From an initial period of intense enthusiasm and apparent acceptance by both patients and dentists, interest has waned in sustained efforts to maintain patients on careful preventive therapy routines. The fact that preventive dentistry concepts may not have the same visibility and credibility among dentists, especially, is unfortunate, *albeit predictable.*

Interest in preventive dentistry, popularized as plaque control, achieved the status of a popular fad; like all fads, it was destined to appeal for a short time only. The histories of medicine and dentistry are full of therapies promulgated as "cure-all's" or "painless treatment." Each had its day—from hysterectomy to penicillin, from air-abrasive drills to audioanalgesia, and from hypnosis to encounter group therapy. Many of these fads in health care have included, at least in part, some sound and useful information or technique, which, if that aspect were retained, would constitute a real contribution to treating human disease. Such is certainly the case for some abused drugs such as penicillin and tranquilizers as well as for overdramatized therapies such as hypnosis and some extensive surgeries.

Motivating the patient to adopt and maintain preventive dental practices can certainly be included as one of those important fads in the field of dentistry where both the underlying concepts are sound and the intended outcomes are highly desirable. Unfortunately, the expectations of dentists were unrealistic in that promised or expected patient behavior changes were not maintained, by and large, over any appreciable period of time.[7,25] This outcome is also highly characteristic of fads—namely, that in the beginning almost everyone claims universal success, and all promises seem to come true; then disenchantment sets in as later returns do not continue to substantiate early findings. Patients were supposed to change to highly specific oral hygiene behaviors (especially those related to brushing and flossing the teeth in a certain way); these changes, however, rarely occurred and/or were maintained.

The "problem" in preventive dentistry—definitions

Preventive dentistry, as a term, seems to have lost most of its general meaning, at least according to its most popular usage in the dental literature. Preventive dentistry seems to have become equated with a series of patient-maintained oral hygiene techniques for controlling the onset of caries and periodontal disease by preventing the initiation of dental plaque. To prevent dental plaque, patients are taught specific toothbrushing methods and techniques for using dental floss. The dentist's responsibility seems largely to "motivate" patients to accept the rationale for new

*See references 1, 3, 4, 6, 7-9, 12, 19, 20, and 27-30.

Table 18-1 □ Scope of preventive dentistry*

Level of prevention	Caries	Periodontal disease	Injury, orofacial defects, malocclusion	Oral lesions	Systemic disease	Occupational hazards
Initiation	Plaque control program Fluorides Dietary control Sealants(?)	Plaque control program Diet Scaling Prophylaxis	Mouth protectors Prenatal care Genetic counseling Retention of primary teeth (caries control)	Education (smoking, irritants, excessive sunlight, alcohol, poor nutrition)		Radiation control Mercury monitoring Noise control Aerosol control Proper office design Hepatitis (transmission control)
← Recall and reinforcement →						
Progression and recurrence	Remineralization Operative dentistry Pulp capping Pulpotomy Endodontics	Root planing Occlusal adjustment Surgical procedures Diet(?) Properly executed restorative dentistry	Habit control Space maintainers Orthodontics Rehabilitative procedures (surgical, mechanical)	Thorough examination Oral cytology(?) Biopsy Removal of irritants	Salivary examination Laboratory tests Referral to physician	
Loss of function	Restorative dentistry, properly executed	Prosthodontics		Irradiation Surgery Chemotherapy	Medical or surgical care	
Loss of life						

*From Mandel, I. D.: J. Prev. Dent. **1**:25, 1974.

methods of brushing and flossing; the patient, however, must do "it." If the patient fails to do "it" regularly, dentists talk about the failure of preventive dentistry and plaque control programs.

In addition to this admittedly oversimplified description and evaluation, we should mention that topical fluoride application, nutritional counseling, and use of occlusal sealants can also be incorporated into a plaque control or preventive program.

It seems fair to conclude, however, that the vast amount of dentist-patient interactions concerning prevention and plaque control have centered on motivating new and long-term brushing and flossing behaviors. Mandel,[23] however, suggests a broader definition and appraisal of prevention. He points out that, to some degree at least, *all* dentistry should be thought of as preventive. Mandel has categorized various levels of prevention and the ways in which preventive concepts might be applied in *all the areas* of clinical dentistry. His definition is summarized in Table 18-1.

The preventive dentistry motivational strategy

In order to change patient behaviors toward more effective dental disease prevention, several prominent authorities have recommended strongly that dentists institute highly structured plaque control programs in their offices. These programs share certain critical ingredients, many of which were discussed in Chapter 13. Proponents of the various plaque control programs contend that the following common principles, if applied according to different patient needs by dentists or trained paraprofessionals, will motivate the patient to initiate and maintain long-term oral hygiene behavior changes:

1. *Information or cognitive clarity.* Provide the patient with a sound rationale for why plaque removal is important and how specific techniques are effective in removing plaque.
2. *Training in new motor behaviors.* Instruct the patient in the psychomotor acts of proper brushing, flossing, self-application of fluorides, and use of disclosing solutions.
3. *Immediate, positive reinforcement and feedback.* Reward the patient with praise and encouragement. Demonstrate how the patient may obtain positive feedback by using disclosing agents and by eliminating undesirable factors such as bleeding gums and bad breath.
4. *Fear arousal.* Point out negative consequences of failure to maintain the plaque control program: "Look under this microscope at the dirty bugs swimming around in your mouth." As we pointed out in Chapter 13, however, fear arousal should be used with caution. High fear arousal for some individuals leads to increased anxiety that disrupts or prevents desirable behavior.
5. *Self-esteem.* Appeal to both enhanced positive self-esteem (look better, feel better, smell better) and diminished negative self-esteem (will not be liked, not a good person).
6. *Personal persuasiveness.* Change the patient's behavior through the force of the personality of the communicator—the "charisma" factor.

These six factors are common to the persuasive strategies associated with current plaque control programs. For the most part, the use of these approaches is absolutely consistent with good psychological theory regarding interpersonal influence. However, although these six factors are common to persuasive strategies, they are not all equally applicable to the same degree for every patient. As we carefully discussed in Chapter 13, "the essential step is to view the attempt to influence the patient from the patient's perspective . . . to stand in the patient's shoes." We want to stress the conscious adaption of dentist strategy to patient needs and likely responses; thus certain levels of fear arousal may be effective with some but, clearly, not with all patients. On the other hand, self-esteem appeals may be more effective with other patients. The principles discussed in Chapters 12 and 13 indicate ways to apply and evaluate these common ingredients in persuasive communications.

Assessment of the status of preventive dentistry

Has preventive dentistry worked? We've already alluded to the disappointment many dentists have experienced in their attempts to change their patients' behavior. We can probably summarize the state of the art as follows:

> Preventive dentistry has become assoicated in the minds of most dentists and many dental educators and researchers with a set of nonclinical activities that might loosely be called patient dental health education. One consequence of the "set" has been to expose dental practitioners and students to a variety of motivational approaches for instilling in their patients new dental health attitudes and behaviors.
>
> Answering the question: "Which efforts of the dentist have been shown to be effective in inducing preventive behaviors in the patient?" Corah forthrightly states that he "knows of no evidence which demonstrates that dentists have any effect whatsoever," by which he means that no data exists to evaluate differential effectiveness of different preventive programs of practicing dentists. The stress on the paucity of evaluation data forms a continuous thread throughout the dental literature. It helps place in proper perspective the proliferation of "how-to" methods now so readily available to the dentist wanting to become more prevention oriented. It is unfortunately true that we simply do not yet know if some of the current approaches to preventive dentistry are having more of an impact than others.*

Toward a personal action philosophy of preventive dentistry

It seems appropriate to make a final comment relating professional behavior and responsibility to disappointment over patient compliance. Throughout this book we have attempted to demonstrate that patients more often than not fail to initiate desirable behavior or to change harmful behavior, even when "it's for their own good." Human behavior is a fantastically complex and barely understood phenomenon. There is no one general theory of behavior that answers our questions about why we behave in the first place and what makes us different from each other. Similarly, there is no one theory of psychotherapy that answers all our questions about how to change behavior to more adaptive forms.

Even superficial analysis reveals that some of the ingredients of effective communication do not always work well. Information is not sufficient to motivate everyone to abandon an undesirable behavior: doesn't every smoker know enough to stop? Moreover, in some cases, fear arousal raises anxiety sufficiently so that the very behavior to be eliminated is, perversely, reinforced—severely frightening a child about the consequences of thumb sucking can lead to more hidden thumb sucking to alleviate the anxiety so aroused.

However, even though progress in changing harmful health behavior has been slow, no one seems disposed to eliminate behaviors that have some effectiveness. For example, warnings on cigarette packages have not been removed, even though cigarette smoking continues to be popular; seat belts are required equipment in every car, but far from all of us use them. Health care professionals need not allow disappointing patient behaviors to serve as a defense (unconscious or otherwise) for the abandonment of their own preventive dental health care programs.

SUMMARY

In this chapter we have focused on the positive interactions that typify most dentist-patient relationships. As we have learned from previous chapters, it is likely that the dentist can modify and reinforce patient behaviors that result in continued or increased oral health, when conditions

---

*From Dworkin, S. F.: Health Educ. Monogr. **2**:236, 1974.

of stress, anxiety, and fear are not allowed to remain high. Desirable patient behaviors such as dependability and acceptance of required treatment are enhanced when the dentist effectively utilizes the reciprocal listening/speaking/performing network described in this chapter. The principles on which this communication process is based are outlined in Chapters 12 and 13.

Prevention was singled out as a set of clinical and behavioral possibilities with which the patient could more dependably identify, accept, and implement. Here, too, the communication of the dentist should deliberately be designed to persuade the patient toward desired health behavior changes that involve achieving improved oral hygiene, better nutrition, and complete dental care.

REFERENCES

1. Arnim, S.: The effect of thorough mouth cleansing on oral health, Periodontics **6:**41, 1968.
2. Barker, L. I.: Listening behavior, Englewood Cliffs, N.J., 1971, Prentice-Hall, Inc.
3. Bass, C. C.: An effective method of personal oral hygiene, J. L. Med. Soc. **106:**101, 1954.
4. Bibby, B. G.: Do we tell the truth about preventing caries, J. Dent. Child. **33:**269, 1966.
5. Bramner, L.: The helping relationship: process and skills, Englewood Cliffs, N.J., 1973, Prentice-Hall, Inc.
6. Cohen, L. K., O'Shea, R. M., and Putnam, W. J.: Toothbrushing: public opinion and dental research, J. Oral Ther. Pharmacol. **4:**229, 1967.
7. Corah, N.: The dental practitioner and preventive health behavior, Health Educ. Monogr. **2:**226, 1974.
8. Dworkin, S. F.: Critique of Corah's paper, Health Educ. Monogr. **2:**236, 1974.
9. Dworkin, S. F., ed.: Persuasive prevention, New York, 1974, Medcom Press.
10. Dworkin, S. F., ed.: Preventive dentistry: state of the art, J. Prev. Dent. (In press.)
11. Enelow, A. J., and Swisher, S. H.: Interviewing and patient care, New York, 1972, Oxford University Press, Inc.
12. Evans, R. I., Rozelle, R. M., Lasater, T. M., Dembroski, T. M., and Allen, B. P.: Fear arousal persuasion and actual versus implied behavioral change, J. Pers. Soc. Psychol. **16:**220, 1970.
13. Froelich, R., Bishop, F. M., and Dworkin, S. F.: Communication in the dental office, St. Louis, 1976, The C. V. Mosby Co.
14. Giddon, D. B., Silberman, S. L., Prasad, L., and Bikofsky, C. G.: A behavioral science analysis of preventive dentistry. In Ward, H. O., ed.: A preventive point of view, Springfield, Ill., 1976, Charles C Thomas, Publisher.
15. Harrison, R.: An introduction to non-verbal communication, Englewood Cliffs, N.J., 1973, Prentice-Hall, Inc.
16. Kegeles, S.: Why people seek dental care: a review of present knowledge, Am. J. Public Health **51:**1305, 1961.
17. Kegeles, S.: Blocks to adequate oral health. In Brown, W., ed.: Oral health, dentistry and the American public, Norman, Okla., 1974, University of Oklahoma Press.
18. Kleinberg, I.: Prevention and dental caries. In Dworkin, S. F., ed.: Preventive dentistry: state of the art, J. Prev. Dent. (In press.)
19. Lindhe, J., and Koch, G.: The effect of supervised oral hygiene on the gingivae of children, J. Periodont. Res. **2:**215, 1967.
20. Loë, H. T., and Jensen, S. B.: Experimental gingivitis in man, J. Periodontol. **36:**177, 1965.
21. MacKinnon, R., and Michels, R.: The psychiatric interview in clinical practice, Philadelphia, 1971, W. B. Saunders Co.
22. Mandel, I. D.: What is preventive dentistry? J. Prev. Dent. **1:**25, 1974.
23. Mandel, I. D.: The medical-dental interface in preventive dentistry, Prev. Med. **5:**377, 1976.
24. Mandel, I. D., and Wotman, S.: The salivary secretions in health and disease, Oral Sci. Rev. **8:**25, 1976.
25. Meskin, L., and Rovin, S.: Do we tell the truth about prevention and treatment of periodontal disease. In Dworkin, S. F., ed.: Preventive dentistry: state of the art, J. Prev. Dent. (In press.)
26. Nizel, A. F.: The science of nutrition and its application in clinical dentistry, ed. 2, Philadelphia, 1966, W. B. Saunders Co.
27. Ramfjord, S. P., et al.: Longitudinal study on periodontal therapy, J. Periodontol **44:**66, 1973.
28. Ramirez, A., Lasater, T., and Anderson, R.: Use of fear appeals on dental health education, J. Am. Dent. Assoc. **83:**1086, 1971.
29. Suomi, J. D., Greene, S., Vermillion, J. R., Doyle, J., and Chang, J.: The effect of controlled oral hygiene procedures on the progression of periodontal disease in adults, J. Periodontol. **83:**1271, 1971.
30. Thornton, A.: Mass communications and dental health behavior, Health Educ. Monogr. **2:**201, 1974.

Chapter 19

LIFE CYCLE CHANGES AND DENTAL CARE

Dentists tend to divide their patients into two age groupings: children and everybody else. At first glance, this division seems both reasonable and adequate. The deciduous dentition is structurally different from adult dentition; hence restorative, endodontic, and orthodontic treatment techniques vary somewhat for the different dentitions. The well-known rapid developmental changes (physical, psychological, and social) that are synonymous with youth also seem to reinforce grouping dental patients into children and adults.

With the emergence of an increasingly older population, however, there has been tremendous interest in the specialized concerns of the so-called older, or geriatric, dental patient. It seems fair to say that many enlightened dentists and dental schools are beginning to conceive of their patients falling into three groupings: the younger dental patient with developing deciduous or mixed dentition; the adult dental patient; and the older dental patient.

In the sociomedical sciences, generally, the trend is not to make such sharp distinctions but to think in terms of *life cycles* and life cycle changes. The notion of life cycle changes calls attention to the seemingly obvious, but largely ignored, observation that human development is a continuous process, wherein a person passes imperceptibly from one stage to another. Certain developmental stages or stages of life have typifying features such as dependency in children or slower reaction times in senility.

Moreover, thinking in terms of life cycle changes encourages consideration of more than just physical attributes, for example, the stage of the dentition. Emotional, interpersonal, economic, and cultural factors seem to be more naturally taken into account when considering how the *person,* not simply the dentition, will tolerate or adapt to treatment alternatives.

OBJECTIVES

The objectives of this chapter are as follows:

1. To explore the concept of life cycles
2. To discuss considerations in working with patients at various stages in the life cycles

CONCEPT OF LIFE CYCLE CHANGES

Different life cycles

Human development seems fully characterized as a series of overlapping life cycles, each composed of many factors in a state of continuous and dynamic change. For purposes of study, it is helpful to label different life cycle stages. The following set of labels may be useful for these stages:

1. Infancy
2. Early, middle, and late childhood
3. Preadolescence and adolescence
4. Young and middle-aged adulthood
5. Old age

Factors operating in each life cycle

Dynamic factors operating continuously, but in more or less characteristic fashion for each life cycle, include the following:

1. Innate (genetic) factors
2. Metabolic factors
3. Environmental factors
4. Maturation factors
5. Aging factors

These parameters of human development can be measured and evaluated in terms of physical growth and development or psychological status.[1,23] Psychological status includes such factors as cognitive abilities, emotional development, mental health, and interpersonal or sociocultural relationships.

In the next two sections we will focus on the younger dental patient, currently the province of pedodontics, and the older dental patient, represented in dentistry by a growing specialized field of study and practice sometimes called geriatric dentistry. Our discussions are, of necessity, brief. We will touch on those aspects of younger and older dental patients that relate to how dentists can or should interact with them. Facets of these life cycle stages that, in our view, have not been presented to dentists with sufficient emphasis will be stressed here.

YOUNGER DENTAL PATIENTS

Perhaps the best example of dentistry's capacity to change behavior patterns on a large scale has been the establishment and acceptance of dentistry for children.[9] As recently as 20 years ago, it was extremely common for parents (well educated and highly health conscious) to question the need for providing young children with routine dental care. "After all," the common argument went, "their teeth are going to fall out soon anyway. So why spend money and time and expose a child to the psychological and physical trauma of having baby teeth filled"? Today the legitimacy of dental care for children is seldom questioned.

The principles and strategies developed throughout this book are applicable here. As a matter of fact, particularly for the younger dental patient, the interaction between perception and motivation is often transparent. For example, the 3-year-old child is more readily stressed by the perceived threat of separation than the 9-year-old sibling. In this section we touch only briefly on two aspects of child development: individual differences and age-appropriate approaches to behavior modification that seem to be consistent with the rest of this book.

Why a specialty of pedodontics?

Pedodontics (the term "pediatric dentistry" is now coming into vogue) developed as a specialized area within dentistry because of dentists' responsibilities for managing diseases of the developing dentition from birth through adolescence and for developing and teaching psychological management of the younger dental patient. Specialized concerns are *growth and development* and *psychological management*. Our interest lies in the development of strategies for the psychological management of the younger dental patient.

It is fairly well acknowledged among dentists that the successful growth of pedodontics as a specialty is in no small part a result of the reluctance of many dentists to treat children. Several reasons are commonly given, which for the most part reflect concerns over the psychosocial aspects of child management rather than the clinical or technical phases of dental treatment. Dentists who are reluctant to treat children often give the following reasons[4,20]:

1. They experience discomfort and anxiety when confronted with children as dental patients. Children's acting out of recalcitrant behaviors such as crying and failure to cooperate have intensified the discomfort many dentists have experienced while treating children.
2. They believe that they are not competent to manage children because of insufficient training and/or experience.

3. They conclude that pedodontics does not yield sufficient compensation, either financial or professional.

The reluctance of dentists to treat children, especially very young children (2 to 4 years of age), is not nearly as prevalent today as it was a decade or two ago. Moreover, increased parental education has led to greater parental acceptance of the need to ensure the natural history of the deciduous dentition. Finally, we must remember that dentistry, historically, has been a source of great fear for children. It is only within the last 2 or 3 decades that typical dental treatment for a child shifted from extraction of an actively infected, painful tooth to preventive, restorative procedures with much attention paid, especially by pedodontists, to managing the emotional behavior of the child. The long-term water fluoridation programs are now having a profound effect on dental treatment for children. It is now abundantly clear that clinical dental practice on children is directly affected by long-term water fluoridation in at least two ways. The most obvious is, of course, the gratifying reduction in the rate of new caries development. The second impact is on the management of children's behavior. Since caries develop less frequently and less rapidly in areas where the water supply is fluoridated, children are less likely to undergo extremely noxious experiences of severe toothache and periapical infection; moreover, with interproximal (smooth surface) caries reduced, treatment visits can be briefer, less frequent, and less complex for the younger dental patient.

The combination of these factors—better training of the dentist, increased parental acceptance, and less traumatic or extensive dental visits—have facilitated the growth and acceptance of dental treatment for children in recent years.

Growth and development of the child

Child growth and development have meant different things over the past 75 years.[1] The study of "normal" physical measurements for children of specified ages was one of the first areas of concern for students of child development. Children were compared with the "normal," or "average," child on the basis of height, weight, circumference, and length of anatomical parts. The limitations of the practical application of information about a specific child's physical measurements soon became apparent: How much was "*too* tall" or "*under*weight"? After what period of time should "delayed" eruption become a cause for concern?

The next step was to measure physical growth and development longitudinally. The longitudinal expression of growth led to identification of individual patterns of development for each child. Predictions about future developmental progress could then be made, at least for physical growth, on the basis of plotted longitudinal data from the present. Aside from problems arising that might interfere with the predictions such as unexpected disease or trauma, the longitudinal expressions of growth still failed to tell enough about how the child could be expected to perform or behave emotionally, intellectually, and socially.

The **total child concept** was introduced into child growth and development to call attention to the need to understand and evaluate the psychological and social adaptive capacities of children as they develop along with physical and systemic functions. It is probably fair to say that the most difficult challenge for health professionals treating children is the interpretation of all aspects of growth and development as individually expressed by the uniqueness of each child. It is now well recognized that treatment recommendations for children must take into account the welfare of the child—the child's ability to tolerate treatment and the receptivity or support for treatment provided through the interpersonal relationships of children with their parents.

Because the growth and development process is inherently a change process, dentists who treat children should be aware of the total child concept. It calls attention to the fact that assuming responsibility for treating a child's teeth carries the additional responsibility of making the treatment fit the child's total milieu; it requires being aware of the longitudinal patterns of physical and psychological growth the particular child represents at the time treatment is provided.

Psychological development—the cognitive-intellectual dimension

The psychological development of children can be studied from the point of view of emotional,[16,23] interpersonal or social,[6] and cognitive or intellectual development.[1,13] Much has been written in all three fields, but the data seem most secure in the area of cognitive-intellectual development. We will briefly discuss this aspect of child development separately, but we will touch on emotional and interpersonal development as part of our later discussion of individual differences, age-specific behaviors, and behavior modification strategies.

Fundamental processes of cognitive development. The term **"cognitive functioning"** refers to higher mental abilities and intellectual processes such as thinking, making abstractions or generalizations, and concept formation. The ability to abstract is necessary to formulate concepts, and the ability to generalize is required to allow a concept to be used once it has been formed.

The most important worker in cognitive development is Piaget. His views should be more widely known among dentists, who need to evaluate the level of language and the kind of comprehension they might use or expect when interacting with children of different ages. Three important processes of cognitive development are accommodation, assimilation, and adaptation.

Accommodation and assimilation. The basic equipment of any "knower," at all stages, consists of a biologically given (that is, inherited) set of operations by which information is processed. Piaget calls these fundamental processes of human intelligence accomodation and assimilation. Accommodation of information refers to a "taking in" process. Assimilation refers to a conversion process during which strange information becomes known to the child. Accommodation and assimilation are continued until new information becomes part of the young organism. An infant will play repetitiously at dropping, then picking up an object given to him or her by an adult. The adult often tires of what becomes a repetitive, boring game, but the infant wants to keep on playing.

Adaptation. When the new information is assimilated, the child is said to have adapted. The adapted infant acts as if no more practice is necessary; the behavior has been mastered.

• • •

The sequence of accommodation-assimilation-adaptation is characteristic of all cognitive-intellectual development. As the child grows older, the process proceeds from simple and gross motor–oriented behaviors to complex, "thinking-oriented" (hence less visible) behaviors.[13]

Periods of cognitive development. The development of intellectual abilities is divided into three large periods: sensory-motor intelligence, preoperational and concrete operational phases, and formal operational thinking.[1,13]

Sensory-motor intelligence: birth to age 2 years. From birth to age 2 years is the period of sensory-motor intelligence. At this time, perceptual-motor coordination begins. Infants learn to distinguish objects as different from themselves. This differentiation of objects, knowledge that things exist "out there," separate from the body, requires perception using the sense of sight. This perception must be integrated with motor activity primarily via the senses of touch and taste.

Preoperational and operational phases: age 2 to 11 years. The period from age 2 to 11 years is divided into a preoperational phase, followed by a concrete operational phase. During the preoperational phase, from age 2 to 7 or 8 years, the first representational activity takes place. Verbal comprehension begins, and attention span increases. In the beginning there is much distortion, concreteness, and egocentrism to the child's attempts at developing internalized representations of the different parts of the world. When entering middle childhood, the child, utilizing his or her intellectual apparatus, uses concrete operations to form representations of the world that are stable and generalizable. The child understands that objects have weight and length, for example; however, concrete behavior is characterized by a here-and-now quality in which the physical properties of objects are dealt with quite literally: this glass has more water than the other because it is taller (for now, never mind that it is also narrower!). Only toward the end of this stage (around age 9 to 11 years) does the concept of conservation become apparent: the amount of water is the same, no matter what the shape of the container.

Formal operational thinking: age 11 to 15 years. From age 11 to 15 years formal operational thinking begins. The child begins to use hypothetical deductive thinking—reasons this from that, organizes information into general propositions, and manipulates symbols in the absence of the object, for example, is ready for algebra and geometry.

Telling children aged 2 to 5 years that plaque is the cause of decay would probably not be too effective. Telling the same children that bugs make holes in teeth is talking their langugage; explaining that careful brushing avoids the need for future dental care is probably more persuasive for the 15-year-old adolescent than the typical 8-year-old child.

Individual differences: maybe they were born that way

Cognitive intellectual development is only one aspect of the unbelievably complex phenomenon of human psychological growth and differentiation. Until recently, one of the largely neglected considerations in this complex phenomenon has been the possibility that innate differences in children account for the wide variety of cognitive, emotional, and social behaviors they exhibit. Fascinating studies with infants and young children now make it clear that children will respond differently to, among other things, intense stimulation, being held, or distraction because, at least in part, they were born that way. These sources of innate difference will be presented subsequently.

The essential individuality of children is often overlooked when personality development is discussed. Innate differences predisposing children to behave in different ways must be considered when interacting with an individual child to reduce anxiety or to gain cooperation. Chess and co-workers[6] have identified the following nine parameters by which children from birth onward manifest individual characteristics in temperament:

activity level From infancy, some infants are spontaneously active. Others lie quietly, some tending to be as physically quiet when awake as when asleep.

regularity Biological functions such as hunger, thirst, and sleep appear with alarm-clock regularity in some neonates and are highly irregular in others.

approach-withdrawal The initial reaction to a new stimulus will be positive for some infants and, apparently, negative for others.

adaptability Neonates differ in the time they require to adjust to new routines and new demands on their developing physiology.

sensory threshold Newborn children differ in their sensitivity to noise, pain, light, etc.

positive or negative mood The predominant emotional quality, even of infants, may be positive or negative.

intensity of response Energy levels achieved when stimulated, whether positive or negative, differ among neonates.

attention span Newborn children differ in their ability to concentrate on novel stimuli.

distractability Newborn children require different amounts of stimulation to interrupt a repetitive behavior.

These nine parameters are of interest to dentists because they reflect the early origins of many behaviors that are not learned —either as a consequence of psychosexual trauma as Freud might contend or through conditioned associations as Pavlov and Skinner might maintain. The dentist attempts to understand but mostly to *work with the patient's behavior*.

As we shall discuss later, it is especially true with children that the dentist's best chances for success seem to be in modifying behavior rather than in changing the child's personality through "understanding." If one accepts the general premise that the younger the child, the less he or she has learned, it becomes clear that to whatever extent individual differences in children's behavior are inborn, the younger the child, the more likely it is that innate or genetic factors will shape his or her behavior, since that behavior is still operating relatively uncontaminated by much learning. It is certainly too simple to attribute the sleeping patterns of a 50-year-old healthy man simply to inborn patterns of activity level or regularity of neurological functioning (for example, a "day" person versus a "night" person). Too many other unknown factors are operating by adulthood, for example, the activity level of his mate. However, it is reasonable to consider that a 2- to 3-year-old child may not be sitting still to the dentist's satisfaction because of individual biological differences in attention span, threshold, or distractability. Consideration of this possibility leads to a willingness of dentists to modify their behavior as one of the strategies required to ultimately modify the child's behavior. Again, the behavior therapy principles discussed in Chapter 14 and applied specifically to children later in this chapter seem to be most effective.

Age-specific behaviors and strategies*

"The why and the how" of behavior, combined with developing intelligence, give rise to behavior that can, more or less, be characterized by chronological age—so-called age-specific behaviors. We are primarily interested in psychological development as it relates to interpersonal relationships between dentist and child and to the dentist's choice of appropriate persuasive strategies.

Infancy: birth to age 2 years[23]

PSYCHOLOGY. Infancy is usually defined as extending from birth to the beginning of articulate speech. The oral cavity is the primary zone of interaction between the infant and the world.

INTELLIGENCE. Sensory-motor intelligence, that is, the ability to coordinate perception with motor activity, begins around age 6 months.

PARENT-CHILD INTERACTION. The infant is completely dependent, physically and psychologically.

INTERPERSONAL RELATIONSHIPS. There is little interest in sustained interaction with others. The infant usually plays alone.

APPROPRIATE BEHAVIOR CHANGE STRATEGIES. Any treatment required at this time should be accompanied by minimal or no separation from the parent. In infants, use secure and consistent physical support, with slow, careful movements. By the time the child is age two years, instructions are often obeyed willingly, especially if accompanied by verbal assurance and praise at the appropriate vocabulary level.

Early childhood: age 2 to 4 years

PSYCHOLOGY. In early childhood, language rapidly improves, and upright locomotion is perfected. By age 3 years, the child becomes more positive and cooperative. Approaching age 4 years, the child develops greater periods of uneasiness and apparent regression.

INTELLIGENCE. Verbal comprehension and attention span increase markedly.

PARENT-CHILD INTERACTIONS. The child evidences aggression, anger, anxiety, and fear.

INTERPERSONAL RELATIONSHIPS. At this age, the child develops social behaviors and enjoys making friends. He or she alternates

*This section is adapted from Dworkin, S. F.: The developing child and persuasion to dental health behavior. In Cheney, H. G., ed.: Handbook of preventive dentistry, Acton, Mass., 1978, Publishing Sciences Group, Inc.

shyness with frankness and cooperative sharing with outbursts of anger. Imagination is used externally in play.

APPROPRIATE BEHAVIOR CHANGE STRATEGIES. There are marked differences in what you should be able to accomplish with the 4-year-old as compared to the 2-year-old child. By age 4 years, the child should respond well to simple explanations, imaginative choice of words, and appeals to fantasy. Children at this age can form sudden and intense, positive relationships with dentists, which alternate with periods of frustration and rejection. Accept the negative behaviors as inevitable for this age group, and do not label the child as recalcitrant or "moody."

Resistance to treatment should be analyzed. It may result from (1) unfamiliar surroundings, persons, and events—a depersonalized anxiety over the unknown; (2) a test of the response of the parent to separation or loss of control; or (3) inappropriate management—indecision or lack of clarity by the dentist or the misjudgment of the cognitive or psychological maturity of the child.

Middle childhood: age 4 to 6 years

PSYCHOLOGY. Middle childhood is a period of great integration that differentiates the child aged 4 to 6 years from the earlier years. Most children begin formal schooling. The child goes through a relatively calm period, when he or she is capable of self-criticism, has a more realistic orientation, and is less amused by fantasy. Questions are asked from an urge to learn. The 6-year-old child's behavior can be markedly bipolar. Openness and gentleness give way to a rebelliousness and difficulty in making up his or her mind.

INTELLIGENCE. Intuitive thinking develops, which represents a growing ability to form concepts and an increasing coordination of logical relations.

PARENT-CHILD INTERACTION. "I can't understand what's come over the child" is a frequent parental comment. Socialization stresses subordination to authorities outside the family. Increasing independence and different levels of expectations are sources of child-parent conflict.

INTERPERSONAL RELATIONSHIPS. The transition from independent play to definite involvement with other children becomes more noticeable. By the beginning of school, there is a clear shift to cooperative play, involving physical activities and talking. The child pays more attention to his or her peers, even in their absence.

APPROPRIATE BEHAVIOR CHANGE STRATEGIES. Children accept benign authority well at ages 5 and 6 years. Utilizing a persuasive approach, the dentist can treat the 5- to 6-year-old child as a "grown-up." Verbal and nonverbal communication should convey your assumption that the child is a young adult. Improved fine motor coordination makes routine oral hygiene practices easier to accomplish and offers opportunities for dental personnel to reward positive achievement.

Late childhood: age 7 to 9 years

PSYCHOLOGY. The beginning of the period of late childhood is tranquil, with few conflicts. The child generally takes a more realistic view of the environment. Imagination is more reflective. By age 9 years, the child is motivated to attack problems of his or her own choosing.

INTELLIGENCE. Thinking is characterized by concreteness which determines the structure of spatial and chronological relations.

PARENT-CHILD INTERACTION. The child works to acquire the family's habits and moral code. Willingness to help and a sense of responsibility appear. The period is generally a quiet one.

INTERPERSONAL RELATIONSHIPS. The period begins with the child as a recipient in his or her social life. Rules of the game are important. A transition toward giving and seeking more relatedness occurs. By age 9 years, the child has achieved a modicum of social maturity represented by stable and better integrated behavior. The child can, however, be highly self-critical and sensitive to the attitudes of parental and other authority figures.

APPROPRIATE BEHAVIOR CHANGE STRATEGIES. The child's growing interest in testing independence, although still requiring support, can be utilized in the dentist's change strategy. In children 7 to 9 years old, benevolent authority can appeal to the child's desire for order, self-initiation, and organization. Long-range behavior change might be reinforced by developing schedules, checkpoints, etc. Especially as the child approaches age 9 years, he or she is willing to repeat tasks and to perfect skills. These tasks represent opportunities for the child to demonstrate maturity and to earn praise and support.

Although children do not need it, they still enjoy appeals to imagination and fantasy as persuasive strategies. However, they are quite aware of the distinction between fantasy and reality.

Preadolescence: age 10 to 12 years

PSYCHOLOGY. The personality reaches a new level of integration and adaptation during the preadolescent period. At ages 11 and 12 years, which are regarded as a happy time, the child anticipates the new adjustments to the grown-up environment.

INTELLIGENCE. The 12-year-old child has established the beginning of hypothetical-deductive thinking and can rely on internalized judgment-making powers instead of needing to refer to actual experience.

PARENT-CHILD INTERACTION. Although this period begins as a relatively relaxed time for both parent and child, by the time the child is 12 years old parents frequently expect him or her to accept responsibility that he or she is not yet ready to take.

INTERPERSONAL RELATIONSHIPS. Social skills are reasonably developed, and there is a great interest in clubs, team sports, and other group activities.

APPROPRIATE BEHAVIOR CHANGE STRATEGIES. The child enjoys being related to as an adult and, if such an approach is used, will accept a great deal of information. He or she is capable of the fine motor coordination necessary to achieve acceptable oral hygiene. As in earlier years, frequent praise goes a long way. However, realistic feedback regarding disappointing performance is well tolerated, especially if accompanied by sustained personal interest.

As is true of all children, behavior in response to any persuasive approach will be cyclical. Periods of acceptance and high motivation will alternate with disappointing loss of interest and abandonment of desired behaviors. Such cycles are to be expected from children (and adults, too). Hopefully, this reality will not discourage or dissuade the dentist from continuing persuasive prevention campaigns. Although recalcitrant periods may look like complete rejection of the dentist's efforts, the child may be curiously testing the dentist's real interest or acting out current needs that temporarily do not leave room for persuasive prevention.

Adolescence: age 12 to 18 years. Rather than attempt to divide the adolescent period into stages, our present purposes are well served by an overview of the period as a whole. Much has been written about the great turmoil, rebellion, and confusion identified with adolescence. There is probably no other developmental period in which so much conflicting advice is available to parents and to adolescents themselves concerning their problems.

In the typical family, problems encountered in child rearing prior to adolescence pale into insignificance compared with the turmoil of the adolescent period. The fundamentals of psychological development are well established by this time, and the patterns for adult intelligence have been developed. The adolescent's major psychological concern relates to changing patterns of personal relationships with peers and parental or external authority.

Dentists treating adolescents are faced with waxing and waning periods of interest in cleanliness, compliance with authority, and acceptance of responsibility. At the same time, many adolescents form personal relationships with the dentist and his or her staff that range from the "teenage crush" to true hero worship. These positive interpersonal relationships should be encouraged but handled with great sensitivity.

Accepting the adolescent patient with his or her mannerisms seems to be the preferred route for sustained relationships. Being too "straight" (that is, like the parents) or highly judgmental about appearance or "kooky" behavior turns this youngster off. The maintenance of viable interpersonal relationships is probably the best lever the dentist has for reaching the adolescent and for keeping him or her coming back for more.

Behavior modification: a summary

Dentists have been most successful with behavior modification strategies for children that use the desensitization concept described earlier.[20] Abundant evidence exists to support the claim that almost any child can receive routine dental treatment in the general practitioner's office, under the conditions of a local anesthetic, if behavior therapy approaches are employed. General anesthetics seem warranted only in extreme dental emergencies. Such cases might involve very young children (around age 2 years) or a patient with severe physical or mental impairment, which precludes the child from being physically *unable* to sit still (as opposed to *not wanting* to sit still). A general anesthetic for children (or for anyone else) for routine dentistry is definitely not required, and there is ample behavioral research and clinical data to support this conclusion.[4,17,27]

OLDER DENTAL PATIENTS

A definition

The so-called older, or geriatric, dental patient is usually defined as someone over 65 years of age.[10] For our purposes, it is useful to divide this patient population into three groups. In the smallest group of those over age 65 years are individuals who are institutionalized, either in a chronic disease hospital, a mental hospital, or some other long-term health facility. A second, much larger group, has serious medical or psychological problems, although not institutionalized. Many of these patients are bedridden or confined to their homes, whereas others are more ambulatory and, with help, can come to the dental office. The third and largest group of persons over 65 years of age are those who are essentially ambulatory, who are not incapacitated, and who can function relatively independently.

This last group is the one seen most frequently in dental offices. The largest group making up the older population is a mobile one (in recent years 150,000 passports per year have been given to individuals over 65 years of age). The accumulation of older persons with long-term illnesses is a factor that does not lend itself toward correction or prevention. It has been suggested that improvements in medical care and preventive medicine have resulted in a lengthening of the average life span, which has resulted in more persons with chronic diseases or diseases of old age.

Health and the aging population: attitudes about health

Older persons generally regard themselves as less healthy than do younger persons. Nevertheless, related to medical evaluations of their conditions, many older persons assess their health quite positively, having perhaps learned to accept certain disabilities and pains as inevitable or unimportant. The older person's self-image tends to reflect the findings from a National Health Survey that only a small minority of individuals aged 65 years and over are too handicapped to carry on their major activity, despite widespread afflictions in old age. Almost half of those persons 65 years of age and over rate their health in general as good or excellent, and although this rating is lower than that for young persons, it is surprising considering the high rates of chronic disease and illness.[15]

For older persons, although there is a correlation between self-evaluation and medical evaluation, self-ratings tend to be more positive. Older persons tend to accept the effects of aging on external bodily features and appearance and are less likely than younger age groups to be concerned about their appearance.

Older persons are more likely than younger persons to believe that ill health and disability are, to a degree, unavoidable. In looking at all age groups, there is an increase by age in the proportions of persons agreeing that an individual has to expect a great deal of illness and some aches and pains, especially when he or she is older. Changing views of health service are correlated with aging, with older persons viewing health care resources more negatively than younger persons. Older persons report they have difficulties communicating with and understanding their physicians.[21]

What do older persons do about their health? Findings for persons age 65 years and over show that older persons are less interested in preventive care than younger persons and that they have a greater tendency to believe they take the best possible care of their own health. In a similar way, the older a person is, the less dissatisfied he or she is with the amount of dental care that is received. In general, positive health care, or the prevention of disease, seems to decline with age. Persons age 60 years and over are less inclined than younger persons to report taking various steps to guard their health. Research on the reasons older persons with reported illness give for not seeing a physician shows that they do not in general stress financial difficulties so much as the presumed unsuitability of medical treatment for many afflictions of old age.[2]

In summary, although the prevalence of illness and impairments is substantial in the older population, much of this is chronic illness of long duration. The data also suggest that older persons seem to take such complaints for granted; they do not consider themselves "sick," and they continue to live a relatively normal life. There is an increasing belief among some professionals dealing with the health of older persons that chronic disease and illness need not be necessary and noncurable concomitants of the aging process. Among these health professionals, there is a growing concern with rehabilitation and preventive health care. However, barriers to success can be found among older persons themselves who take illness for granted and among professionals who hold the same view or are simply not interested in treating older persons.

Since the perception of health is an important determinant of one's beliefs and practices in the areas of medical and preventive care, the implications of this perception are significant. It is difficult to motivate most older persons to seek medical care for the many ailments that are not severely handicapping. It is even more difficult to attempt to make preventive service meaningful.[14]

Dental needs of older patients

Relatively little attention has been paid to the dental needs of older persons, including the need for changes in the dental health beliefs and behaviors of older persons , their oral health needs, and the need for trained practitioners to work with them.

Need for changes in the dental health beliefs and behaviors of older persons. The oral cavity, like any other part of the human body, suffers the same problems of chronic disease that are correlated with the aging process. Some of these problems are inherent in the aging process itself, but many others are more causally related to attitudes about the believed consequences of aging and the resulting patterns of behavior. Many of the chronic oral problems of the aged represent conditions of poor oral health that can be rehabilitated or prevented. The need for good oral health in older persons has been documented. This need is important for the health of the individual in terms of nutrition, freedom from infection, comfort, speech, taste, and social acceptance. Compared to studies in medicine, attitudinal studies about aging and oral health have been limited.

There is less dental care and less concern for preventive care in the older person than in the younger one. Although not adequately documented, there is corollary evidence that the facial and oral changes resulting from poor oral health are believed by older adults to be a concomitant of the aging process. It has been suggested that older persons do not manifest care for their bodies because, with a delimited life space, there is little "payoff" for doing so.[15] It follows that there would be little desire on the part of the elderly to alter certain superficial aspects of their bodies. A change in facial appearance, for example, would be less needed or wanted by an older person because there is little advantage to which such an alteration could be turned.

Although there is a correlation between aging and dental disease, this is not necessarily a causal one. An increasing number of dentists and dental researchers are arguing for a rehabilitative-preventive approach to the oral health problems of the aged. These professionals catalog problems of diseased and missing teeth, ill-fitting or partial dentures, periodontal disease and other diseases of the soft tissues, bone deterioration, and other oral health problems of the elderly as capable of being rehabilitated, if not prevented. Moreover, this approach views the consequences of poor oral health in terms of poor diet leading to malnutrition, pain, infection, and even social malfunctioning.

A major problem creating barriers to proper rehabilitation and preventive care for older persons is the dental disease attitudes of the elderly themselves. These attitudes are not adequately researched, but what findings there are suggest that older persons believe that poor oral health is a concomitant of aging and that nothing can be done. Chronic dental disease is accepted as a consequence of the aging process by the older person. Therefore restorative and preventive dental care, even care for acute conditions, are not sought as much by older as by younger persons. Even when free care is offered, many older persons do not take advantage.

Perceived need has been found to be important in determining these dental behaviors. Low perceived need with a high actual need for dental care is not uncommon among elderly poor persons. The beliefs that one is susceptible to dental disease and that disease will have serious effects are necessary before individuals will seek dental care.

Oral health needs. The oral health problems of the elderly have been documented. Hollingstead, for example, found that, for a selected older population in England, the lower a patient's social, educational, and income status, the less likely he or she was to appreciate the value of natural teeth and the more likely he or she was to have them extracted and replaced by dentures.[12] This same individual, because of his or her lower valuation of the importance of oral health, would be likely to retain ill-fitting dentures for long periods of time. Korduner and Marken found that there was frequently a deterioration within a short time of fitting dentures, and patients tended to overly adapt to the changes, resulting, for example, in dentures being worn well beyond their useful life. In a sample of elderly edentulous patients in Australia, it was found that 90% showed some form of irritation of the denture-bearing tissues. In short, geriatric dental problems result from aging in combination with some form of self-imposed or involuntary neglect.[11,12,14]

Several surveys of elderly populations in the United States reveal high incidences of pathological conditions.[21] In one study of 785 older institutionalized persons[12] who had no subjective symptoms and who were under optimal care, the soft tissues revealed 19 different types of disease ranging from innocuous areas of pigmentation to early squamous cell carcinoma.

An additional consideration relates to diet. The older person with poor dental health will tend to select a diet that fails to support bodily requirements, resulting in physical deterioration. Older persons with poor teeth tend to consume a diet low in protein and high in carbohydrates and fats.

Dental and other health needs of the older population are many and complex. These needs are highlighted by the increasing numbers of older persons and by recent vocal demands for quality health care as a right. The number of persons 65 years of age and over was 3.1 million in 1900. By 1940 the number had tripled to 9.0 million. It more than doubled again to 20.2 million by 1970. In the year 2000 there are expected to be about 29 million persons in this age category. The number is rising about 3 to 4 million persons every decade, or roughly 300,000 to 400,000 persons per year.[21]

Older persons are known to have low availability of preventive services and high frequency of long-term illness and impairment. The older population suffers from a tendency for health providers and medical and dental schools to give low priority to their needs and from weak efforts to deliver and coordinate comprehensive health services of a high quality. Oral health is an integral component of the older person's total well-being. In like manner, dental services cannot be logically separated from the comprehensive set of health services required to render the life of the older person as healthy and meaningful as possible. The dental problems of the older person must be seen as part of his or her total life experiences and the aging process.

Need for trained practitioners to work with older persons. The dentist typically practices in a severely circumscribed physical and social environment. As with younger patients, some dentists may feel unable to provide adequate dental care to a patient group that they do not understand or that is located in settings (for example, homes or institutions) outside the familiar private practice setting. Few dentists have received adequate exposure to geriatric dentistry and gerontology. Of 56 dentists graduated from schools of public health from 1969 to 1975, none have specialized in chronic disease or mental health. And yet at the same time, some 556 dentists were working in long-term care institutions and another 600 were employed in mental hospitals. Few of these dentists have received specialized training in the provision of dental services to our older population. Moreover, the educational programs of other health-related professions do not include dental problems in courses dealing with geriatrics.

The attitude of dentists who believe, or are trained to believe, that older persons are not candidates, or are poor candidates, for dental rehabilitation and preventive care constitutes a barrier to effective treatment. The major cause of this attitude is a lack of understanding about the nature and processes of human aging and their relationship to oral health. This attitude is further exacerbated by the failure of dentists to communicate adequately with older persons and to understand their social and economic situations. It has been suggested, also, that in chronic illness, older persons seem to have an awareness that physicians may not be anxious to be consulted about difficulties they may consider minor or about patients whose illness no longer presents a challenge to them. Physicians have been warned never to attribute any illness in older persons to the aging process, as is common among health professionals. Prompt treatment given in minor episodes may be a vital factor in the prevention of later invalidism associated with old age.

It seems evident, from a review of the medical and dental literature, that the attitudes physicians and dentists have about their patients influence the kind of care they deliver and the treatments they prescribe. In the field of dentistry, no studies have methodically analyzed the attitudes of dentists toward the older person and, in turn, the effect these attitudes have on treatment planning and, ultimately, on the dentist-patient relationship. Further, no studies have been carried out assessing the knowledge of practicing dentists about the aging process and its effect on the oral health of older persons.

This is not to understate the problem of chronic illness and physical changes in older persons as a special population of patients. Older individuals can and do present unique problems requiring special knowledge and understanding on the part of dentists. In particular, the problems that make the older person different from other patients are as follows:

1. Medical disorders that interfere with effective dental care
2. Physical disabilities that limit their capacity to benefit from dental care
3. Lack of motivation
4. Inability to adapt to essential routines or to use prescribed appliances
5. Difficulties in communication

There is a need for specialized training of dentists to meet these problems.

Psychological considerations in understanding the behavior of older patients*

Optimal dental health in older persons is a complexly determined combination of physiological and psychological factors. Consideration must be given to how treatment will be tolerated and to determining a prognosis that is both desirable and likely. Although these considerations are true of every diagnostic and treatment decision a dentist makes, the point bears special emphasis for the older patient. Unique physical, psychological, and economic concerns may lessen the room for error or the choices available to the dentist and patient.

There are many psychological factors that should be considered in deciding what is optimal dental treatment for older patients. Some problems are well known: Do older persons feel neglected? Do they believe their culture and society value them less after their long lives than when they were young and productive? How are they reacting to the loss and illness of those peers and loved ones whom they have known for so many years? One hardly need be a psychiatrist to cite everyday problems and considerations that are powerful factors in the aging process.

Psychiatric problems associated with growing older. In addition to these factors drawn from common experience, there are some psychiatric problems specifically associated with growing old. Three general psychiatric syndromes associated with aging represent the most common problems to the health practitioner treating geriatric patients. These are organic brain disease, the senile psychosis, and the involutional psychosis. These clinical labels might imply to the layman powerful incapacitating mental conditions, which they often are. However, dentists typically see older patients who exhibit milder or, perhaps earlier, forms of these disturbances in their cognitive-intellectual, emotional, and interpersonal behavior.

The distinction between organic brain disease and the senile psychosis is difficult to make, even for neurologists and psychologists. The precise differential diagnostic label is probably not critical to the dentist anyway. *The dentist's best source of data for arriving at management decisions should be the patient's verbal and nonverbal behavior during the dentist-patient interaction.* The danger in prematurely deciding to use the label "organic brain damage" is the negative implication it carries for many health professionals. In general, ascribing a concrete physiological base as an explanation of behavior tends to limit the number of times a dentist will try different strategies with a patient. If a patient is prematurely labeled as brain damaged, we do not really test how much the patient can understand or how cooperative he or she will be. Instead we blame the behavior on a damaged nervous system, and we decide that we cannot expect anything better. This is a great injustice to many older persons. It is exactly the way they are treated by too many other persons, including their own families. When they are treated in such a manner, older individuals are more likely to act out the limited role that everyone has been willing to assign them.

Behavioral symptoms common to organic brain disease and senile psychosis. There are behavioral symptoms common to both organic brain disease and senile psychosis. In general, aging brings a slowing down of psychomotor reaction time and

*This section is adapted from Dworkin, S. F.: Dent. Assist. **39**(Nov.):22, 1970.

of mental intellectual processes such as the abilities to form associations and to comprehend quickly. Also, aging brings a fading memory but most often a memory that fades first for recent events, while still retaining vivid recollections of earlier life experiences. Accompanying these processes are a decline of responsiveness and a waning of initiative and creative imagination. A narrowing of interest and an increase in egocentricity also seem to be among the most common psychological changes.

Changes in behavior along the directions indicated may range from mild absent-mindedness to extreme mental and emotional impoverishment that is characteristic of senility. There is no agreement as to when someone has crossed the border from mild (and more or less expected) changes in functioning into senility or senile psychosis. However, extreme loss of contact with or interest in the environment; extreme depression or agitation; abundance of paranoid symptoms, usually of persecution, and very often localized around the "bad treatment" the patient believes he or she is receiving are important signs that the patient has deteriorated markedly.

Behavioral symptoms common to involutional psychosis. Involutional psychosis is of interest because, although it occurs earlier in life, that is, frequently around menopause in women (in the late 40s) and frequently a little later in men (in the 50s), some of the behavioral manifestations are similar to the senile psychosis. The predominant effect, behaviorally, is to make individuals older than their chronological age. The involutional psychosis, which also represents a broad spectrum of behaviors, is associated with the involutional period of life, that is, a period of decrease in the functional activity of endocrine and reproductive glandular systems. How large a part the actual physiological changes play in determining behavioral changes is not exactly known. We frequently see marked depression as well as paranoid and delusional behaviors associated with a conviction that life is not worth living. Most people, even at 45 or 50 years of age, believe they are "over the hill." They become convinced that the dreams of their youth are never to be fulfilled, and they lose interest in themselves and the world around them.

Regardless of where they originate or how they are labeled, these psychological facts of older life lead to similar classes of behavior that have direct implications for dental treatment.

Determining optimal treatment for older patients

In general terms, a characteristic of senescent behavior is that persons behave more like themselves, that is, there is an intensification of the kind of life-style displayed in earlier years. This change means that the older person is predisposed to respond to stress of any kind such as experiencing pain or even encountering new persons and new situations in an exaggerated, albeit characteristic, way. This predisposition to fall back on familiar styles automatically reduces options for behavior and gives much of the behavior of older persons a flavor often described as rigid.

Behavioral considerations. The following three important behavioral characteristics of the older patient should be examined to help determine optimal treatment for this individual:

1. Relative rigidity/flexibility
2. Relative irritability/agreeableness
3. Relative ability to comprehend what is being said

After spending a few minutes exploring where the patient stands on each of these three dimensions, dentist-patient interactions can be modified to accommodate both dentist and patient needs. Behavior and dentistry should be suited not only to the chronological age of the patient (perhaps the least important consideration) but also to his or her psychological age.

Dentists and dental paraprofessionals cannot presume to conduct in-depth inquiries into the older person's psyche. However, by spending a few minutes in conversation, one can evaluate the possible degree of cooperation and acceptance that is probably present. Intelligent decisions need to be made regarding how the patient will maintain a prosthetic appliance, undergo restorative procedures, or maintain a program of oral hygiene. Such simple things as observing changes in the recall patterns of older patients, noting changes in oral hygiene habits, or observing a reluctance to accept what was previously viewed as routine can be clues to underlying problems. Testing the willingness to consider a new idea can indicate whether "optimal treatment" for this patient is simply the relief of pain and the establishment of a clean mouth or more extensive and even elaborate restorative work.

It is also important to observe specifically how the patient tolerates what his or her own body is doing or becoming. Whether or not the patient expects that the body can take recommended treatment is a crucial factor in any prognosis. Often the older patient believes that no one can help and, therefore, nothing matters, not even getting teeth fixed. In such cases, all concerned should recognize the difficult hurdle to be overcome before successful treatment can be accomplished.

Medical history considerations. In stressing some of these aspects of the psychology of aging, it is not intended that one have an oversimplified view of what older persons are all about. Especially, it is not intended that the importance of physiology be denied when evaluating how to most helpfully respond to older individuals. The ramifications of the aging process are crucial determinants in any treatment or prognosis. Indeed the most important early clues can be objectively obtained from a careful review of the patient's medical history. Both the patient's current medical state and the rate at which change or deterioration has taken place in the past are critical. Certainly, the prognosis for any treatment plan has to be more guarded in cases where there is evidence of rapid physiological deterioration than in those where patients have apparently reached a plateau and has maintained themselves for quite some time at the current level of physiological functioning.

Everybody's growing older—even the dentist!

This discussion has implications for the dentist and the staff, also. Dentists grow older, too. They are not immune to the effects of aging: a slowing of functioning, seeing their world depeopled of long-time friends and loved ones, etc. It is extremely important for the dentist to take into account his or her own reaction to growing older. How flexible, agreeable, and understanding is he or she lately? We can hardly expect more of our patients than we can demonstrate ourselves. This leads to a final point, which is a suggestion for what might be called **preventive geriatrics.**

We cannot prevent ourselves or others from growing chronologically older. We can, however, do some things at earlier ages that may delay the age at which we become psychologically old. Broadly speaking, we can attempt to fill our earlier and most productive years with a wide variety of experiences and interests. We can examine ourselves for unduly rigid or defensive behaviors, which may become the predominant mode of behaving in later years. We can seek to avoid reinforcing, through nonthinking repetition, those behaviors that we even now recognize as deleterious to ourselves and to our relationships with others.

The practically unanimous decision of everyone working with the older patient is that those who grow older gracefully are those who do not think of themselves as older simply because their years have increased. Those who have had sufficient interests and experiences arrive at a time of diminished physical activity still wanting to maintain an interest in the world, not merely in themselves. Because of their earlier experiences, they can still find the world an interesting place to be. Such individuals are less likely to fall into stereotyped behavior. They are more likely to maintain friends. These recommendations apply to you and me no less than they apply to our patients. They are, of course, easier to write down and read about than they are to execute. But that does not change the fact that we have a responsibility to ourselves, our families, and our patients to understand as much as possible about the implications of the aging processes.

REFERENCES

1. Baldwin, A.: Behavior and development in children, New York, 1955, Holt, Rinehart, & Winston, Inc.
2. Banting, D. W.: Dental care for the aged, Can. J. Public Health **62:**503, 1971.
3. Bettelheim, B.: The empty fortress, New York, 1967, Macmillan, Inc.
4. Chambers, D. W.: Managing the anxiety of young dental patients, J. Dent. Child. **37:**363, 1970.
5. Cheney, H. G., ed.: Handbook of preventive dentistry, Acton, Mass., 1978, Publishing Sciences Group, Inc.
6. Chess, S., Thomas, A., and Birch, H.: Your child is a person, New York, 1965, The Viking Press, Inc.
7. Davidoff, A., Winkler, S., and Lee, M.: Dentistry for the special patient: the aged, chronically ill and handicapped, Philadelphia, 1972, W. B. Saunders Co.
8. Dworkin, S. F.: The developing child and persuasion to dental health behavior. In Cheney, H. G., ed.: Handbook of preventive dentistry, Acton, Mass., 1978, Publishing Sciences Group, Inc.
9. Dworkin, S. F., ed.: Persuasive prevention, New York, 1974, Medcom Press.
10. Dworkin, S. F.: Psychological aspects of aging: implications for dentistry, J. Dent. Assist. **39**(Nov.):22, 1970.
11. Ettinger, R. L.: An evaluation of the attitudes of a group of elderly edentulous patients to dentists, dentures, and dentistry, Dent. Pract. Dent. Rec. **22:**85, 1971.
12. Fishman, N., and Bikofsky, C., ed.: Proceedings of the conference on dentistry and the geriatric patient. Boston, 1972, Harvard School of Dental Medicine.
13. Flavell, J.: The developmental psychology of Jean Piaget, Princeton, N.J., 1963, D. Van Nostrand Co.
14. Fredman, J. W.: Dentistry in the geriatric patient, Geriatrics, **23:**98, 1968.
15. Gergen, K., and Bakk, K. W.: Aging and the paradox of somatic concern. In Simpson, I., and McKinney, J., eds.: Social aspects of aging, Durham, N.C., 1966, Duke University Press.
16. Graziano, A., ed.: Behavior therapy with children, Chicago, 1975, Aldine Publishing Co.
17. Kohlenberg, R., Greenberg, D., Reymore, L., and Hass, G.: Behavior modification and the management of mentally retarded dental patients, J. Dent. Child. **39:**61, 1972.
18. Kramer, M., Taub, K., and Ridick, R.: Patterns of use of psychiatric facilities by the aged. In Eisdorfer, C., and Lawton, D., ed.: The psychology of adult development in aging.
19. Kutscher, A., and Goldberg, I., ed.: Oral care of the aging and dying patient, Springfield, Ill., 1973, Charles C Thomas, Publisher.
20. Machen, B., and Johnson, R.: Desensitization, model learning and dental behavior of children, J. Dent. Res. **53:**83, 1974.
21. National Clearing House on Aging: Facts about older Americans, 1976, DHEW Pub. No. (OHD) 77-20006, Washington, D.C., 1976, U.S. Government Printing Office.
22. Read, W.: Personal communication, 1977.
23. Rexford, E., Sander, L., and Shapiro, T.: Infant psychiatry, New Haven, Conn., 1976, Yale University Press.
24. Riley, M., and Foner, A.: Aging and society, vol. 1, New York, 1968, Russell Sage Foundation.
25. Shoben, E., and Borland, R.: An empirical study of the etiology of dental fears, J. Clin. Psychol. **10:**171, 1954.
26. Shock, N. W., ed.: Perspectives in experimental gerontology, Springfield, Ill., 1966, Charles C Thomas, Publisher.
27. Wright, G. Z., and Alpern, G. D.: Variables influencing children's cooperative behavior at the first dental visit, J. Dent. Child. **38:**60, 1971.

INDEX